617.
102
7
BAH

...edicine and Science
...Injury Prevention

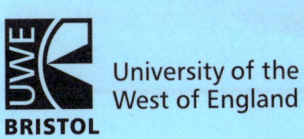

70004677

University of the West of England BRISTOL

Library Services
Learning Resources Centre
Hartpury Campus
Hartpury
Gloucester
GL19 3BE

14 DAY LOAN

Please ensure that this book is returned by the end of the loan period for which it is issued.

UWE, BRISTOL R7518 02.08
Printing & Stationery Services

-8 DEC 2009

4 Oct 2010

24 hours Telephone Renewals (automated) 0117 328 2092

Handbook of Sports Medicine and Science
Sports Injury Prevention

EDITED BY

Roald Bahr MD, PhD

Department of Sports Medicine and
Oslo Sports Trauma Research Center
Norwegian School of Sport Sciences
Ullevål Stadion, Oslo, Norway

Lars Engebretsen MD, PhD

Orthopaedic Center
Ullevaal University Hospital and Faculty of Medicine
University of Oslo
Oslo, Norway
Department of Sports Medicine and Oslo Sports Trauma Research Center
Norwegian School of Sport Sciences
Ullevål Stadion
Oslo, Norway

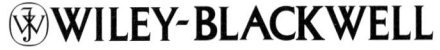

A John Wiley & Sons, Ltd., Publication

This edition first published 2009, © 2009 International Olympic Committee

Published by Blackwell Publishing

Blackwell Publishing was acquired by John Wiley & Sons in February 2007. Blackwell's publishing program has been merged with Wiley's global Scientific, Technical and Medical business to form Wiley-Blackwell.

Registered office: John Wiley & Sons Ltd, The Atrium, Southern Gate, Chichester, West Sussex, PO19 8SQ, UK

Editorial offices: 9600 Garsington Road, Oxford, OX4 2DQ, UK
The Atrium, Southern Gate, Chichester, West Sussex, PO19 8SQ, UK
111 River Street, Hoboken, NJ 07030-5774, USA

For details of our global editorial offices, for customer services and for information about how to apply for permission to reuse the copyright material in this book please see our website at www.wiley.com/wiley-blackwell

The right of the author to be identified as the author of this work has been asserted in accordance with the Copyright, Designs and Patents Act 1988.

All rights reserved. No part of this publication may be reproduced, stored in a retrieval system, or transmitted, in any form or by any means, electronic, mechanical, photocopying, recording or otherwise, except as permitted by the UK Copyright, Designs and Patents Act 1988, without the prior permission of the publisher.

Wiley also publishes its books in a variety of electronic formats. Some content that appears in print may not be available in electronic books.

Designations used by companies to distinguish their products are often claimed as trademarks. All brand names and product names used in this book are trade names, service marks, trademarks, or registered trademarks of their respective owners. The publisher is not associated with any product or vendor mentioned in this book. This publication is designed to provide accurate and authoritative information in regard to the subject matter covered. It is sold on the understanding that the publisher is not engaged in rendering professional services. If professional advice or other expert assistance is required, the services of a competent professional should be sought.

The contents of this work are intended to further general scientific research, understanding, and discussion only and are not intended and should not be relied upon as recommending or promoting a specific method, diagnosis, or treatment by physicians for any particular patient. The publisher and the author make no representations or warranties with respect to the accuracy or completeness of the contents of this work and specifically disclaim all warranties, including without limitation any implied warranties of fitness for a particular purpose. In view of ongoing research, equipment modifications, changes in governmental regulations, and the constant flow of information relating to the use of medicines, equipment, and devices, the reader is urged to review and evaluate the information provided in the package insert or instructions for each medicine, equipment, or device for, among other things, any changes in the instructions or indication of usage and for added warnings and precautions. Readers should consult with a specialist where appropriate. The fact that an organization or Website is referred to in this work as a citation and/or a potential source of further information does not mean that the author or the publisher endorses the information the organization or Website may provide or recommendations it may make. Further, readers should be aware that Internet Websites listed in this work may have changed or disappeared between when this work was written and when it is read. No warranty may be created or extended by any promotional statements for this work. Neither the publisher nor the author shall be liable for any damages arising herefrom.

Library of Congress Cataloging-in-Publication Data

Sports injury prevention : Olympic handbook of sports medicine / edited by Roald Bahr and Lars Engebretsen.
       p. ; cm. — (Handbook of sports medicine and science)
    Includes bibliographical references and index.
    ISBN 978-1-4051-6244-9 (alk. paper)
 1. Sports injuries—Prevention—Handbooks, manuals, etc. 2. Sports medicine—Handbooks, manuals, etc. I. Bahr, Roald, 1957– II. Engebretsen, Lars, 1949– III. IOC Medical Commission. Sub-Commission on Publications in the Sport Sciences. IV. Series.
    [DNLM: 1. Athletic Injuries—prevention & control. 2. Sports Medicine—methods. QT 261 S76482 2009]
    RD97.S745 2009
    617.1′027—dc22
                                                                    2008039504

ISBN: 978-1-4051-6244-9

A catalogue record for this book is available from the British Library.

Set in by Charon Tec Ltd (A Macmillan Company), Chennai, India
Printed and bound in Malaysia by Vivar Printing Sdn Bhd.

1 2009

Contents

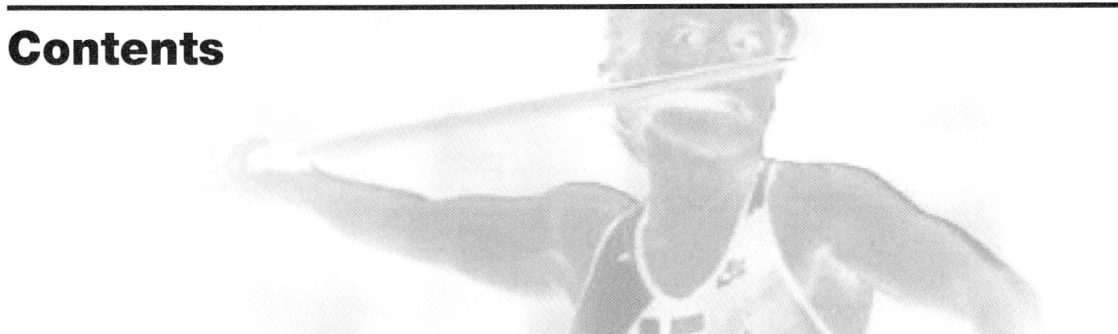

List of Contributors, vi
Foreword, viii
Preface, ix

1 Why is injury prevention in sports important? 1
 Lars Engebretsen and Roald Bahr

2 A systematic approach to sports injury prevention 7
 Willem Meeuwisse and Roald Bahr

3 Developing and managing an injury prevention program within the team 17
 Andrew McIntosh and Roald Bahr

4 Preventing ankle injuries 30
 Jon Karlsson, Evert Verhagen, Bruce D. Beynnon and Annunziato Amendola

5 Preventing knee injuries 49
 Timothy E. Hewett, Bruce D. Beynnon, Tron Krosshaug and Grethe Myklebust

6 Preventing hamstring injuries 72
 Geoffrey M. Verrall and Árni Árnason, Kim Bennell

7 Preventing groin injuries 91
 Per Hölmich, Lorrie Maffey and Carolyn Emery

8 Preventing low back pain 114
 Adad Baranto, Tor Inge Andersen and Leif Swärd

9 Preventing shoulder injuries 134
 Michael R. Krogsgaard, Marc R. Safran, Peter Rheinlænder and Emilie Cheung

10 Preventing elbow injuries 153
 Mark R. Hutchinson and James R. Andrews

11 Preventing injuries to the head and cervical spine 175
 Paul McCrory, Michael Turner and Andrew McIntosh

12 Preventing tendon overuse injuries 187
 Jill Cook, Mads Kongsgaard, Karim Khan and Michael Kjær

13 Implementing large-scale injury prevention programs 197
 Randall W. Dick, Claude Goulet and Simon Gianotti

14 Planning for major events 212
 Michael Turner and Jiri Dvorak

Index, 229

List of Contributors

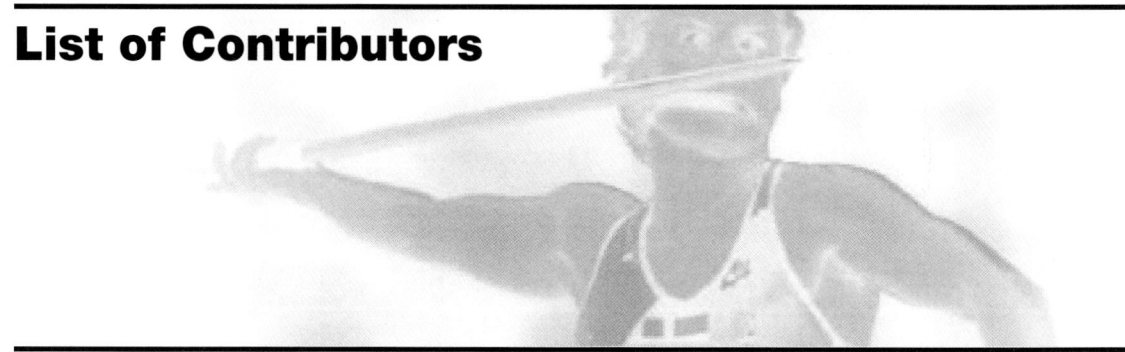

Annunziato Amendola MD
Department of Orthopaedic Surgery and Rehabilitation, University of Iowa Sports Medicine Center, University of Iowa, Iowa City, IA, USA

Tor Inge Andersen PT
National Center of Spinal Disorders, National Center of Pain and Complex Disorders, Trandheim University Hospital, St Olar, Norway

James R. Andrews, MD
Medical Director, American Sports Medicine Institute, Birmingham, Alabama, USA; Andrews Sports Medicine Institute, Gulf Breeze, FL, USA

Árni Árnason PT, PhD
Department of Physiotherapy, University of Iceland, Reykjavik, Iceland

Roald Bahr MD, PhD
Department of Sports Medicine, Oslo Sports Trauma Research Center, Norwegian School of Sport Sciences, Ullevål Stadion, Oslo, Norway

Adad Baranto MD, PhD
Department of Orthopaedics, Sahlgrenska University, Göteborg, Sweden

Kim Bennell BAppSc (Physio), PhD
Centre for Health, Exercise and Sports Medicine, School of Physiotherapy, University of Melbourne, Australia

Bruce D. Beynnon PhD
Department of Orthopaedics and Rehabilitation, McClure Musculoskeletal Research Center, The University of Vermont, VT, USA

Jill Cook PhD, B App Sci (Phty)
Centre for Physical Activity and Nutrition Research School of Exercise and Nutrition Sciences, Deakin University, Melbourne, Australia

Randall W. Dick MS, MS
Research/Injury Surveillance System National Collegiate Athletic Association, Indianapolis, IN, USA

Jiri Dvorak MD
FIFA Medical Assessment and Research Center (F-MARC), Schulthess Clinic, Zurich, Switzerland

Carolyn Emery BScPT, PhD
Sport Medicine Centre, Faculty of Kinesiology; Community Health Sciences, Faculty of Medicine, University of Calgary, Calgary, Canada

Lars Engebretsen MD, PhD
Orthopaedic Center, Ullevaal University Hospital and Faculty of Medicine, University of Oslo, Oslo, Norway; Department of Sports Medicine and Oslo Sports Trauma Research Center, Norwegian School of Sport Sciences, Ullevål Stadion, Oslo, Norway

Simon Gianotti BCA
Institute of Sport and Recreation Research New Zealand, Faculty of Health and Environmental Science, AUT, Auckland, New Zealand

Claude Goulet PhD
Department of Physical Education, Laval University, Québec, Canada

Timothy E. Hewett PhD
The Human Performance Laboratory, Departments of Pediatrics, Orthopaedic Surgery, Biomedical Engineering and Rehabilitation Sciences, The Sports Medicine Biodynamics Center, Cincinnati Children's Hospital Medical Center, University of Cincinnati College of Medicine, Cincinnati, OH, USA

Per Hölmich MD
Department of Orthopaedic Surgery, Orthopaedic Research Unit, Amager University Hospital, Copenhagen S, Denmark

Mark R. Hutchinson MD
Department of Orthopaedics, University of Illinois at Chicago, IL, USA

Jon Karlsson MD, PhD
Professor of Sports Traumatology, Department of Orthopaedics, Sahlgrenska University Hospital, Göteborg, Sweden

Karim Khan MD, PhD
Professor, Center for Hip Health and Mobility, University of British Columbia, Vancouver, Canada

Michael Kjær MD, DMSci
Department of Rheumatology, Institute of Sports Medicine, Bispebjerg Hospital, University of Copenhagen, Copenhagen, Denmark

Michael R. Krogsgaard, MD, PhD,
Associate Professor, specialist in Orthopaedic Surgery
Department of Orthopaedic Surgery, Copenhagen University Hospital Bispebjerg, Denmark

Tron Krosshaug PhD
Oslo Sports Trauma Research Center, Norwegian School of Sport Sciences, Oslo, Norway

Lorrie Maffey BMRPT, Dip
Faculty of Kinesiology; Community Health Sciences, Faculty of Medicine, University of Calgary, Calgary, Alberta, Canada

Paul McCrory MBBS, PhD
Centre for Health, Exercise and Sports Medicine, University of Melbourne Parkville, Australia

Andrew McIntosh PhD, MBiomedE, BAppSci (PT)
School of Risk and Safety Sciences, The University of New South Wales, Sydney, Australia

Willem Meeuwisse MD, PhD
Professor and Chair,
Sport Injury Prevention Research Centre Faculty of Kinesiology and Faculty of Medicine,
University of Calgary,
Alberta, Canada

Grethe Myklebust PT, PhD
Oslo Sports Trauma Research Center, Norwegian School of Sport Sciences, Oslo, Norway

Peter Rhein Iegature
Clinic for Physiotherapy, Frederiksberg, Denmark

Marc R. Safran MD
Department of Orthopaedic Surgery, Stanford University, Stanford, CA, USA

Leif Swärd MD, PhD
Department of Orthopaedics, Sahlgrenska University, Göteborg, Sweden

Michael Turner MBBS, MD
Chief Medical Adviser, The British Horseracing Authority and Lawn Tennis Association; formerly CMA to British Olympic Association and Snowsport, UK

Evert Verhagen
Department of Public and Occupational Health, EMG Institute, VU University Medical Center, Amsterdam, The Netherlands

Geoffrey M. Verrall MBBS
Sports Medicine Clinic, Adelaide, Australia

Foreword

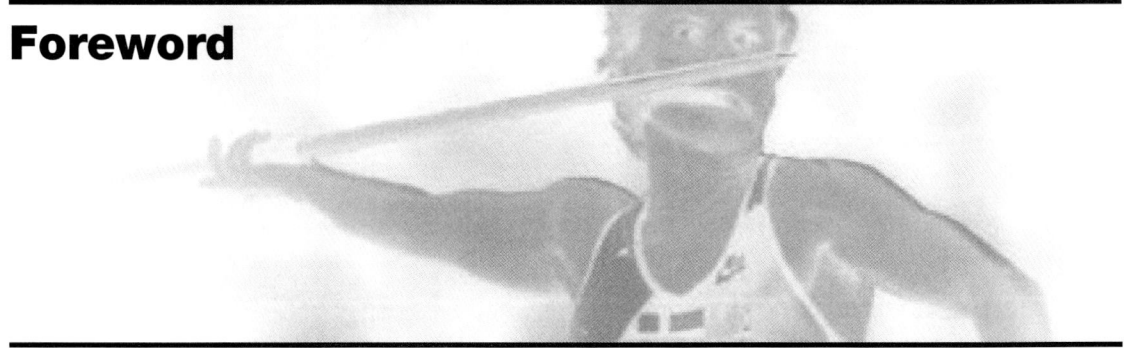

The objective established in 1991 by the IOC Medical Commission for the Handbook series was the presentation in a clear style and format of basic clinical and scientific information regarding the sports of the Olympic Summer Games and the Olympic Winter Games. Each of the handbooks that have been published during the intervening years was developed by a team of authorities coordinated by editors who had earned international respect and recognition in the areas of sports medicine and the sport sciences.

Since the appearance of the first publication, handbooks have appeared that have dealt with 10 Olympic sports as well as the general topics of strength training and nutrition for athletes. Sections dealing with sports injuries have appeared throughout these handbooks. Two volumes of the other IOC Medical Commission series, Encyclopaedia of Sports Medicine, have been devoted completely to injuries in sport.

The protection of the health of the athletes is one of the IOC's priorities. Therefore, the understanding of injuries and their prevention became one of the focuses of the Medical Commission and the Medical and Scientific Department of the IOC.

The principal objective of this Handbook on Sports Injury Prevention is a comprehensive review of the information currently available regarding the identification of the risk factors for specific injuries in each sport, the understanding of the injury mechanisms, the appropriate conditioning of athletes for the particular sport, and the risk management appropriate to each activity.

The Handbook on Sports Injury Prevention constitutes the most comprehensive review of the preclusion of the occurrence of injuries presently available and each section presents highly practical information based on published science. We welcome this splendid contribution by Roald Bahr, MD, PhD, Lars Engebretsen, MD, PhD, and 36 contributing authors to the literature of sports medicine and sports science.

Preface

In sports, injuries happen. Sometimes they happen by chance, sometimes by intent. Sometimes they are difficult, even impossible, to explain. But frequently there are clear patterns. And when there are patterns, there are also opportunities for reducing the risk of injury.

The objective of this book is to describe those opportunities – for the benefit of everyone playing sports. Although it may be expected that the main readership will be physicians, trainers and physical therapists working with sports teams, the coaching staff is an even more important target group. And although it is assumed that the reader has a basic knowledge of human anatomy and physiology, ultimately the main audience is of course the athlete. With these target groups in mind, we have attempted to create a work that is at once comprehensive in approach, practical in content, and accessible in delivery.

Our intention is to describe a practical approach to the prevention of sports injuries. The first three chapters describe the general principles of injury prevention. Chapter 1 discusses why injury prevention in sports is important, including perspectives on short- and long term consequences for health and performance. Chapter 2 describes the basis for intervention, how information on risk factors and injury mechanisms can be used to identify patterns. Such patterns can be used to identify athletes with a higher risk for injury or situations with a propensity for injury; information which is critical to be able to target and develop preventive programs. Chapter 3 describes how an injury prevention program can be developed and implemented within the team. In this context, a team can also mean a team of athletes competing in individual sports, such as a team of alpine skiers.

One choice we faced when planning this book, was whether to organize the contents per sport or per body part/injury type. One advantage of describing sports-specific programs is that it would be possible to detail measures particular to that sport, for example equipment-related measures such as alpine ski bindings. However, partly because some such information is available already (e.g. vol. V of the Encyclopedia of Sports Medicine series: Clinical Practice of Sports Injury Prevention and Care, ed. P.A.F.H. Renström), we felt that a region-specific approach would be more appropriate. Chapters 4 through 12 therefore describes how the most common sports injury types can be prevented; ankle, knee, hamstring, groin, low back, shoulder, elbow, head and cervical spine injuries. The final two chapters discusses how tendon overuse injuries, which represent a major problem across sports and body region, can be prevented (ch. 12) and how large-scale injury prevention programs can be implemented (ch. 13).

Each of the region-specific chapters includes an introduction outlining how relevant each injury type is in each of the main Olympic sports. In contrast to previous works on sports injury epidemiology, we have attempted to keep this section brief and to the point, answering the key questions:

How common is the injury in question? What is the risk – in my sport? The next section attempts to describe the key risk factors for the injury in question – how to identify athletes at risk. This includes a description of the various internal and external risk factors suggested for the injury in question, emphasizing modifiable risk factors and how the coach/medical team can identify players at risk of injury. In some cases, simple tests or screening methods which can be applied to a team setting are described. This section is followed by a description of the typical injury mechanisms for the injury in question, not just the biomechanics of injury, but also the circumstances leading to injury, such as player behavior, opponent behavior, the playing situation, or other relevant factors. We have also asked all authors to provide a section identifying risks in the training and competition program, a risk analysis to document the parts of the season when athletes are at the greatest risk for sustaining injuries as a result of the training or competitive programs. For some injury types, this type of analysis could be an important basis for planning preventive measures, particularly for the purpose of avoiding overuse injuries during transitional periods. The final – and most important – section of each of these chapters is the section on prevention methods. This section discusses possible ways to prevent the injury in question, and although these may be relevant across sports, the text provides examples from sports where injury prevention has been successful. We have tried to make this section as practical as possible, with examples of take-home ready-to-use programs wherever possible, complete with illustrations of exercises used.

This book is the first of its kind. Never before has anyone attempted to provide a guide to injury prevention – to be applied across different sports. This represents a significant challenge, since there is no model available to guide us in the development of the contents. We wish to thank the authors, who have worked hard to not just provide an up-to-date description of injury prevention methods relevant to their region and injury type, but also to develop a text consistent in content and format across the various chapters. If we have succeeded, the credit belongs to this group of dedicated professionals. If not, the responsibility is ours.

Oslo, September 2008
Roald Bahr & Lars Engebretsen

Chapter 1
Why is injury prevention in sports important?

Lars Engebretsen[1] and Roald Bahr[2]

[1] Orthopaedic Center, Ullevaal University Hospital and Faculty of Medicine, University of Oslo, Oslo, Norway
[2] Department of Sports Medicine, Oslo Sports Trauma Research Center, Norwegian School of Sport Sciences, Ullevål Stadion, Oslo, Norway

This book is a result of the IOC Medical Commission's increasing emphasis on prevention of sports injuries. The numerous health benefits of physical activity have been well documented, resulting in public health support of regular physical activity and exercise. Although beneficial, exercise and sports also have corresponding risks, including that of musculoskeletal injuries. However, at a time when there is an abundance of medical meetings, journals, and papers, some might argue that the last thing we need is a new book focusing on yet another field of research and clinical practice. What would justify such an emphasis on a new and developing field in medicine? First, it must ask important questions not answered by others. Second, the new research field should have the potential to create truly new knowledge, lead to new ways of thinking and lay the foundation for improved health for our patients. This is usually not possible without a multidisciplinary approach, involving a mixture of basic scientists and clinicians. Third, research results from the new field should be publishable in respected journals, recognized and cited by peers, presentable at high-quality meetings, and fundable on competitive grant review. Let us examine each of these issues to see if there is sufficient merit in sports injury prevention research.

Is injury prevention important?

First, is injury prevention important? Epidemiological studies show that of injuries seen by a physician, in Scandinavia, every sixth is sustained during sporting activity (Bahr et al., 2002). Among children, every third hospital-treated injury is the result of sports participation (Bahr et al., 2002). During 1997 and 1998, in the United States, annually there were an estimated 3.7 million sports- and recreation-related emergency department visits annually in the United States, representing approximately 11% of all injury related emergency department visits; 2.6 million visits were among persons aged 5–24 years. The medical charges for these visits were estimated at 500 million US$ annually.

The risk of injury clearly differs between sports, as documented by a study initiated by the IOC Medical Commission in team sports during the 2004 Olympic Games in Athens (Junge et al., 2006). As shown in Table 1.1, while a soccer and handball player suffered one injury every 10th match he or she play, a volleyball player at the elite level only had an injury every 100th match on the average. Not all of these injuries are serious; in fact only about half of all the injuries recorded were

Sports Injury Prevention, 1st edition. Edited by R. Bahr and L. Engebretsen Published 2009 by Blackwell Publishing ISBN: 9781405162449

Table 1.1 Injury risk in selected team sports during the 2004 Olympic Games in Athens.

Sport	Total injury rate[1]	Rate of time-loss injuries[2]
Football		
Men	109 (85–133)	44 (29–60)
Women	105 (74–136)	44 (24–64)
Handball		
Men	89 (64–114)	40 (23–57)
Women	145 (110–180)	36 (18–53)
Basketball		
Men	64 (40–89)	29 (12–45)
Womenv	67 (42–91)	24 (9–39)
Field hockey		
Men	55 (37–72)	24 (12–36)
Women	17 (5–29)	4 (0–10)
Baseball (men)	29 (15–43)	13 (3.2–22)
Water polo (men)	30 (16–44)	9 (1.1–16.3)
Volleyball (men)	11 (1.4–21)	9 (0.2–17)

Source: Junge et al. (2006).
[1] Injury rate is reported as the number of injuries per 1000 player matches (with 95% confidence intervals).
[2] Rate of time-loss injuries is reported as the number of injuries expected to lead to time loss from further training and competition.

expected to cause the player not to continue with subsequent training or match time. Nevertheless, when taking injury severity into account, a research group within the English Football Association found that the overall risk to professional athletes is unacceptably high—approximately 1000 times higher among professional football players than for high-risk industrial occupations (Drawer & Fuller, 2002) (Figure 1.1). Although football and handball rank highest in injury rates of the team sports included in the Olympic summer program, there are actually other sports where the injury rate is considerably higher, for example, ice hockey and the other football codes: American football, rugby, and Australian rules football.

Some injury types, such as serious head and knee injuries, are a particular cause of concern. Head injuries are known to have a high incidence among alpine skiers and snowboarders, especially among snowboarders, and the frequency increases year by year in this group. Head injury is the most frequent reason for hospital admission and most common cause of death among skiers and snowboarders with an 8% mortality rate among those admitted to hospital with head injuries. Among injuries related to football, 4–22% are head injuries. The reported incidence during matches—1.7 injuries per 1000 player hours—incorporates all types of head injuries including facial fractures, contusions, lacerations, and eye injuries (Andersen et al., 2004). The estimated incidence of concussion—0.5 injuries per 1000 match hours—probably represents a minimum estimate due to the problem of defining and grading concussions (Andersen et al., 2004). Although most athletes with head injuries recover uneventfully following a single concussive episode, repetitive mild head trauma may be implicated in the development of cumulative cognitive deterioration. Based on paper and pencil tests, cumulative effects of repeated concussions have been found to cause deterioration in neuropsychological function among athletes in other sports such as American football and boxing, as well as in non-athletes.

The highest incidence of anterior cruciate ligament (ACL) injuries is seen in 15- to 25-year-old athletes in pivoting sports such as football, basketball and handball. This incidence is three to five times higher among women than men (Griffin et al., 2006). In 1970, Kennedy stated that "the anterior cruciate ligament is the most common cause of the exathlete." In other words, the treatment offered at the time did not permit athletes to go back to sport. This is no longer the case, at least in the short term, thanks to the advances in sports medicine research, with major improvements in surgical techniques and rehabilitation programs. Today, most elite athletes are initially able to resume their sports career, should they wish to do so. And although the retirement rate may be higher among athletes with a previous ACL injury compared with healthy athletes, the main concern is the dramatically increased risk of long-term sequelae—like abnormal joint dynamics and early onset of degenerative joint disease. Importantly, we still lack evidence to suggest that reconstructive surgery of either menisci or cruciate ligaments decrease the rate of post-traumatic osteoarthritis (OA). After 10 years, approximately half of the patients display signs of OA, and it appears that the majority of the patients will have osteoarthrosis after 15–20 years (Figure 1.2) (Myklebust & Bahr, 2005). Thus, whereas

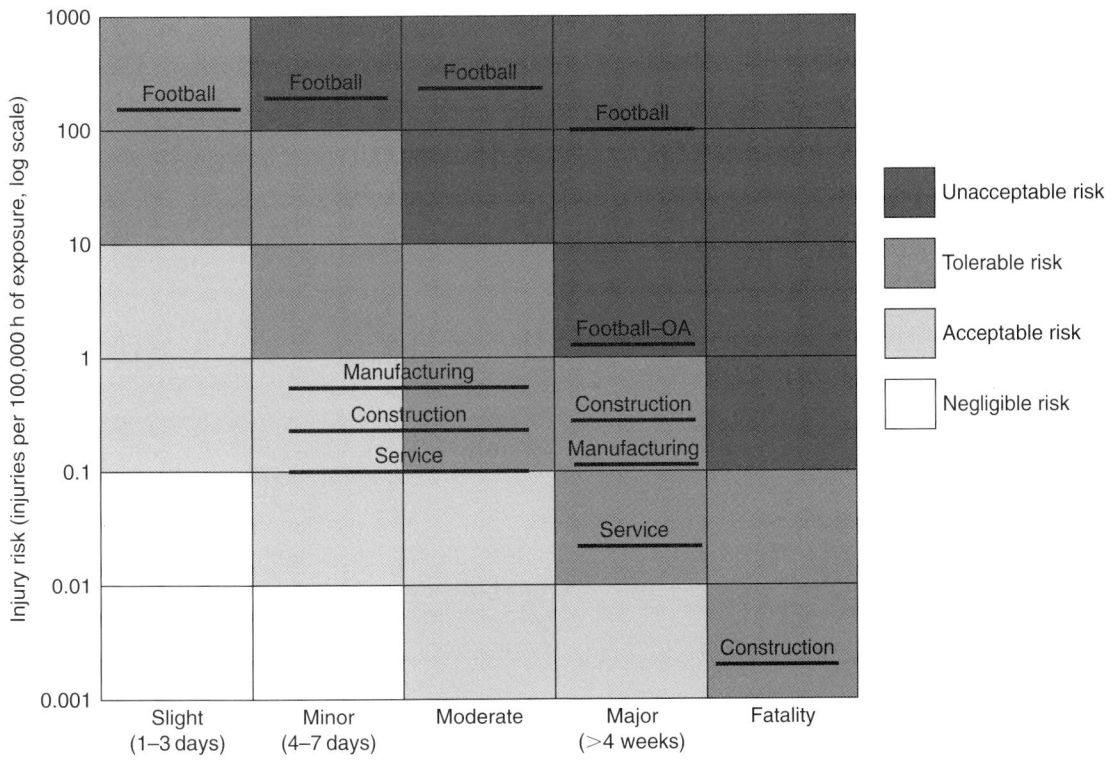

Figure 1.1. Comparison between injury risk (shown on the logarithmic vertical axis as the incidence per 100,000 h of player exposure) and injury risk (shown on the horizontal axis as the duration of absence from work/play, from slight through minor, moderate and major to fatalities) in professional football (Premier League), along with data from the manufacturing, construction and service industries for comparisons. Also, the dark gray areas are classified as unacceptable risk when using industrial standards for risk management. Reproduced with permission from Drawer and Fuller (2002)

developing improved treatment methods for injuries, in general, and ACL injuries, in particular, remains an important goal, it may be even more important to prevent injuries.

Is there an evidence base for injury prevention?

The second issue relates to the potential for new ideas and improved health outcomes. In May 2000, a PubMed search revealed that out of 10,691 papers on athletic injury, there were only six randomized controlled trials (RCTs) on sports injury prevention (Table 1.2). However, a similar search of the literature in December 2007 revealed that sports injury prevention research is emerging as a new field in medicine. While the number of studies on athletic injuries has increased by 43% over the last 7 years, clinical studies and RCTs related to sports injury prevention has increased by 200–300% (Table 1.2). Gradually, congresses in sports medicine, orthopedics, and traumatology include an increasing number of symposia, lectures, and instructional courses on injury prevention issues. Research is also improving in quality, not only in quantity. For example, recent issues of high-impact general medical journals such as the *British Medical Journal* and the *Journal of the American Medical Association* have included several papers related to injury prevention; two case-control studies among

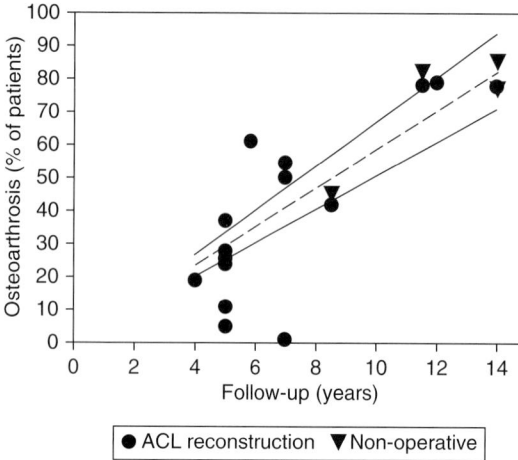

Figure 1.2. Anterior cruciate ligament (ACL) follow-up studies and Osteoarthritis (OA) prevalence. The data illustrate the prevalence of radiographic OA after reconstructive surgery with bone-patella-tendon-bone graft or hamstring graft and after non-operative treatment. The dashed line indicates the forced regression (y = 6.0t; r = 0.85) between time (t) and OA prevalence (y), with the 95% confidence intervals shown by thin solid lines. Reproduced with permission from Myklebust and Bahr (2005)

Table 1.2 Results of PubMed searches on sports injury research related to treatment and prevention.

Search terms	May 2000	December 2007	Increase (%)
Athletic injury	10,691	15,347	43
& treatment	6,606	9,774	48
& Limit: Clinical trials	182	359	97
& Limit: RCT	87	180	107
& prevention	2,064	3,319	61
& Limit: Clinical trials	29	125	330
& Limit: RCT	21	70	233

Note: Results are shown as the number of items resulting from the search terms shown.

skiers and snowboarders indicating a significant reduction in the risk of head injury with helmet use (Hagel et al., 2005; Sulheim et al., 2006), an RCT demonstrating a 47% reduction in knee and ankle injuries from a structured program of warm-up exercises in adolescent team handball players (Olsen et al., 2005), and an ecological study of a nationwide educational injury prevention program indicating a reduced frequency of spinal cord injuries in rugby (Quarrie et al., 2007). Many major public health and specialty journals are currently publishing new studies in this field. The publication of these studies in highly respected medical, physical therapy and nursing journal illustrates that sports injury prevention is an important public health issue.

Is sports participation healthy?

Sports participation is important from a public health perspective. There is no longer any doubt that regular physical activity reduces the risk of premature mortality in general, and of coronary heart disease, hypertension, colon cancer, obesity, and diabetes mellitus in particular. The question is whether the health benefits of sports participation outweigh the risk of injury and long-term disability, especially in high-level athletes? A study from Finland has investigated the incidence of chronic disease and life expectancy of former male world-class athletes from Finland in endurance sports, power sports, and team sports (Sarna et al., 2000). The overall life expectancy was higher in the high-level athlete compared to a matched reference group (75.6 versus 69.9 years). They also showed that the rate of hospitalization was lower for endurance sports and power sports compared to the reference group (Kujala et al., 1996). This resulted from a lower rate of hospital care for heart disease, respiratory disease, and cancer. However, the athletes were more likely to have been hospitalized for musculoskeletal disorders. A follow-up study revealed that former team sport athletes had a higher risk of knee OA, and other studies have documented an increased risk of hip and knee arthritis among former football players. Thus, the evidence suggests that although sports participation is beneficial, injuries are a significant side effect. To promote physical activity effectively, we have to deal professionally with the health problems of the active patient. This does not only involve providing effective care for the injured patient, but also developing and promoting injury prevention measures actively.

Injury prevention is a complex process. To prevent injury, scientists must first correctly identify one or several risk factors, the mechanisms of injury, devise an effective intervention to modify it, implement the intervention with sufficient compliance, and study the outcome of the intervention with a method that is sensitive enough to detect reductions in the injury rate which are clinically meaningful. When prevention is successful or fails, it may not always be clear which step in this chain of events was deficient. This complexity makes injury prevention difficult, but not impossible. A number of interventions have shown a reduction in injury rates, that is, ACL injuries in team handball and soccer; ankle injuries in soccer, basketball and volleyball; head injuries in hockey and skiing; wrist injuries in snowboarding; and hamstrings injuries in Australian Rules football and soccer. The list is increasing year by year for the benefit of the athlete and the sports.

The future of injury prevention

Do we need to further develop prevention programs in the future? Year by year we seem to have more information about risk factors and their relative roles. If the relative additional risk of having specific risk factors is known, some individuals should probably be advised against participation in certain sports where the risk factor cannot be eliminated. On the contrary, if the effect of eliminating one risk factor after another is known, individuals may be able to participate in sports with low risk if they are compliant with their specific training program. The goal must be to reach a stage where the risk factors are known and where we can assign a relative risk of an injury to individuals. During the preseason examination, individuals with risk factors can then be assigned training programs that have been validated. Even at this stage, future research in this field is necessary. The nature of sports is always changing—becoming faster and generally more demanding. Just think of the difference in alpine skiing over the last 25 years. In almost any sports the same increase in pace is seen. Thus, research on risk factors and injury mechanisms must be ongoing and intervention studies crucial.

In an evolving field such as this, international cooperation is critical. The involvement of the IOC, which highlights sports injury prevention research in this book, improves the dissemination of information around the world. In addition, this book initiative has been supported by all of the major sports and sports medicine organizations, which bodes well for the future.

References

Andersen, T.E., Árnason, A., Engebretsen, L., Bahr, R. (2004) Mechanisms of head injuries in elite football. *British Journal of Sports Medicine* **38**, 690–696.

Bahr, R., van Mechelen, W., Kannus, P. (2002) Prevention of sports injuries. In M. Kjær, M. Krogsgaard, P. Magnusson, L. Engebretsen, H. Roos, T. Takala & S.L.Y. Woo (eds) *Textbook of Sports Medicine. Basic Science and Clinical Aspects of Sports Injury and Physical Activity.* pp. 299–314. Blackwell Science, Oxford.

Drawer, S., Fuller, C.W. (2002) Evaluating the level of injury in English professional football using a risk based assessment process. *British Journal of Sports Medicine* 36, 446–451.

Griffin, L.Y., Albohm, M.J., Arendt, E.A., Bahr, R., Beynnon, B.D., Demaio, M., Dick, R.W., Engebretsen, L., Garrett Jr., W.E., Hannafin, J.A., Hewett, T.E., Huston, L.J., Ireland, M.L., Johnson, R.J., Lephart, S., Mandelbaum, B.R., Mann, B.J., Marks, P.H., Marshall, S.W., Myklebust, G., Noyes, F.R., Powers, C., Shields Jr., C., Shultz, S.J., Silvers, H., Slauterbeck, J., Taylor, D.C., Teitz, C.C., Wojtys, E.M., Yu, B. (2006) Understanding and preventing noncontact anterior cruciate ligament injuries: a review of the Hunt Valley II meeting, January 2005. *American Journal of Sports Medicine* **34**, 1512–1532.

Hagel, B.E., Pless, I.B., Goulet, C., Platt, R.W., Robitaille, Y. (2005) Effectiveness of helmets in skiers and snowboarders: case-control and case crossover study. *British Medical Journal* **330**(7486), 281.

Junge, A., Langevoort, G., Pipe, A., Peytavin, A., Wong, F., Mountjoy, M., Beltrami, G., Terrell, R., Holzgraefe, M., Charles, R., Dvorak, J. (2006) Injuries in team sport tournaments during the 2004 Olympic Games. *American Journal of Sports Medicine* **34**, 565–576.

Kujala, U.M., Sarna, S., Kaprio, J., Koskenvuo, M. (1996) Hospital care in later life among world class athletes. *Journal of the American Medical Association* **276**, 216–220.

Myklebust, G., Bahr, R. (2005) Return to play guidelines after anterior cruciate ligament surgery. *British Journal of Sports Medicine* **39**, 127–131.

Olsen, O.E., Myklebust, G., Engebretsen, L., Holme, I., Bahr, R. (2005) Exercises to prevent lower limb injuries in youth sports: cluster randomised controlled trial. *British Medical Journal* **330**(7489), 449.

Quarrie, K.L., Gianotti, S.M., Hopkins, W.G., Hume, P.A. (2007) Effect of nationwide injury prevention programme on serious spinal injuries in New Zealand rugby union: ecological study. *British Medical Journal* **334**(7604), 1150.

Sarna, S., Sahi, T., Koskenvuo, M., Kaprio, J. (2000) Increased life expectancy of world class athletes. *Medicine and Science in Sports and Exercise* **25**, 37–44.

Sulheim, S., Holme, I., Ekeland, A., Bahr, R. (2006) Helmet use and risk of head injuries in alpine skiers and snowboarders. *Journal of the American Medical Association* **295**, 919–924.

Further reading

Bahr, R. (2003) Preventing sports injuries. In R. Bahr & S. Mæhlum (eds) *Clinical Guide to Sports Injuries*, pp. 41–53. Human Kinetics, Champaign.

Caine, D.J., Caine, C., Lindner, K. (1996) *Epidemiology of Sports Injuries*. Human Kinetics, Champaign.

Caine, D.J., Maffulli, N. (eds) (2005) *Epidemiology of Pediatric Sports Injuries. Individual Sports. Medicine and Sport Science*. Vol. 48. Karger, Basel.

Khan, K., Bahr, R. (2006) Principles of sports injury prevention. In P. Brukner & K. Khan (eds) *Clinical Sports Medicine*. pp. 78–101. McGraw-Hill, Sydney.

Maffulli, N., Caine, D.J. (eds) (2005) *Epidemiology of Pediatric Sports Injuries. Team Sports. Medicine and Sport Science*. Vol. 49. Karger, Basel.

Renström, P.A.F.H. (ed) (1994) *Clinical Practice of Sports Injury Prevention and Care: Olympic Encyclopaedia of Sports Medicine*. Vol. 5. Blackwell Publishing, Oxford.

Chapter 2
A systematic approach to sports injury prevention

Willem Meeuwisse[1] and Roald Bahr[2]

[1] University of Calgary Sport Medicine Centre, Calgary, Alberta, Canada

[2] Department of Sports Medicine, Oslo Sports Trauma Research Center, Norwegian School of Sport Sciences, Ullevål Stadion, Oslo, Norway

Injury prevention in sport has numerous benefits. These include greater health of the individual; longevity in the activity; and reduced costs to the individual, the sport, the health care system, and society. An obvious benefit is the potential for better performance through injury prevention. This may be particularly relevant when trying to motivate athletes, coaches, and sports teams to focus on injury prevention. The likelihood of success is greater if all the best players on the team are available for team selection. And the chance of success is nil if you are injured when the Olympics start!

Prevention can be grouped into three broad categories of primary, secondary, and tertiary prevention. Primary prevention is the goal of most prevention activity, and is what most people think of when they consider prevention. That is, primary prevention involves the avoidance of injury (e.g., ankle braces being worn by an entire team, even those with no history of previous ankle sprains). If primary prevention activities are successful, an individual will not sustain injury in the first place.

This differs from secondary prevention which involves appropriate early diagnosis and treatment once an injury has occurred. The aim here is to ensure that the injury is optimally cared for to limit the development of disability, and is what most people think of as treatment (e.g., early RICE treatment of an ankle sprain).

Finally, tertiary prevention is the focus on rehabilitation to reduce and/or correct an existing disability attributed to an underlying disease; what most people think of as rehabilitation (e.g., in the case of a patient who has had an ankle sprain, this would involve balance board exercises and wearing an ankle brace while gradually returning to sport).

Sequence of injury prevention research

In 1992, van Mechelen outlined a sequence of injury prevention research (Figure 2.1). This conceptual model can be successfully applied by sports medicine staff, as well. First, according to the research model, the magnitude of the problem must be identified and described in terms of the incidence and severity of sports injuries. If you are responsible for a team, this would involve monitoring injury risk on a continuous basis by recording all injuries within the squad, as well as training and match participation (often called "exposure"). As a second step in injury prevention research, the risk factors and injury mechanisms must be identified that play a part in causing sports injuries to occur. For the medical team and coaching staff, this could involve systematic steps to examine the athletes and their training and competition program. The third step is to introduce measures that are likely to reduce the future risk and/or severity of injuries. Such measures should be based on information about the risk factors and the injury mechanisms as identified in

Sports Injury Prevention, 1st edition. Edited by R. Bahr and L. Engebretsen Published 2009 by Blackwell Publishing ISBN: 9781405162449

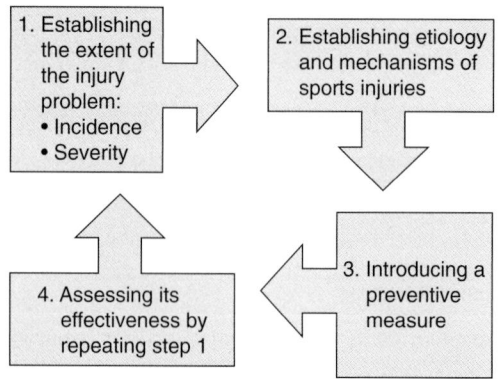

Figure 2.1. A model of injury prevention research—the four steps in sports injury prevention (van Mechelen et al., 1992)

the second step. Finally, the effect of the measures must be evaluated by repeating the first step. From a researcher's standpoint, it is preferable to evaluate the effect of preventive measures by means of a randomized controlled trial. For the team staff, continuous surveillance of the injury pattern within the team will reveal whether the changes occur in the injury risk (providing the medical staff realize that changes in patterns of injury over time in a single team can be due to many different factors).

Injury surveillance

The object of surveillance is to enumerate the extent of injury in a given group or population. In this book, the rate of specific injury types across different sports will be reported. Based on surveillance data from previous studies, we can learn which injury types should be targeted when considering injury prevention in different sports. Surveillance within a specific team, league, or sport organization can also highlight potential areas of prevention that might be unique to that group. A soccer coach may want to focus on hamstring strains, knee and ankle sprains, whereas a baseball coach may decide to consider shoulder and elbow problems when planning his training and competition program. However, injury rate is not the only factor to be considered. Injury severity is also an important concern. For example, serious knee injuries or head injuries may warrant particular attention, not based on injury rate alone, but because they can potentially result in permanent disability and even death.

However, when comparing results between studies in different sports and different sports settings, there are a number of important characteristics of surveillance that must be considered, including the injury definition. There is also the question of diagnostic coding or classification of injury and issues surrounding the count of injury and reinjury, and assessment of severity.

Injury definition

Defining what constitutes an injury is not as easy as it may seem at first glance, and there have been many different approaches to injury definition in the past. A consensus statement was issued in 2006 in the sport of football (soccer) stating that the broadest definition of injury would be any event occurring as a result of participation in sport (Fuller et al., 2006). Injury was then further classified into *medical attention injuries*; those that required assessment or treatment by a medical practitioner. A further sub-division was *time-loss injuries*; those causing a player to miss one or more practices or games or sessions. The important point in any research regarding injury surveillance is that one must know in advance exactly what will be counted, and this must be consistent across all people and all groups recording injury. This is important to ensure consistency both within a given period of surveillance and over time between different periods of surveillance.

Injury classification

Similarly, consensus has been achieved regarding the classification of injury into various body regions and injury types (Fuller et al., 2006). These can be refined more fully within the context of sport through the use of diagnostic coding systems that are tailored specifically for sport.

Injury severity

Injury severity can be classified on the basis of the level of tissue damage, the type of structure injured, or the nature of the injury itself. However, within the context of sport the most meaningful measure is likely the amount of time an individual is unable to participate in their customary activity of training or competition. Obviously, career-ending injuries or injuries causing permanent disability, or even death, are a particular concern. The "time lost" can be counted in days or sessions (games or practices) missed. The total time lost from injury within a team can be used to monitor the quality of not only the efficiency of the medical team in diagnosing and treating injuries, but also the injury prevention program within the team.

Injury recurrence

In counting injuries, it is important to realize that all injuries are not isolated events. That is, some injuries are a recurrence of something that has happened previously, either pre-dating or during the same period of data collection. Fuller et al. (2007) have recommended that recurrence be grouped into "exacerbations" and "reinjuries." Exacerbations should not be counted as a new injury event, but any time missed should be attributed to the first injury. In contrast, reinjuries should be counted as a separate injury event with their own time loss. If injury surveillance within a team reveals an unusually high rate or proportion of recurrences, this could mean that injury rehabilitation is insufficient or that athletes are allowed too early return to play after previous injuries.

Exposure

With injury surveillance one can look at numbers of new injuries over a period of time. However, within the context of sport where there is varying degrees of participation (and therefore exposure to the potential of injury), it is more meaningful to capture injuries in reference to the amount of time that a given individual participates. Participation can be counted in hours or sessions. From this, an injury rate, or incidence rate, can be calculated. In this book injury incidence is typically reported as the number of injuries per 1000 hours of player exposure. This allows injury risk to be compared between different sports and different groups.

Determining the causes of injury

If one is to prevent injury, the causes of injuries must be determined. First, one must identify those factors associated with an increased risk of injury ("risk factors").

Risk factors

Although all individuals possess certain characteristics or factors, they are considered risk factors if they increase the chance of an injury occurring. However, the assessment of risk can be complex, since most factors in sport do not act in isolation. A risk factor may be part of a collection of other factors that, together, produce a picture of "sufficient cause" for an injury to occur. Sometimes, one specific risk factor is necessary and without this factor, an injury will not occur (Meeuwisse, 1994; Meeuwisse et al., 2007).

There are many factors that impact on the potential occurrence of injury. There are internal or intrinsic risk factors that are part of an athlete's make up that may make them predisposed to injury. Then, they begin to participate and are exposed to external or extrinsic factors, which may make them susceptible to injury. These risk factors (often in combination) will determine whether a specific event or force will produce an injury (Figure 2.2).

In some cases the risk factor that is being evaluated is not the cause of injury. Interestingly, if the factor is shown to be associated with an increased risk of injury it is considered a risk factor. This allows this factor to be a valid predictor or marker of injury. However, removing the risk factor may not necessarily prevent injury if a causal relationship does not exist.

Etiology

In some instances the immediate cause (or etiology) of injury is obvious. However, all is not always what it appears to be. Even in the most obvious examples, there is often more than one factor that has led to the injury. In the case of a macro-traumatic injury, such as a kick to another player's leg resulting in a muscle contusion, there

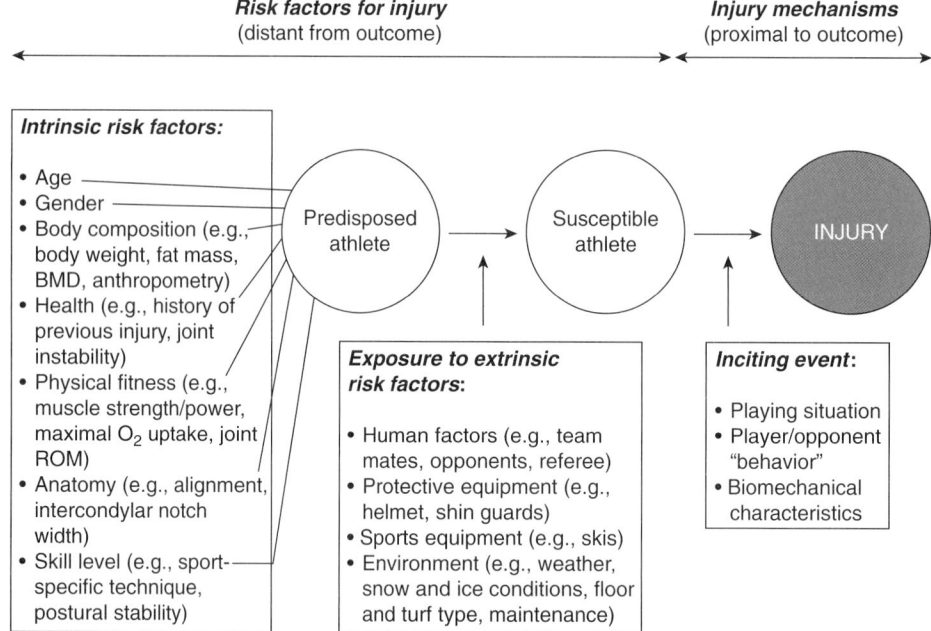

Figure 2.2. A model of injury causation (Meeuwisse, 1994; Bahr & Krosshaug, 2005)

may have been factors related to the injured player, the opponent, the equipment, the playing environment, etc., which all could have contributed to the injury occurring, or its severity. Therefore, it is important to take a more encompassing view of etiology or causation.

A model has been developed in the past to account for a number of different variables that may contribute to injury. Meeuwisse (1994) outlined a model wherein an athlete begins with a certain set of characteristics (Figure 2.2). These are typically referred to as intrinsic risk factors or internal factors which may predispose the athlete for injury. This includes athlete characteristics: factors such as age, maturation, gender, body composition, and fitness level. One factor that consistently has been documented to be a significant predictor is previous injury—almost regardless of the injury type studied. Intrinsic factors such as these interact to predispose for injury, or in other cases protect from injury. Examples of factors which may make an athlete less predisposed to some, but not all, injury types include fitness-related factors such as muscle mass, strength, balance, and neuromuscular control.

An athlete then begins to participate in sport within a certain environment and is exposed to extrinsic risk factors. These may include equipment and field conditions, for example, floor friction in indoor team sports, snow conditions in alpine skiing, a slippery surface (running track), very cold weather, or inappropriate footwear. Extrinsic factors may also reduce injury risk, such as the wearing of protective equipment. Exposure to such external risk factors may interact with the intrinsic factors to make the athlete more or less susceptible to injury. When intrinsic and extrinsic risk factors act simultaneously, the athlete may be at far greater risk of injury than when risk factors are present in isolation.

The final link in the chain is the inciting event, which is usually referred to as the injury mechanism—what we see when watching an injury situation. Each injury type and each sport does have its typical patterns, and for team medical and coaching staff it is important to understand the typical injuries and mechanisms in their sport (Bahr & Krosshaug, 2005).

It has been recognized more recently that this process should not be seen as linear and static.

That is, it does not have a clear starting and ending point in the context of sport. Athletes participate in sport over typically a long period of time and bring with them characteristics of prior training as well as other sport experience and injury. Moreover, they carry their intrinsic risk factors with them into repeated exposure to extrinsic risk factors and many potentially inciting events, most of which never result in injury.

Therefore, one limitation of the model is that it is not obvious how the athlete's training routine and competitive schedule can be taken into consideration as potential causes, and the model has therefore traditionally mainly been used to describe the causes of acute injuries. For overuse injuries, the causative factors can sometimes be distant from the outcome. For example, for a stress fracture in a long distance runner the inciting event is not usually the single training session when pain became evident, but the training and competition program he or she has followed over the previous weeks or months.

Another limitation is that repeated exposure may produce adaptation, either in the course of normal training or as a consequence of being exposed to potentially injurious events. Overuse or gradual onset injuries are typically produced as a result of high training loads over a period of time. In some athletes, these training loads will result in adaptation and the athlete will actually become stronger and therefore have an improved (reduced) set of intrinsic risk factors. In other athletes, this may result in tissue breakdown and microtraumatic changes that would worsen (increase) their intrinsic risk factors.

Ultimately, this happens on a cyclical basis for every single participation in sport (Meeuwisse et al., 2007). As athletes are exposed to the playing environment and face different events, some of those will become an inciting event and therefore a mechanism for injury. Others, however, produce no injury but rather adaptations in the athlete, which may be biomechanical, structural, behavioral, etc. Then, these athletes repeatedly participate in sport, creating a dynamic cycle wherein repeat participation can result in either injury or no injury.

Therefore, it is important to keep in mind that risks will change under repeated participation. This is not just because of external changes such as differences in weather or playing surfaces or equipment worn. Internal risk factors can also change as a result of participation. Specifically, an athlete's susceptibility to tissue-level damage may be reduced as strength improves with repeated use or as technique becomes adapted in a positive manner. At the same time, repeat participation can produce microtrauma that weakens tissue and increases susceptibility to injury. In addition, athletes may change their behavior, their style of play or even their choice of protective equipment based on a perceived susceptibility or risk of injury. These circumstances do not tend to remain constant even within one player over the course of time. Rather, adaptations or changes may occur during a season through both training and competition. The behavior of these factors have been described in more detail by Meeuwisse et al. (2007).

Modifiable and non-modifiable risk factors

Assuming that a risk factor is a cause of injury, the best way to prevent injury is to change the risk factor. For example, a risk factor of muscle weakness can be overcome with a strengthening program, or a risk factor of poor proprioception can be improved by balance re-training. In addition, if artificial turf were a risk factor, it could be minimized by playing on grass.

However, in some cases, the risk factor cannot be changed, eliminated, or modified. Even so, non-modifiable factors (such as gender) may be equally important in injury prevention if they can be used to target intervention measures to those athletes who are at increased risk. For example, anterior cruciate ligament (ACL) injuries have been shown to be four to six times more common among female athletes than male athletes in some sports, such as soccer, basketball, and handball. Based on this, female athletes should be the primary target group for ACL injury prevention programs in these sports.

The mechanism of injury

In some cases, the key to injury prevention may lie with the injury mechanisms, not with the risk factors. For example, one may consider being struck in the face by a hockey puck or stick as a completely random event, which could occur regardless of intrinsic or extrinsic risk factors. If defenders and attackers are hit as often as goalies, it may not be possible to identify the player at risk. And even if the chance of being struck were twice as high for goalkeepers, a face mask would be the obvious preventive measure and the key question would be how to design such a mask, and not who should wear it.

To fully understand the inciting event, and the ultimate chain in the factors leading to injury, it is helpful to use a comprehensive model, which accounts for the events leading to the injury situation (playing situation, player, and opponent behavior), as well as includes a description of whole body and joint biomechanics at the time of injury (Bahr & Krosshaug, 2005). Ideas for preventive measures may originate from each category of information, depending on the injury type in question.

For some injury types, the key to prevention may lie with the events leading to the injury situation (e.g., the playing situation, player behavior, or opponent behavior). For example, to prevent head injuries in soccer the first obvious question is: What strikes the head? The ball? Or is it a head-to-head clash with an opponent in a heading duel? Or the opponent's arm or elbow? Or do head injuries typically result when falling and hitting the ground? Recent studies from elite male soccer on the national and international level have shown that the commonest mechanism involved heading challenges and the use of the upper extremity with elbow to head contact. In the majority of the elbow to head incidents, the elbow was used actively at or above shoulder level (Figure 2.3). From these findings stricter rule enforcement and even changes in the laws of the game concerning elbow use can be made to reduce the risk of head injury.

In other sports, it may be more important to have detailed knowledge of the biomechanics. For example, to design an appropriate hockey helmet, it is necessary to have an accurate estimate of the impact forces involved in the game, such as when a falling player hits the ice. Other examples of factors which may be important to understand

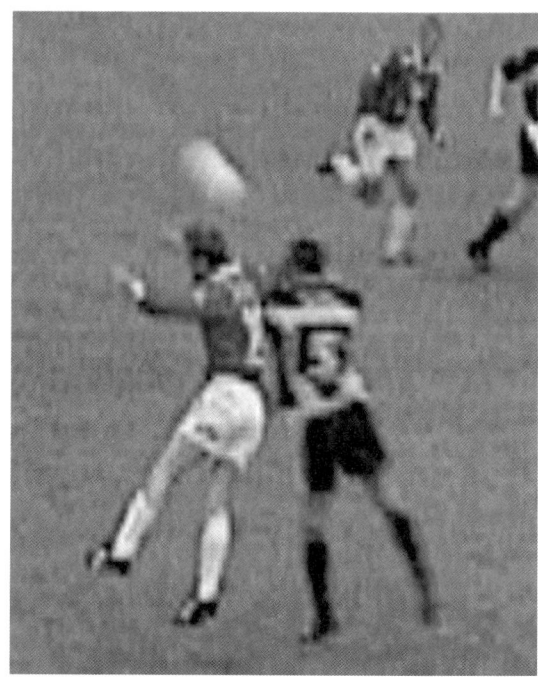

Figure 2.3. Typical mechanism for head injuries in soccer. Elbow to head contact in a heading duel. The player on the left uses his right elbow actively above shoulder level to prevent the opponent player from reaching the ball. Reproduced from Bahr and Krosshaug (2005) with permission

and describe the injury mechanisms are shown in Table 2.1. Such information can be obtained from a variety of research methods, each with its own strengths and limitations. These include interviews of injured athletes, analysis of video recordings of actual injuries, clinical studies (where the clinical joint damage findings are studied to understand the injury mechanism through examination, diagnostic imaging, or surgical exploration), in vivo studies (measuring ligament strain or forces to understand ligament loading patterns), cadaver studies, mathematical modeling and simulation of injury situations, or measurements/estimation from "close to injury" situations. For most injury types, one research approach alone will not be sufficient to describe all aspects of the injury situation. A broader and more precise understanding could be attained by combining such research approaches as athlete interviews, video analysis,

Table 2.1 Categories of injury mechanism descriptions with examples of elements and descriptions.

Category	Elements	Examples of factors describing the injury mechanism			
		Non-contact ACL injury in basketball	ACL injury in a mogul skiing jump landing	Knockout in boxing	Lower leg stress fracture in football
Playing (sports) situation	Team action	Fast break	Course steepness	Uppercut, Hook	Exposure to matches and training (total load)
	Skill performed prior to, and at, the point of injury	Zone defense	Jump elements (e.g., twist, helicopter)	Counterattack	Midfielder with defensive and offensive tasks (i.e., many runs in matches/training)
	Court position Player position	Charging Cutting	Jump height and length	Foot work Forced into the corner/to the ropes	Hard working team Frequency of duels
	Ball handling	Setting up for a shot Defensive rebound Man-to-man defense		Ring-side referee decision Inter-boxer distance	
Athlete/opponent behavior	Player performance	Effort	Rhythm and balance prior to the jump	Awareness	Effort
	Opponent interaction Player attention	Perturbation by opponent Intention Foot firmly fixed to the floor Intention Technical foul	Concentration Balance Boot-binding release Visual control Jumping technique Over-rotation Falling technique	Aggressiveness Punching power Punching speed Balance	Toe/heel runner Jumping technique Duel technique
Whole body biomechanics	Description of whole body kinematics and kinetics	Sideways translation	Linear and angular momentum	Center of mass velocity	Stride length
		Rotation of the body around the fixed foot Speed at impact	Energy absorption Center of mass to the rear	Punching force Punching direction	Stride frequency Vertical excursion
		Foot in front of center of mass		Weight distribution on the legs Energy transfer	Ground reaction forces Knee flexion angle Bending moment
Joint/tissue biomechanics	Detailed description of joint/tissue kinematics and kinetics	Valgus moment	Shear forces	Head acceleration	Shear forces
		Pivot shift of the tibia relative to the femur Notch impingement	Anterior drawer Intercondylar lift-off Loading rate	Pressure distribution and localization	Surface/shoe dynamics

Reproduced from Bahr and Krosshaug (2005) with permission.
ACL = anterior cruciate ligament.

and clinical studies, or by combining video analysis and studies using cadavers, dummies, or mathematical simulations. The multifactorial nature of sport injuries is important to consider in these studies to understand why certain forces lead to injury in some cases, but not in others. Examples will be presented in the subsequent chapters dealing with specific injury types.

Developing intervention methods and programs

The third stage in van Mechelen's approach is the introduction of prevention measures. The development of injury intervention programs depends to a large extent on the previous step wherein causes of injuries are identified. Strategies for injury control have been developed from other research areas, particularly from research on motor vehicle accidents. One such model, the injury prevention matrix, has two dimensions (Table 2.2). One dimension relates to whether the measure is designed to avoid accidents altogether (pre-crash measures), to avoid injury even if an accident occurs (crash measures), or whether it aims to minimize the consequences of an injury (post-crash measures). The other dimension relates to whether the measure targets the individual, the environment, or perhaps equipment used. Other categories are also possible along this dimension. Although Haddon (1980) originally developed the injury prevention matrix for motor vehicle accidents, it represents a useful approach for analyzing potential injury prevention methods when applied to sports.

Pre-crash measures

Measures related to the pre-crash stage have been developed to counteract potential injury-causing situations by preventing accidents altogether. In sports, examples of *athlete*-related pre-crash measures include ensuring adequate, sport specific, physical conditioning of athletes, increasing their skill level, and improving neuromuscular control and agility to avoid situations where they might get injured. Psychosocial variables may be addressed in an effort to influence the athletes' resiliency and injury vulnerability. In addition, sport-specific screens may help identify athletes at risk for injury and modify their risk prior to participation. Examples of *environmental* pre-crash measures include modifying the friction of the playing surface (too high may lead to twisting injuries to the lower extremity, too low may lead to slipping and falling injuries) or changing regulations to avoid dangerous plays. *Equipment*-related pre-crash measures include modifying shoe friction and choosing cleat length according to the playing surface and weather conditions. All of these measures are based on modifying risk factors that have been shown to be a cause (or part of a cause) of injury.

Crash measures

Measures related to the second stage, the crash stage, have been developed to protect the athlete against injuries if a potentially harmful situation arises. These measures mainly focus on assisting athletes to withstand the forces involved when a collision or a fall occurs. *Athlete*-related crash measures could involve, for example, a general strength-training program, flexibility program, or falling techniques. *Environmental* crash measures include safety nets to avoid falling alpine skiers from flying into the crowd or soft mats protect gymnasts failing to dismount or falling down from an apparatus. There are many examples of *equipment*-related crash measures in sports, such as release bindings for alpine skiing, helmets

Table 2.2 Haddon's matrix applied to sport injury prevention: Measures introduced to prevent sport injuries.

	Pre-crash	Crash	Post-crash
Athlete	Technique, Neuromuscular function	Training status, Falling techniques	Rehabilitation
Surroundings	Floor friction, Playing rules	Safety nets	Emergency medical coverage
Equipment	Shoe friction	Tape or brace, Ski bindings, Leg padding	First-aid equipment, Ambulance

and pads for various sports, taping and braces for joints, shin guards, and eye protection.

Post-crash measures

Post-crash measures are designed to minimize the damage resulting from an injury and the risk of reinjury (which is a strong risk factor for sports injuries), and mainly relates to the chain of medical treatment provided after an injury. Post-crash measures in sports may include providing adequate medical services during sports events (personnel and equipment); training athletes and coaches to provide adequate on-field first aid, including quick evacuation procedures to a hospital in the case of severe injuries, adequate rehabilitation programs for injured athletes and ensuring appropriate medical clearance before they return to competition.

Active versus passive measures

Injury prevention measures can also be categorized as active or passive (Haddon, 1974). Examples from motor vehicle accident prevention are seat belts (active) which require the individual to fasten them, and air bags (passive) which do not require the operator to take any action. In between these extremes there are measures which require some action by individuals. An example is where specific safety gear is required in the rules of the sport; that is, this requires some action by the individual, but this action is a prerequisite to be allowed to participate. This is the case for helmet wear in ice hockey and competitive skiing and snowboarding. In contrast, among recreational skiers and snowboarders, helmets are still not required by most skiing resorts. In this setting, helmet use must be considered an active measure, dependent on education and attitudes with significant barriers in terms of cost and availability.

The distinctions are not merely classifications. They have direct, practical relevance. Historically, passive approaches, when available, have a spectacularly more successful record in injury prevention outside of sport. This is also the case within the sports context, where there is a long tradition for mandating safety equipment, and specific safety standards for sports venues. For example, in leagues where the type of facial protection in ice hockey is optional, players at the varsity/college level have been shown to choose the minimum level mandated. There is an inherent level of risk that athletes appear to be willing to absorb, which may be a barrier to adopting active measures.

Implementing injury prevention programs

Once methods with a potential for prevention have been identified, there is a need to carefully develop the prevention measures, assess them under ideal conditions, and consider the implementation context (Finch, 2006).

An important part of the development of interventions is first testing their *efficacy*. This means that under ideal conditions, they are tested to determine if the intervention works. This is typically done in a controlled research setting with extensive monitoring and measurement of compliance with the intervention. This differs from *effectiveness*, which is where an intervention is implemented in a broader context, often in a community or sport setting, where the degree of attention to the program and monitoring is much less.

If we use the analogy of a drug, efficacy would be the question of whether the drug works under controlled conditions of ideal use. Effectiveness would measure whether the drug worked in a given patient, who may be affected by side effects, convenience of use, etc. Therefore, the culture of sport has a major influence on the effectiveness of intervention programs. Specifically, attitudes and behaviors or historical biases within the sport may prove to be either incentives or barriers to effective implementation of injury prevention programs. To build on our earlier example, the move to mandate full facial protection in adolescent ice hockey was initially resisted due to concerns from sport administrators that the nature of the game would be altered, and from medical personnel that such changes could lead to an increase in neck injuries.

Therefore, the development of injury prevention programs must take into consideration more than the biomechanics of injury or their specific immediate causes. It must also engage stakeholders within the sport and/or community to understand some of the behavioral aspects and norms of the environment in which sport and injury occur. If a prevention program is biologically appropriate, but not appropriate within the context of the sport, it has little hope of being adopted and therefore little chance of being effective.

References

Bahr, R., Krosshaug, T. (2005) Understanding injury mechanisms: a key component of preventing injuries in sport. *British Journal of Sports Medicine* **39**, 324–329.

Finch, C. (2006) A new framework for research leading to sports injury prevention. *Journal of Science and Medicine in Sport* **9**, 3–9.

Fuller, C., Ekstrand, J., Junge, A., Andersen, T.E., Bahr, R., Dvorak, J., Hägglund, M., McCrory, P., Meeuwisse, W. (2006) Consensus statement on injury definitions and data collection procedures in studies of football (soccer) injuries. *Clinical Journal of Sport Medicine* **16**(2), 97–106.

Fuller, C., Bahr, R., Dick, R., Meeuwisse, W. (2007) A framework for recording recurrences, re-injuries and exacerbations in injury surveillance. *Clinical Journal of Sport Medicine* **17**(3), 197–200.

Haddon Jr., W. (1974) Strategy in preventive medicine: passive vs. active approaches to reducing human wastage. *The Journal of Trauma* **14**, 353–354.

Haddon, Jr., W. (1980) Advances in the epidemiology of injuries as a basis for public policy. *Public Health Report* **95**, 411–421.

Meeuwisse, W. (1994) Assessing causation in sport injury: a multifactorial model. *Clinical Journal of Sport Medicine* **4**(3), 166–170.

Meeuwisse, W., Tyreman, H., Hagel, B., Emery, C., (2007) A dynamic model of etiology in sport injury: the recursive nature of risk and causation. *Clinical Journal of Sport Medicine* **17**(3), 215–219.

van Mechelen, W., Hlobil, H., Kemper, H. (1992) Incidence, severity, etiology and prevention of sports injuries—a review of concepts. *Sports Medicine* **14**(2), 82–99.

Further reading

Andersen, T.E., Árnason, Á., Engebretsen, L., Bahr, R. (2004) Mechanisms of head injuries in elite football. *British Journal of Sports Medicine* **38**, 690–696.

Bahr, R. (2003) Preventing sports injuries. In R. Bahr & S. Mæhlum (eds) *Clinical Guide to Sports Injuries*, pp. 41–53. Human Kinetics, Champaign.

Khan, K., Bahr, R. (2006) Principles of sports injury prevention. In P. Brukner & K. Khan (eds) *Clinical Sports Medicine*, pp. 78–101. McGraw-Hill, Sydney.

Meeuwisse, W., Wiley, J. (2007) The sport medicine diagnostic coding system. *Clinical Journal of Sport Medicine* **17**(3), 205–207.

Rae, K., Orchard, J. (2007) The orchard sports injury classification system (OSICS) version 10. *Clinical Journal of Sport Medicine* **17**(3), 201–204.

Chapter 3
Developing and managing an injury prevention program within the team

Andrew McIntosh[1] and Roald Bahr[2]

[1]School of Risk and Safety Sciences, The University of New South Wales, Sydney, Australia
[2]Department of Sports Medicine, Oslo Sports Trauma Research Center, Norwegian School of Sport Sciences, Ullevål Stadion, Oslo, Norway

We are all aware how important it is to manage risks. Most of us have insurance in case something goes wrong. Many people who play sport will have health insurance or sports injury insurance through their club or association. This is certainly important and will assist in managing the consequences of injury, but does not contribute greatly to injury prevention on an individual or team basis. This chapter will describe the components, activities, and strategies required to develop and manage injury risks in a team setting. The "team setting" not only denotes the team of players that run out onto the field. It also includes teams of athletes in individual sports, such as a swimming team or an alpine skiing team, and includes the support team—manager, coach, trainer, physiotherapist, and doctor. Communication and coordination within the support team and between it and the athletes is a requisite feature of risk management in sport.

Principles of risk management

The principles of risk management applied to the sports setting have been described in detail by Fuller (2007). Risk management is the overall process

Sports Injury Prevention, 1st edition. Edited by R. Bahr and L. Engebretsen Published 2009 by Blackwell Publishing ISBN: 9781405162449

of identifying, assessing, and controlling risks. It can be applied within and across sport in the upper levels of policy and administration, in a team, and by an individual.

Injury risks have been identified in most sports. This process is often general, for example, participants in contact sports experience head injuries. Risk assessment is a more formal process of measurement and/or estimation of hazards and risks to athletes on a team. This means measuring the incidence and severity of injuries, associated injury risk factors, and injury mechanisms, as described in Chapter 2. Risk evaluation involves determining the significance and acceptability of the risks to all stakeholders; including the athletes, the coaches, and the club.

Risk control is the process of identifying and implementing methods to control the level of exposure to hazards and/or the consequences. There are four options for risk control: eliminate, retain and manage, outsource, and insure. All options could be in play, each addressing a range of risks. In sport, controls are largely restricted to retain and manage, and insure. There is the presumption that the team has decided to participate in the sport, so elimination of the sporting activity is not an option, although under some circumstances a team may decide not to participate in a specific event. For example, in recent years there has been discussion about teams touring in countries where there has been recent political unrest, war, or terrorism. Teams might agree to cancel a round due to adverse weather, thereby eliminating all sports injury risks on that day. From a team's perspective, it might be possible to outsource medical services and management of venues. A sports team could not be outsourced, whereas a cleaning function in a company could be outsourced to contractors. The two choices that are most often faced are either to accept a risk or reduce a risk. Risk acceptance implies that an informed decision has been made to accept the consequences and/or likelihood of an injury. These risks may be mitigated through insurance, to cover any losses. This approach does allow all stakeholders to continue their program unchanged in the knowledge that their insurance will cover their loss in case of injury, but does not provide much incentive for injury prevention programs. In professional sports many clubs approach the injury issue simply by employing extra players for each position when injuries occur, which represents another form of risk acceptance.

Although participants may appear to accept the level of risk associated with a sport, this is often the result of ignorance of the actual levels of risk involved. This is clearly an important issue, because it is difficult for a participant to accept risks about which they have no knowledge. In most cases, acceptable levels of risk in sport are determined more by the risk perceptions of the participants than by actual data on the risks involved. Another difficulty lies in the fact that, in contrast to other occupations, there are no accepted standards to which risks can be compared.

Risk reduction, on the other hand, involves developing and applying methods to prevent injuries and/or reduce their consequences. In addition to the obvious benefits to the individual athlete, there is also a financial incentive for sports teams through reduced insurance costs and less need to employ extra players. In recreational and youth sports, risk reduction approaches may assist in maintaining or developing the sport's viability through retaining fit participants and promoting the sport as being safe.

Risk identification and assessment

The establishment of a risk management program in a team setting might be driven from the top or from the grass roots. The first task is to identify the injury risks in the sport and bring these to the attention of the team in its various shapes and sizes. In many sports there is already a strong recognition of injury risks. Simply having good on- and off-field medical treatment and rehabilitation is not injury risk management.

The basic steps that will identify injury risks include:
- reviewing injury reports from at least one season;
- reviewing player turnover and availability within one or more seasons;
- reviewing the literature on injury risks in the specific sport.

The person or group who identifies the risks may then need to be advocates within the team or club for risk assessment and control. This will ideally form the basis of a risk management program that is adopted and managed by the club or team.

As mentioned earlier, risk assessment is the formal process of measuring hazards and risks and reviewing these. It may be necessary to undertake prospective studies of injury rates, patterns, and potential risk factors within a team. Some of the major sports have developed guidelines for injury surveillance. Several leagues, such as the National Hockey League, have established systems where every patient's record recorded by the medical team is linked to a central database. In this way the league can monitor injury trends and every team can assess their own injury rates and compare themselves to the league average. Other examples are the International Skiing Federation (FIS), which has established an injury surveillance system to record all injuries during their World Cup; the FIS Injury Surveillance System (FIS ISS); and the National Collegiate Athletic Association (NCAA), which developed its injury surveillance system in 1982 to provide current and reliable data on injury trends in US intercollegiate athletics. Injury and exposure data are collected yearly from a representative sample of NCAA member institutions and the resulting data summaries are reviewed by the NCAA Sport Rules Committees and by the NCAA Committee on Competitive Safeguards and Medical Aspects of Sports. The web-based system also allows individual schools to have a real-time electronic injury record of their specific injuries. The goal of both of these

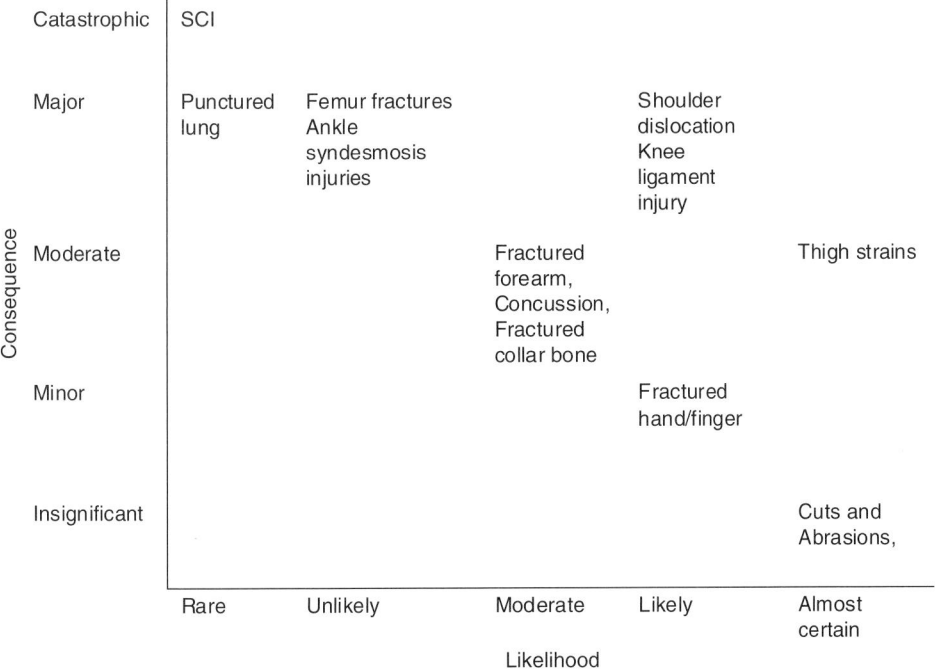

Figure 3.1. Qualitative risk matrix in community rugby; relationship between injury severity (consequence) and injury frequency (likelihood)

surveillance systems is to reduce injury rates through suggested changes in rules, protective equipment, or coaching techniques based on data provided.

A key element is that injury surveillance is a continuing process. Not only are there seasonal changes, but injury data may assist in identifying the level of success of injury prevention strategies. A formal survey, perhaps using a questionnaire or interview, of the player cohort might also be helpful in assessing risks and provide results without the need to wait for one year. As discussed in Chapter 2, there may also be a number of risk factors, internal and external, that should be assessed (Figure 2.2).

Risk control: injury prevention

Once there is a clear understanding of hazards and risks, and preferably a quantifiable level of risk, decisions are required about interventions to control those risks. Many controls exist and there is a continuous development of new methods. The difficulty faced by many is gaining access to this information and staying abreast of the developments; it is time consuming and often highly technical. Often the existence of effective controls, for example, breakaway bases in softball and baseball, take many years to be recognized and adopted.

The "hierarchy of controls" (Figure 3.1) should be followed, but it is recognized that in sport, engineering controls might be difficult to apply. The hierarchy is in the descending order of effectiveness: elimination, substitution, engineering controls, administrative controls, training, and personal protective equipment. The following are examples of each of these controls in skiing.

Once there is a decision to participate in a specific sport, it may be very difficult to eliminate all hazards and risks. Let's consider a pole on a ski run that serves the function of supporting a video camera that provides an important view of the skier. A pole is a collision hazard in a high kinetic energy sport. The pole could be eliminated and no

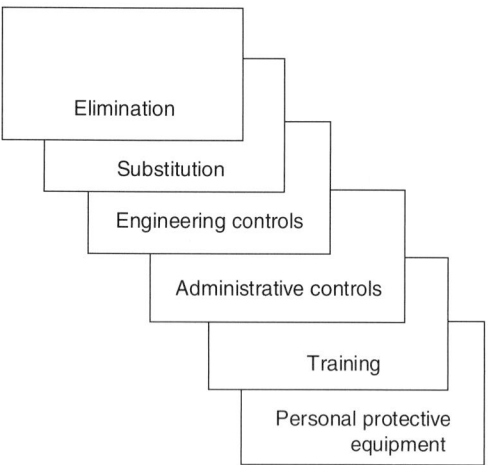

Figure 3.2. Hierarchy of controls

video recorded. The pole could be eliminated and a camera far removed from the ski run installed with lenses to substitute for the proximity. The pole could be substituted by a crane or wires that suspend the camera at the site. An engineering solution might be to manufacture a frangible pole that breaks away during a collision at a force lower than that which would cause injury. Administrative procedures could be implemented to determine where poles could be placed and a process for inspecting the ski run adopted. The skier could be offered personal protective equipment, for example, a helmet and a padded suit, to protect the skier if collision occurs. An additional administrative control would be to mandate the use of that equipment. Finally, the skier could be trained not to collide with poles while skiing competitively. However, we know that even the most skillful athletes err.

Sport has often restricted itself to the less effective controls—personal protective equipment, training individual and team skills plus fitness, and rules. It may also be difficult to implement controls on a team basis because rules of the game, including those that govern protective equipment use and infrastructure, are determined at a national or international level. Disagreements might arise within a competition if, for example, a team decided to prepare its home ground to be slow in order to reduce injury.

Another way of looking at hazards, risks, and controls is through the injury prevention matrix, where injury prevention methods (related to host, agent, physical environment, and social environment) are categorized based on their ability to prevent accidents altogether (pre-crash), to prevent injury even when there is an accident (crash), or prevent disability even when there is an injury (post-crash) (Table 2.2). This approach has been described in more detail in Chapter 2. Clearly training of the support staff's response to a serious injury will assist post injury, as will provision of vehicle access to the ground (post-crash). Whereas, team skill training will hopefully prevent unintentional impacts between players within a team (precrash). Improving personal protective equipment function will assist in preventing the injury (decreasing the risk) during the event (crash). Administrative controls that mandate PPE and education are preevent interventions.

Reaching agreement

Agreement on injury prevention within the team, between teams and within a competition is important. Agreed objectives for the season might be a 30% reduction in lost time injuries or 100% compliance with equipment use protocols, or return to play guidelines. Objectives need to be realistic, important, and common from the players to the officials.

The following discussion will focus on two areas. First, it will discuss the various steps and activities which may form part of a risk management program, focusing on the potential roles of medical staff. Second, it will discuss the importance of equipment and facilities in injury prevention.

The roles of the medical staff

Although not all teams have medical staff as part of the support structure, this section will discuss the potential involvement of team medical staff (physicians, physiotherapists, athletic trainers, etc.) in the development of a risk management program. These include:
• recording of injury and participation data to develop an injury surveillance program;

- season analysis—review of training and competition program;
- preseason screening of physical and behavioral capabilities, limitations, and injury;
- monitoring "at risk" team members, for example fitness, technique, and behavior;
- education regarding injury management and prevention;
- coordination of injury risk management;
- identification of emergency management requirements;
- synthesis of "best practice" and emerging trends from professional and scientific literature.

Access to team physicians, physical therapists, athletic trainers, and other health professionals is mainly available at the elite and professional levels of sport. Nevertheless, many of the risk management functions listed earlier can be performed by coaching staff, parents, or the athlete.

Note that there are privacy issues related to management of individual injury/medical information. There is a need for strong trusting relationships within the team. Guidelines are available which define appropriate lines of communication so that medical staff can maintain a confidential relationship with a player, but still provide pertinent information to team management (Anon., 2000).

Developing an injury surveillance program within the team

Risk management is based on continuous risk assessment. To assess risk within a team, it is necessary to establish a system to monitor injuries and exposure. For medical staff, recording injuries should represent one of the easiest tasks in risk management; they are required to keep accurate records of all assessments and treatment provided to their patients. Thus, establishing a surveillance system only involves analyzing information that is already there. To make this task even easier, excellent electronic tools are available, where the necessary statistical tools have been integrated in software which helps to maintain patient's records. Nevertheless, even at the highest levels of sport, this is rarely done on a routine basis.

Another task is to establish a system to record individual training and competition exposure within the team. This represents a challenge for the medical team, since they are not always present during practices or on road trips, and therefore this task is often done by the coaching staff. Many of the injury recording software programs also have the capability of recording exposure data, which can then be entered based on the coaching records. Exposure data is necessary to calculate risk as described in Chapter 2, and the standard method for calculating injury incidence rates is the number of injuries per 1000 hours of exposure, which is typically used in football codes. For some sports and specific player positions, for example, a pitcher or a bowler, injuries per balls delivered may be a more powerful measure from the perspective of identifying relationships between injury and exposure. It may also be relevant to record exposure in relation to external risk factors, such as turf type (e.g. training on grass, gravel, artificial turf), use of personal protective equipment, and whether the exposure is during competition or training.

Interpretation of injury data is difficult unless exposure data are collected. Consider the example where there is an increase in the number of match injuries from one season to the next. If the number of matches increases by 30%, there would be no increase in injury incidence.

If no medical team is available, it is still possible to develop useable systems to record valuable injury information. In its simplest form, the coach or assistant coach could keep attendance records and simply note absences due to injury throughout the season (and the injury type in question). At the end of the season, the coaching staff would then be able to calculate the number of injuries and the number of days of absence attributable to injury, as well as the main descriptors of injury.

As described in Chapter 2, injury risk is not just a question of injury incidence. The severity of injury must also be taken into account, and most often severity is expressed as the number of days of absence from sports because of an injury. Based on this, the total injury risk to a team can be calculated as the product of injury incidence and injury severity. This is shown in Table 3.1, using

Table 3.1 Variations in the observed values of incidence, severity, and risk for injuries sustained in rugby union matches. Reproduced with permission from Fuller (2007).

Injury type	Incidence (injuries/1000 player hours)	Severity (days/injury)	Risk (days/1000 player hours)
Cervical facet joint injury	2.00	10	20
Foot fracture	0.42	44	18
Foot stress fracture	0.12	151	18
Thigh hematoma	8.00	6	48
Lateral ankle ligament injury	4.20	12	50
Wrist/hand fracture	1.10	43	47
Medial knee ligament injury	3.10	31	96
Shoulder dislocation/instability	1.30	81	105
Anterior cruciate ligament injury	0.42	258	108

a range of injuries sustained by players during rugby union matches as an example. This example shows that in terms of risk, thigh hematomas represent much less of a concern than anterior cruciate ligament injuries do, even if they are 16 times more common!

Injury data can also be illustrated by a risk matrix that highlights risks in terms of likelihood and consequences. This is an appropriate and powerful tool for presenting injury risk data. The example shown in Figure 3.2 is derived from rugby union. It suggests that injury reductions in the areas of shoulder dislocation and knee ligament injury are priorities, as it is in spinal cord injury prevention. By examining factors that contribute to the causation of shoulder and knee injuries, strategies to reduce injury rates can be formulated.

At the highest levels of play, teams may even want to monitor injury mechanisms using match tapes. In professional sports, first-class video recordings are available from all matches and sophisticated software has been developed to analyze play-by-play performance of players. This represents an opportunity to index and analyze all injury situations, as well. Such analyses may reveal whether there are certain situations with a high propensity for injury, or improper technique or inadequate tactical responses on the part of the injured athlete. Even if more sophisticated analysis of the inciting event is laborious, and perhaps better left to scientists, it is possible that large professional teams can develop their own expertise in understanding the injury mechanisms involved. This information may be used to improve coaching and individual player skills. At the community level these expensive resources are absent.

When assessing data from injury surveillance, it is important to recognize that within a team, it is very unlikely that a sufficiently large sample size exists through which the benefit of a single or multiple interventions can be assessed. Therefore, "success" or "failure" in few individuals should not be considered justification for a complete overhaul of the team's training and injury prevention programs. In the same way, seasonal variation in sports injury may simply be due to chance. Often the media report a number of similar catastrophic sports injuries over a period of a few weeks which gives the impression that a problem is out of control. There is no need to panic or overreact, especially if there has been continuing injury surveillance.

Season analysis: review of training and competition program

One helpful method to manage risk in sports is a formal review of the training and competition program to identify risks *prior to* the start of the season. The method of season analysis therefore is fundamentally different from injury surveillance, where data on injuries are collected as they happen. Season analysis represents an attempt to identify risks before they occur (Figure 3.3).

Risks in the program can be related to the competition schedule, the training program, the

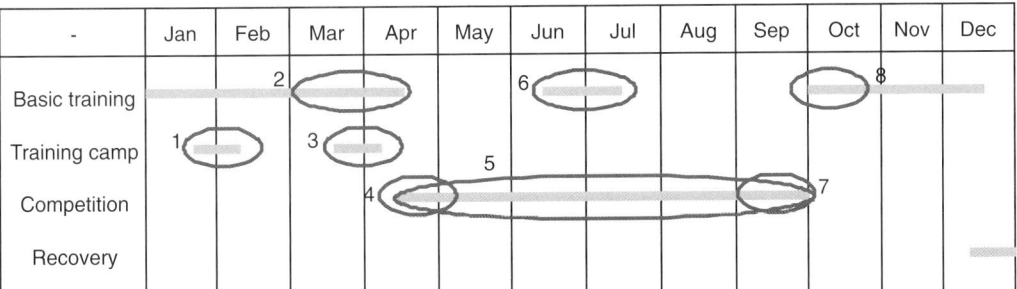

1. Change of surface, climate, and running tempo during training camp in Portugal. Athletes should not increase the amount or intensity of training too much.
2. Transition to higher training volume and high intensity of training, combined with several practice games indoors and on artificial turf.
3. New training camp to polish form before the competitive season, with occasional practice games on hard grassy playing fields on Cyprus. Competition for a spot on the team leads to increases in intensity during competition and training.
4. The beginning of the competitive season. A higher tempo and a packed competitive schedule to which the athlete is unaccustomed. Change of surface to soft grass.
5. High risk of acute injuries during the competition season and a toughpacked competitive schedule at full intensity.
6. Interposed period of hard basic training, strength exercises to which the athlete is not accustomed, and more training for running than usual.
7. The end of the competitive season. Worn out and tired players?
8. Transition to basic training period with running on gravel.

Figure 3.3. Season analysis and profile. Examples of periods of the season when an increased risk of injuries to a senior-level soccer team exists. Comments concern the risk periods that are circled

possibilities for athlete recovery, travel, or other issues. Although health care personnel responsible for teams or training groups may have to initiate this type of analysis, it is strongly recommended that the process is done in collaboration with the coaching team and, if at all possible, the athletes. Professional contracts deal with athlete availability and player associations to advocate maximum levels of competition and schedules. The inclusion of coaches and athletes will enable them to draw on their past experiences with the team, which is especially important if there are no injury surveillance data available from the past. If injury surveillance data are available, the season analysis is an opportunity to review formally the past experiences and discuss whether the injury patterns seen may be related to the training and competition program. For example, a surge in stress fractures on a soccer team may be attributed to a simultaneous increase in the volume of running and a change from a soft to a hard running surface.

Due to the multi-factorial nature of injury causation in sport, identifying risks in sports programs—over a season or during a tournament—is complicated. In other words, season analysis represents an attempt to predict what may happen—and as such, a form of guesswork. Nevertheless, through discussions between coaches, athletes, and medical staff, it is possible to recognize when athletes are at the greatest risk of sustaining injuries as a result of the training or competitive programs. Examples of situations in which injury risk is higher are when athletes switch from one training surface to another (e.g., from grass to gravel) or to new types of training (e.g., at the start of a strength training period). Figure 3.3 illustrates how a team may be at particular risk of different injury types at different stages of the season. Other examples of key program events which could be correlated with injury incidence include:
- poor sleep due to tight schedule or time differences;
- change over from heavy preseason training to competition;
- return to play after mid-season pause;
- beginning of final rounds;

- increased training and competition load associated with representative duties;
- change in training volume;
- change of climate, for example, move from a summer training camp in "Mediterranean" climate to "Northern" climate;
- selection time for important matches, for example, representative schedule (a player may hide early symptoms of an injury, thinking this may prevent selection).

This type of analysis may be particularly important to avoid overuse injuries. The analysis is based on the idea that the risk of injuries is greater during transitional periods and that each stage has certain characteristics that may increase risk. The risk profile usually varies from sport to sport, which underlines how important it is for a medical staff to be intimately familiar with the characteristics of the sport they cover.

Based on the principles of risk management, once a particular element in the team's program has been identified to represent a high risk for injury there are two possible solutions: (i) risk acceptance and (ii) risk mitigation. The coaching staff may decide that this particular element is unavoidable, critically important to the success of the team, and therefore must be accepted. However, this is not a decision that should be taken without those at risk, that is the athletes. If a high risk is identified, the coaches should not decide to accept it on behalf of the players (or anyone) without appropriate consultation. Preferably, it may be possible to reduce risk, for example, by a more gradual change in running surface than was originally planned.

Preseason screening: the preparticipation or annual examination

An obvious responsibility of the medical team is the medical screening of athletes. Preseason or preparticipation examinations are routinely done on hundreds of thousands of athletes around the world every year, in some cases required by sports regulations, or even by law. However, the value of doing routine physical exams on athletes is questionable. If done properly, they can represent a key ingredient in the risk management program of the team. If they are done simply to clear athletes for participation, their value in injury prevention is limited. Unfortunately, this is commonly the case.

Preseason examinations are done for a variety of reasons other than to prevent injuries. Most are done for medico-legal reasons; to ensure that the participant is healthy. In other words, the objective is to clear the athlete for participation and verify that there is no sign of injury or illness which would represent a potential medical risk to the athlete (and risk of liability to the sports organization). There are also special cases, for example, when professional teams trade players, where the purpose of the medical screening exam is to protect their investment.

It follows from this that the general screening examination may include a number of different conditions, such as:

- Musculoskeletal injuries
- Cardiovascular disease and risk
- Asthma and pulmonary function
- Eating disorders
- Cognitive deficits related to mild traumatic brain injury.

The factors included in the general screening examination can be tailored to the sport in question, by focusing on conditions known to be particularly prevalent (e.g., low back problems in rowers, eating disorders among female gymnasts, pulmonary function among cross-country skiers) or where the physical requirements of the sport implies a higher risk of certain conditions (e.g., Marfan's syndrome among basketball or volleyball players).

Depending on the sport and, consequently, the profile of the conditions of interest, screening examinations may involve:

- Examination by a medical practitioner or specialist
- Examination by a physiotherapist or trainer
- Completion of surveys or validated questionnaires regarding the psychology of the player, injury history, expectations, and issues
- Assessment of nutrition and diet
- Neuropsychological assessments
- Assessment of individual and team skills by coaching staff
- Self-reporting of performance deficiencies by players
- Family history, for example diabetes, cardiac disease, and depression.

However, if the purpose is to prevent injuries, the value of doing routine examinations alone is limited. For screening exams to serve a purpose in risk management there are some additional requirements. First, the exam must be designed to identify athletes with risk factors relevant to the sport in question. Second, there must be a plan to follow up athletes with measures intended to reduce risk, if risk factors are identified. Third, the screening exam and follow-up must be planned and led by the medical and coaching staff of the team. Let us consider each of these requirements in turn.

The first requirement, that the exam is designed to identify athletes with risk factors relevant to the sport in question, is rarely met in current practice. In fact, in most cases, the same screening exam is used across sports. This is inappropriate. There can be no single recipe for all sports, as injury patterns and risk factors differ significantly. In the following chapters, Chapters 4 through 11, the incidence of the most important injury types across sports are described. The same chapters also describe the main risk factors for each of these injury types. To design a screening program for one particular sport, it is, therefore, necessary to define the key injury types (based on data from the literature on incidence and severity and preferably also surveillance data as described earlier), and then to define the key risk factors (for these injuries). Based on this information, the screening exam can be tailored to the sport.

Even if the key risk factors have been defined, a key task remains; to select appropriate methods to screen for these risk factors. Screening methods should be valid, accurate, sensitive, and specific. Valid means that the testing method measures the factor you wish to measure. For example, if low hamstrings strength is a risk factor for muscle strains, what method should be used to measure this best? The test is accurate (reliable) means that it will yield the same result each time. A testing method with high sensitivity will identify all players with that factor. A test with high specificity will identify only players with that factor. If the sensitivity is poor then an injured player might be permitted to participate in competition, and if specificity is poor then a fit player might be excluded from the competition. Finding valid and accurate tests to measure relevant risk factors with adequate sensitivity and specificity can be difficult.

The second requirement is that if the presence of a known injury risk factor is identified, an appropriate course of action can be taken to control the risk. If strength is inadequate, it should be followed up with a strength training program. If balance is poor, a training program should be designed and implemented to rectify this. This might be on an individual level, but could be at a team level too. The presence of common risk factors across the team might point to failures in player selection and management, or medical/rehabilitation management.

The third requirement is that the medical and coaching staff of the team must be intimately involved in the screening exam and follow-up of the results. In community level sport, it may be tempting for a club or school to enlist the assistance of local sports medicine personnel to screen their athletes. This is only advisable if they can establish a mechanism to communicate the results to the team, and there are resources to follow up athletes with risk factors. Also, the specialist must be up to date with screening methods for the sport in question and their interpretation.

Monitoring "at risk" team members or team, for example fitness, technique, and behavior

The screening of all players preseason may flow into within season monitoring of a subset of "at-risk" players. The questions that will be answered by this screening include: Are players fit to resume normal local competition following representative competition or international travel? Has a player recovered physical capacity following resolution of a medical condition; is a player returning too early following injury or masking symptoms to continue playing? Is there improvement in a player's technique following identification of a deficit and a training program? If the preseason screening identified a player with a history of inappropriate on- and/or off-field behavior, have appropriate steps been taken and are there changes? Is the athlete attending rehabilitation sessions? Is the athlete wearing the specific item of protective clothing correctly and on all occasions. The same principles apply here, as with preseason monitoring; the measures need to be valid and reliable, and intervention and follow-up is required.

Return to play following injury

The captain of the Australian cricket team responded to a media inquiry as to whether a specific player was returning to a competition too early following injury by saying that the player was fit, that the team did not wish to field an unfit player as he would be less competitive, and the player did not wish to hurt his chances of further selection by playing poorly due to injury. It is clear that it is in the team's interest for all members to be fit prior to their complete return to competition. The team, in its broad context, can foster a culture whereby safety is paramount. A player will clearly perform to their best and over a longer time (seasons) if injuries are managed well. The team can let it be known that players' positions in the team are not in jeopardy while they are recovering from injury. Unfortunately, this is often not the case.

Supervised injury management programs are very helpful, and can be established even at the community and youth levels where resources are limited. A recent study from Swedish amateur soccer illustrated this (Hägglund et al., 2007). Their program was implemented by team coaches and consisted of information about risk factors for reinjury, rehabilitation principles, and a 10-step progressive rehabilitation program including return to play criteria. An analysis of their data showed a 66% reduction in reinjury rate in the intervention group compared to a control group for all injury locations and a 75% for lower limb injuries.

The 10-step rehabilitation program was intended to serve as a guide for the coaches with structured assessment during the functional rehabilitation of players and to assist in return to play decisions. Although the program was designed primarily for lower extremity injuries, coaches were instructed to use it for all injuries. The program was introduced to injured players when they were able to walk without limping and without pain. The program contained various exercises with a gradually increased load. Progress through the program was allowed when the player was able to comply with the exercises without pain and swelling at the injured site. If a player experienced pain or swelling, he returned to the previous symptom-free level and resumed the progress at a later session. No specific time limit or number of repetitions were set for the progress, but coaches were instructed to evaluate symptoms both when exercises were performed as well as the day after. The final step was return to competitive play, and an injured player was not eligible for first team selection until he had been able to participate fully in team training without pain and swelling at the injured body site. The required number of pre-match training sessions varied based on the severity of the injury.

This study illustrated that it is possible to establish programs to guide return-to-play decisions in a structured manner, and that such programs are beneficial in preventing reinjury. At lower levels of play, building relationships with the local doctors and physiotherapists can assist in establishing injury management systems, but this requires more than just providing easy access for injury assessments and emergency care.

Specific guidelines for return to play are being published, challenged, and revised continuously. In the area of mild traumatic brain injury, where there remains controversy over the "right" time to return to play, the process of making that decision is evidence-based (McCrory et al., 2005). Similar evidence-based guidelines are being developed for other injury types.

Education regarding injury management and prevention

Educating the team, including the medical and coaching staff, regarding injury management and prevention is necessary. This will at least raise awareness of specific topics, such as symptoms that might be related to concussion, and may assist in compliance with injury management and injury prevention programs. Specific sessions can be conducted preseason and within season. A preseason session provides an opportunity to present a summary of the findings from the previous season's injury surveillance program, observations from other groups or sports, injury prevention initiatives in the new season, and an overview of the injury management procedures for the team. The preseason session permits discussion and debate on injury management and prevention, with opportunities for all members of the team to contribute. The rules may have been changed since last season or substantial changes made in equipment and facilities, the background to these changes and the implications for the team can be presented. During the season, opportunities arise in team meetings to present updates and reminders on relevant topics. The need may arise to run education sessions within season prior to embarking on an international tour or before a tournament. All the activities described here and in other sections of this chapter assist in developing a *safety culture* in the team.

Identification of emergency management requirements

Emergency management is an integral part of risk management. Emergency management cannot prevent the initial injury, but it can prevent subsequent injury and reduce the level of impairment. There are some very good documents on emergency planning and management in sport (see Chapter 14 for details on coverage for large events). The first step is to identify the team's requirements. Again, injury surveillance and risk assessments will identify the nature and extent of the emergency management responses required. Common emergencies are spinal injury, head injury, heat stress, and cardiopulmonary disease. The appropriate level of specialist medical care required at the venue for large events is discussed in Chapter 14. For smaller events it may be appropriate to ask whether the injury risk is greater than in day-to-day living. While there might be a risk of spinal injury or heart attack in a junior tennis tournament, it is probably not necessary to have specialist care on-site. A level of medical coverage and a plan for obtaining specialist care if necessary is required; that is, a list of phone numbers for ambulances and local doctors. In contrast, in all contact sports, high velocity sports, and martial arts, the risk of head and spinal injury is sufficient to warrant making emergency equipment easily available, for example, to immobilize and transport athletes, and possibly the presence of a trained emergency physician over and above the basic level of medical support required by the team or teams at the event. The emergency management plan will address people, equipment, and processes. Training and practice are essential for the successful implementation of an emergency management plan.

Coordination of injury risk management

All the activities described in this section could be bundled together into a safety management system. This requires coordination and planning. The system can also be audited for compliance and completeness. The process requires:
1. Assessing the team's needs
2. Setting goals and objectives
3. Development of policies, strategies, programs and actions aimed at achieving goals
4. Implementing programs and policies, including education
5. Providing resources to implement programs
6. Establishing a system for review and evaluation

Each stage needs to be documented. The activities presented so far in this section feed into this process, especially injury surveillance. Within this system responsibilities are defined for everyone in the team. The implementation of a safety management system can promote a cycle of continued improvement leading to injury reduction and possibly on field improvements. Ideally a team approach is taken and a small management group established with representation from athletes, coaching, and medical staff. This is consistent with the statutory requirements for occupational health and safety committees in large places of work. In a recreational football club, this would be best done for the club, or if the club is sufficiently large, for defined age groups or division, for example, youth and seniors. The seasonal nature of sport provides a natural opportunity in the off-season to review and evaluate the injury risk management program. Revisions can be implemented during preseason training and competition. The review process must consider the resources available and methods for increasing those resources, for example applying for funds, fund raising, or donations, are useful avenues to explore.

Equipment and facilities

International and national standards for equipment and facilities

There are numerous national, international, and sport specific equipment and facility standards and guidelines. Examples are:
- Helmets: National Operating Committee on Standards for Athletic Equipment (NOCASE); Canadian Standards Association (CSA); American National Standards Institute (ANSI), Snell Foundation; Standards Australia (SA); and International Standards Organisation (ISO)
- Playing surfaces: ASTM International and the International Association for Sports Surfaces Science
- Shin guards: NOCSAE
- Gymnastics facilities and crash mat characteristics—the Federation Internationale de Gymnastique

Research shows that there are differences in the performance of equipment that meets the same standard. The reality is that equipment standards set minimum performance requirements and some products might just meet these, while others exceed the requirements and offer more protection to the user. There may also be no requirement in a country that a specific piece of equipment meets a relevant standard to be offered for sale. Where possible, a team should seek further information prior to deciding on equipment. The team or club is in a much better position to inquire about this than an individual and should advise the athletes or their families accordingly.

In youth and community team sport deleterious situations arise with equipment when the "one size fits all" approach is taken. Sizing and good fit are very important. Therefore, the team kit should contain equipment that covers the sizing requirements of the whole team.

Surprisingly, standards do not exist for some equipment. There is no standard for padding for goal posts, for example. However, checking whether the padding extends to a sufficient height on the posts can be done. There are some gaps in facility and equipment specifications, for example, the International Ice Hockey Federation provides very clear guidelines and advice regarding the development of an ice hockey arena, but details of what constitutes "protective glass" and "padding" are unclear. The International Gymnastics Federation (FIG) provides guidelines regarding size and stiffness of crash mats and equipment design.

Behavioral adaptation

Behavioral adaptation or risk compensation are terms which have been used to describe a possible change in behavior in an athlete when they use protective equipment. The theory is that the person will assess the level of risk and, if they assess that the protective equipment reduces that risk, they will simply undertake more extreme activities to return the risk to a level they are comfortable with. Whether this theory is true generally or only for some individuals remains unknown and it is controversial. Regardless, athletes should be informed and educated about the injury risks in sport and the known effectiveness and limitations of protective equipment and other controls; as described earlier. The results of studies of the effectiveness of sports equipment in preventing injury are being published regularly. Further, if an athlete appears to become more reckless wearing protective equipment, the coaching staff should monitor this and intervene. Ideally athletes should be trained while wearing protective equipment so that they become familiar with the limitations. With some equipment the safety performance can compromise athletic performance. For example, ideally ski bindings will release at a load less than that fracturing the tibia. If the bindings are set with a very large margin of safety, they may release when a skier is safely executing a successful high-speed turn. If the bindings are set not to release easily, the same skier may end up executing the turns successful but during an accident suffer serious lower limb injury. Consideration for experience, performance, skill, and competition level is required.

Inspection and maintenance of facilities and equipment

The issue of duty of care arises when facilities and equipment are discussed. All members of the broad team are responsible for the equipment and facilities. Certainly it is not possible for a player to re-surface an area, but the player might alert team management to those concerns.

The facilities and equipment (fixed and mobile) can be inspected regularly to identify hazards and compliance with the relevant standards or guidelines. Damage or wear and tear might create hazards for players and officials. A protocol for routine inspection of facilities and equipment should be a part of a risk management plan. Organizations such as FIS provide guidelines for the set up and inspection of facilities used in FIS events. There are also private contractors and technical organizations that offer services to measure facility performance, for example friction, impact energy attenuation, and thermal properties.

Training

As stated earlier, it is important that teams are trained to use equipment. Training might consist of advising on the level of protection offered by particular equipment, the correct use, adjustment and care of equipment, and equipment misuse. As a note of warning, it might be necessary to explain the limits of protection conferred by specific equipment and provide feedback or supervision with fit and adjustment. Training drills while wearing equipment are important too as they help athletes become accustomed to wearing equipment and issues, such as communication, can be identified and resolved.

References

Anon. (2000) The British Olympic Association's position statement on athlete confidentiality. *Journal of Sports Science* **18**, 133–135.

Fuller, C.W. (2007) Managing the risk of injury in sport. *Clinical Journal of Sport Medicine* **17**, 182–187.

Hägglund, M., Waldén, M., Ekstrand, J. (2007) Lower reinjury rate with a coach-controlled rehabilitation program in amateur male soccer. A randomized controlled trial. *American Journal of Sports Medicine* **35**, 1433–1442.

McCrory, P., Johnston, K., Meeuwisse, W., Aubry, M., Cantu, R., Dvorak, J., Graf-Baumann, T., Kelly, J., Lovell, M., Schamasch, P. (2005) Summary and agreement statement of the 2nd International Conference on Concussion in Sport, Prague 2004. *British Journal of Sports Medicine* **39**, 196–204.

Further reading

Australian Master OHS & Environment Guide, 2nd Ed (2007) CCH Australia

AS/NZS 4360:2004 Risk management and HB 436:2004 (Guidelines to AS/NZS 4360:2004) Risk Management Guidelines Companion to AS/NZS 4360:2004, SAI Global.

Caine, D.J., Maffulli, N. (eds.). (2005) Epidemiology of pediatric sports injuries. Individual Sports. *Medicine of Sport Science* **48**.

Federation Internationale de Gymnastique http://www.fig-gymnastics.com/

International Ski Federation http://www.fis-ski.com/uk/home-page.html

Maffulli, N., Caine, D.J. (eds.) (2005) Epidemiology of pediatric sports injuries. Team sports. *Medicine of Sport Science* **49**.

McClure, R., Stevenson, M., McEvoy, S. (eds.) (2004) *The Scientific Basis of Injury Prevention and Control*. IP Communications, Melbourne.

McIntosh, A.S., Janda, D. (2003) Evaluation of cricket helmet performance and comparison with baseball and ice hockey helmets. *British Journal of Sports Medicine* **37**, 325–330.

National Operating Committee on Standards for Athletic Equipment http://www.nocsae.org/

Peltz, J.E., Haskell, W.L., Matheson, G.O. (1999) A comprehensive and cost-effective preparticipation exam implemented on the World Wide Web. *Medicine and Science in Sports and Exercise* **31**, 1727–1740.

Chapter 4
Preventing ankle injuries

Jon Karlsson[1], Evert Verhagen[2], Bruce D. Beynnon[3] and Annunziato Amendola[4]

[1] Professor of Sports Traumatology, Department of Orthopaedics, Sahlgrenska University Hospital, Göteborg, Sweden
[2] Department of Public and Occupational Health, EMGO-Institute, VU University Medical Center, Amsterdam, The Netherlands
[3] Department of Orthopaedics and Rehabilitation, McClure Musculoskeletal Research Center, The University of Vermont, VT, USA
[4] Department of Orthopaedic Surgery and Rehabilitation, University of Iowa Sports Medicine Center, University of Iowa, Iowa, USA

Epidemiology of ankle injuries in sports

Ankle injuries

It is well known that across all sports the most common location of injury is the ankle. It has been estimated that about 25% of all injuries across all sports are ankle injuries (Tik-Pui Fong et al., 2007). Thereby, it is important to have a clear focus on ankle injuries, the associated risk factors, as well as the methods of prevention. Ankle injuries can be classified as either acute or chronic, with ligamentous injury by far being the most common acute diagnosis. About 85% of all ankle injuries involve the lateral ankle ligaments, that is, ankle sprains. Chronic injuries are often related to, or sequelae of acute sprains, or overuse syndromes of the surrounding soft tissues. In view of the predominance of ankle sprains, this chapter will focus on ligamentous injuries, in particular lateral ligament injuries.

The lateral ankle ligaments are the more important structures that hold the ankle bones and joint in position. In doing so, these ligaments protect the ankle joint from abnormal movements, especially from excessive twisting, turning, and rolling of the foot. It is these movements that cause an ankle sprain, that is, when the foot twists, rolls, or turns beyond its normal motions. This causes the ligaments to stretch beyond their normal range in an abnormal position, leading to overstretching or rupture of one or more lateral ankle ligaments. It is not surprising that particularly contact sports, indoor sports, and sports with a high jump rate have a high incidence rate of ankle sprains (Table 4.1). In volleyball it has even been estimated that half of all acute injuries are ankle sprains.

In general an ankle sprain causes an individual to refrain from sports participation at least for 1 day. A side effect of an ankle sprain is the high risk of re-injury to the same ankle, which can result in disability and can lead to chronic pain or instability in 20–50% of these recurrent cases. The relatively high rate of ankle sprains across all sports and the potentially negative consequences of ankle sprains on future sports participation, motivates specific attention for preventive measures against this type of injury.

Sport-specific injury epidemiology: soccer

It has been estimated that 50–60% of all sports injuries in Europe and, as a result, 3.5–10% of all hospital treated injuries are related to soccer. Soccer has also become one of the fastest growing sports in North America. Because of its popularity, soccer injury epidemiology has been the topic of frequent reports. Table 4.1 summarizes the findings of several published studies on soccer injuries. The lower extremity was the most common site of injury regardless of the skill or age level of all the participants, ranging

Sports Injury Prevention, 1st edition. Edited by R. Bahr and L. Engebretsen Published 2009 by Blackwell Publishing ISBN: 9781405162449

Table 4.1 Risk of ankle sprains in different sports. The numbers reported are average estimates based on the studies available.

Sport	Competition incidence[1]	Overall incidence[1]	Rank[2]	Comments
Team sports				
Volleyball	1.8–5.5	0.6–2.0	1 (32–49%)	
Soccer	0.4–26.7	0.1–5.0	1 (15–41%)	
Team handball	1.32	0.4–1.6	2 (11–14%)	
Basketball	1.2–5.4	0.9–4.7	1 (13–27%)	
American Football	5.0–13.0	0.5–3.9	2 (12–21%)	
Australian Football	3.9–4.9	1.3–2.3	3 (9–14%)	
Indoor soccer	10.1–10.3	NA	1 (19–25%)	
Individual sports				
Orienteering	3.8	0.82	1 (27–32%)	
Badminton	NA	0.6	1 (19–24%)	
Gymnastics	NA	0.06–0.31	2 (11–21%)	

[1]Incidence is reported for adult, competitive athletes as the number of injuries per 1000 h of training and competition.
[2]Rank indicated the relative rank of ankle within each sport, as well as the proportion as a percentage of the total number of acute injuries within the sport.
NA: Data not available.

65–90% of all recorded injuries. Ankle injuries were the most common in all studies, ranging 15–41% of all injuries, and the majority of these were sprains.

American football and rugby

One of every fourteen teenager presenting to the emergency room following a traumatic event has a sports-related injury, and American football is the most common precipitating athletic activity in the United States. In a recent review of high school and collegiate football injuries, the most commonly injured body sites were the knee and lower leg/ankle/foot. The majority (~70%) of lower leg/ankle/foot injuries were to the ankle (15.2% of all injuries). The most common cause of knee and ankle injury was ligament sprains (53.2% for knee and 88.0% for ankles). Rugby has a larger incidence of head, neck, and spine injuries as well as fractures. Ankle sprains represent 9.1% of all injuries.

Running, jogging, and hiking

Running has become one of the major recreational and competitive sports. Generally, injuries encountered in these sports are overuse or repetitive stress type from accumulative impact loading. Location of injury is overwhelmingly found in the lower extremity and the greatest prevalence of injuries, one-third, is around the foot and ankle. Orienteering/long distance running are variants of running sports. Running is the major training exercise for orienteers and likely the reason for the majority of injuries are from overuse. In a prospective study of elite orienteers, 94% of the injuries occurred during running and 53% of those occurred while running on uneven ground. Almost 90% of the total injuries occurred in the lower extremity and almost two-thirds of the total injuries occurred in the lower leg, ankle, and foot regions. The most common traumatic injury was a sprain of the ankle and usually occurred during running in forest or uneven ground.

Basketball

In numerous studies in basketball players, professional and amateur, the lower extremity was most commonly injured; the ankle and sprains as the most common type of injury. The ankle and knee injuries were also the most severe with the greatest time lost from participation. An alarmingly high rate of residual symptoms, up to 50%, is seen in athletes with a history of ankle sprains.

Volleyball

In most studies involving high level volleyball players, the ankle is the most common overall site of injury, with ankle sprains as the most common injury. Most of the injuries occur at the net, with ankle sprains resulting from landing on another player's foot.

Gymnastics

Women's gymnastic injury rates have consistently been among the highest seen across sports. The lower extremity accounts for one-half to two-thirds of all reported injuries in gymnastics. Sprains and strains appear to account for over half of these injuries. Although many reports stress that the ankle is one of the most commonly injured joints in gymnastics, one study comparing gymnasts to age-matched controls found that the prevalence of ankle complaints was the same, 27% in both groups.

Racquet sports

Common racquet sports include tennis, badminton, squash, and racquetball. Although one may associate these activities with upper extremity problems, for example, tennis elbow and wrist pain, from epidemiological studies available, the lower extremity is still one of the most common sites of injury. Most published studies indicate that over 50% of injuries in these sports occur in the lower extremities. Of these, ankle sprains appear to be the most common injury. In the constrained racquet sports, such as racquetball and squash, which have a significantly higher rate of facial injuries, ankle sprains are the most frequent of the non-facial injuries, accounting for more than 25% of total injuries.

Key risk factors: how to identify athletes at risk

Previous ankle ligament sprain

Of the many risk factors suggested for lateral ankle ligament sprains (Table 4.2), perhaps the most important is a previous sprain. The rationale for this is that disruption of a ligament compromises an important biomechanical stabilizer of the ankle and creates partial deafferentation that can compromise neuromuscular control of the ankle (Hertel, 2000). Studies of soccer athletes, volleyball athletes, basketball athletes, and military recruits undergoing basic training found that they were all at a twofold risk for lateral ankle ligament injury after suffering a prior ankle injury. It is important to identify these players with previous injury and/or impaired neuromuscular control, in order to provide proper treatment and medical guidance.

Postural sway

Postural sway is closely linked to a previous ankle sprain occurrence (Willems et al., 2005a, b). A sprain affects neuromuscular control of the ankle, subsequently leading to an increased risk of re-injury. Recognizing that an athlete's center of gravity constantly changes position during upright posture (i.e., postural sway), and that this is under the control of both the central and the peripheral nervous system, many different approaches have been used to characterize postural sway and this outcome appears to be related to the risk of suffering an ankle injury. Postural sway is generally characterized in a practical approach that involves measurements of the duration of time that a subject can maintain a single leg stance without touching down to recover balance. Athletes, who are able to maintain a single leg stance for at least 15s are considered to have normal posture, whereas those that touchdown to regain balance within the 15s test are considered to have abnormal posture (Figure 4.1). Several studies have shown that athletes with abnormal posture suffer more ankle sprains as compared to athletes with normal sway.

Gender

Among female athletes, the risk of suffering a first time ankle ligament tear is associated with the sport they participate in. Several studies have shown that the risk of suffering a first time ankle ligament injury appears to be highest for female basketball athletes, who are estimated to have a 25% higher risk than male basketball athletes.

Table 4.2 Internal and external risk factors for ankle sprains in different sports. The numbers reported are average estimates based on the studies available.

Risk factor	Relative risk[1]	Evidence[2]	Comments
Internal risk factors			
Previous ankle sprain	2	++	Increased risk for recurrence during 12 months post-injury
Postural sway	NA	+	
Gender	125	+	Risk is higher for females
Range of motion of the ankle	NA	+	
Height and weight	NA	+	
Anatomic foot type	NA	+	
Foot width	NA	+	
Generalized joint laxity		0	No known association
Ankle joint laxity	NA	+	
Muscle strength	NA	+	
Limb dominance	NA	+	
External risk factors			
Shoe type		++	No association
Play in game versus practice	2–44	++	Higher risk during games
Player position	1–5	++	Relative risk depends upon sport

[1] Relative risk indicates the increased risk of injury to an individual with this risk factor relative to an individual who does not have this characteristic. A relative risk of 1.2x means that the risk of injury is 20% higher for an individual with this characteristic. NA: Not available.

[2] Evidence indicates the level of scientific evidence for this factor being a risk factor for ankle sprains: ++ —convincing evidence from high-quality studies with consistent results; + —evidence from lesser quality studies or mixed results; 0—expert opinion without scientific evidence

In contrast, there is evidence that suggests the risk of suffering repeated ankle ligament sprains is similar for females and males for jumping sports such as volleyball. Additional research that focuses on the effect of gender on the risk of suffering a first time ankle ligament injury is needed in other high risk sports that produce ankle ligament injuries.

Range of motion of the ankle

A decrease in dorsiflexion range of motion of the ankle has been associated with an increased risk of suffering an ankle sprain (Willems et al., 2005a, b; de Noronha et al., 2006). The relationship between decreased dorsiflexion and increased risk of ankle ligament injury may be produced by a tight gastrocnemius muscle–tendon complex, which could place the ankle–foot complex in greater plantar flexion during activity. This would unlock the talus from the ankle mortise, and place the ankle at an increased risk of abnormal inversion and internal rotation. This finding suggests that athletes that are predisposed to ankle ligament injury because of decreased dorsiflexion range of motion may realize some benefit in terms of reduction of ankle ligament injury risk by participating in stretching programs that are designed to increase dorsiflexion motion.

Height and weight

Height and weight have been implicated as risk factors because when a athlete is in an at-risk position for inversion ankle trauma, an increase in either height or weight proportionally increases the magnitude of the inversion torque that must be resisted by the ligaments and muscles that span the ankle complex; however, there is little consensus in the literature with regard to how these outcomes are related to risk of ankle ligament injury. There are studies that demonstrated that height and weight are not independent risk factors for ankle sprains. In contrast, from soccer, American football, and the military there are other studies, reporting that athletes of greater height and weight (and increased body mass index (BMI)) are at increased ankle sprain risk. The different findings between the investigations may be explained, at least in part, by the different sports which were studied.

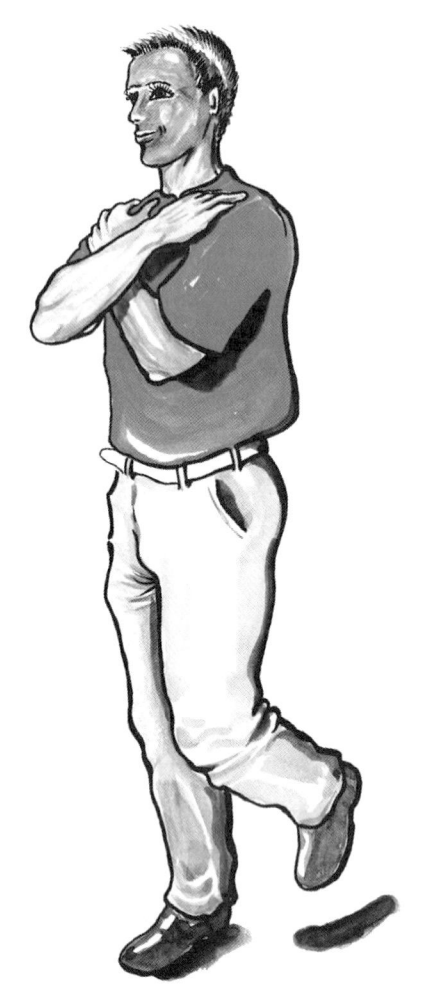

Figure 4.1. Balance test. The patient stands on one leg with the other leg slightly flexed and hanging straight down. He crosses his arms over his chest and looks at a point straight ahead. If he can balance for 1 min with his eyes open, he closes his eyes and balances for another 15 s

Limb dominance

Limb dominance has been implicated as a risk factor for lower extremity trauma because most athletes place a greater demand on their dominate limb and as a consequence produce an increased frequency and magnitude of moments about the knee and ankle, particularly during high demand activities that place the ankle and knee at risk. However, the literature is divided with regard to limb dominance as a risk factor for suffering an ankle ligament sprain. Contrasting findings in the literature are most likely produced by different study designs, differences in the sample sizes, the different sports studied, or the methods used for data analysis.

Foot type, foot size, and anatomic alignment of the lower extremity

Anatomic foot type, when classified as pronated, supinated, or neutral, does not appear to be a risk factor for ankle sprains. It is important to point out that the use of the classification system, which characterizes anatomic foot type as pronated, supinated, or neutral, may be inadequate for identifying abnormalities in foot biomechanics. Indeed, the definitions of different foot types are vague and not scientifically based. This approach has not been related to musculoskeletal abnormalities, as it does not have the specificity and sensitivity to identify abnormalities in foot biomechanics, and it is evaluated while a subject is standing barefoot (sometimes in a laboratory) and not during a situation when the lower extremity is at risk for injury. Therefore, specific and sensitive measurements of foot contact mechanics that can be used during dynamic, at-risk activity need to be developed and used to determine if they are capable of identifying an ankle at risk for an inversion sprain. Studies revealed that dynamic pes planus, pes cavus, and increased hind foot inversion are associated with an increased risk of suffering a sprain of the lateral ankle ligaments (Morrison & Kaminski, 2007). The same goes for an increased foot width, which can be explained, at least in part, by the fact that during an inversion injury, an increased foot width is associated with an increased moment arm and corresponding inversion moment in comparison to a narrow foot.

Ankle joint laxity and generalized joint laxity

To most involved in diagnosis and treatment of ankle injuries, increased laxity of the joint would be considered a "sure bet" as a risk factor for an ankle injury, because it indicates that a soft tissue restraint may have been compromised along with its contribution to stability (laxity restraint) and neural intervention of the ankle complex. However, the literature presents conflicting findings with regard to the relationship between joint laxity and ankle ligament injury. The discrepancy between the available evidence may derive from the use of the clinical examination and a grading system to evaluate joint laxity. Indeed, accurate and reproducible clinical examination is not easy. Another reason might be an inadequate sample size with too few subjects with increased ankle laxity included. It is important to appreciate that increased ankle joint laxity may be highly correlated with prior ankle ligament injury which by itself is an established risk factor for ankle ligament re-injury. From this perspective, if a study includes joint laxity as an outcome, an increase in this outcome may simply serve as a surrogate for prior injury. There appears to be a consensus in the literature that generalized joint laxity has no predictive value for ankle sprains. This is the case when considering men and women athletes as a group, and men and women as separate groups.

Muscle strength

While most would consider it intuitive that lower extremity strength is related to the risk of suffering an ankle ligament sprain, only a few investigations have studied this with a prospective design and accurate equipment and there is little consensus between the studies. An increased risk of ankle ligament injuries has been observed for collegiate female athletes participating in soccer, field hockey, and lacrosse when they have higher peak torque ratios between the invertors and evertors of the ankle. A study of male physical education students reported that decreased strength of the muscles that dorsiflex the ankle was associated with an increased risk of suffering an ankle ligament injury (Willems et al., 2005b). In contrast, a study of male military recruits found no relationship between muscle strength and the likelihood of suffering an ankle ligament injury.

Shoe type

An extrinsic risk factor, which has been well investigated, is the shoe type. Although most would agree that current athletic shoes offer limited support to an ankle in response to inversion trauma, it is important to recognize that little is known about the effect of athletic shoes and how they are related to ankle injury. Specific characteristics of the shoe may either reduce the risk of injury (e.g., certain design characteristics may provide increased proprioceptive input) or increase the risk of injury (e.g., restricted ankle range of motion, abnormal foot-shoe, and shoe-surface traction, or increase the inversion moment arm about the ankle complex). There is little information on the effect that different characteristics of athletic shoes have on the risk of ankle injury. It is more likely that the newness of the shoe plays a more important role than its height in preventing ankle sprains.

Play setting

There is a general consensus that across all sports the risk of injuries in general is higher during competition than during training. It seems logical to assume that this also goes specifically for ankle sprains. This logical assumption is backed up by sound evidence from soccer, basketball, as well as volleyball. The main reason for this difference in injury risk lies in different play modes between competition and training. During competition athletes are more prone to take "risks" in order to win. During training, logically, taking risks is minimized and most play consist of short well controlled bouts of sports specific drills. In short, the playing environment during training is more controlled and thereby safer.

Playing position

Volleyball athletes are at increased risk when they play the front row positions, by landing under the net after a jump for a spike or block. However, in sports such as basketball and soccer which also involve jumping, planting, and cutting, the risk of ankle ligament injury appears to be similar between positions. Nevertheless, at least for soccer, it is known that most injuries occur when an athlete has to play outside his or her usual playing position, for example, a striker making a defensive action, or a defensive player moving toward the opponent's goal. Therefore, while in certain sports ankle sprain risk may not be directly associated with playing position, an athlete at a specific playing position may be so well adjusted to his or her tasks that changing roles on the team increases risk.

Take-home message

In recent years considerable research has focused on risk factors related to ankle sprains. This has resulted in a number of potential risk factors, of which most are surrounded by conflicting findings from scientific studies. The only well documented, and probably by far strongest risk factor for an ankle sprain, is a history of a previous similar injury, especially an injury during the past year. Therefore, it is important to map previous injury and test proprioceptive ankle function by means of a postural sway test. This latter method has been proved to be able to detect athletes at risk. Although preventive measures should be advocated to all athletes, especially this subgroup of previously injured athletes should be targeted with preventive measures, such as proprioceptive training, taping, or bracing.

Injury mechanisms for ankle sprains

Anatomical and biomechanical aspects

Before describing the injury mechanisms leading to an ankle sprain, a short description of the ankle complex is required. The ankle is a so-called hinge joint, bringing the lower leg (tibia and fibula) and the foot (talus) together. The hinge allows dorsiflexion (pulling the ankle up to make the toes face up) and plantar flexion (stretching the ankle and make the toes face down). These movements occur in varying degrees between 50° and 90°. The talus is wider in the front, making it a wedge-shaped bone. Due to its shape the talus provides maximum stability in dorsiflexion but minimal stability in plantar flexion. Although there is room for some inversion and eversion movement (turning the foot inward or outward respectively), the range of motion of these movements is limited. This limitation in movement is primarily restricted by the capsule surrounding the ankle, which is reinforced by both medial and lateral ligaments. The lateral ligaments, the area of interest here, are the anterior talofibular ligament,

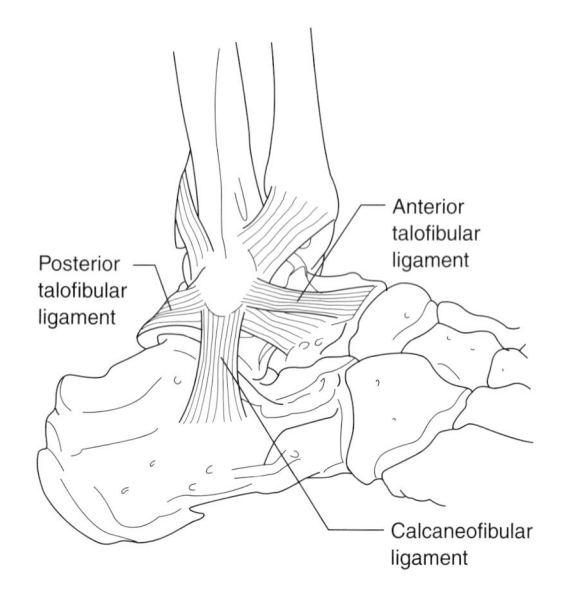

Figure 4.2. The lateral ankle ligaments

the calcaneofibular ligament, and the posterior talofibular ligament (Figure 4.2).

When sitting with a relaxed ankle, the ankle tends to hang in a slight plantar flexed inversed position, that is, the toes are slightly facing the floor and pointing slightly inward. This is the "neutral" position of the ankle. This can also be seen when inspecting worn shoe soles. The initial point of impact is on the outside of the heel, showing in the fastest wear on that side of the sole. What happens is that when walking, in the swing phase the ankle moves to its "neutral" position. Although this is the "neutral" ankle position, it is also a position that puts the ankle at risk for inversion injuries, that is, ankle sprains. As said, in this ankle position the bony stability provided by talus is low, and most of the laxity restraint is provided by the lateral ligaments. Although the ankle is in perfect balance in the "neutral" position, a slight interference moving the ankle in to a further plantar flexed inversion position, results in forces which the lateral ligaments can't handle. As a result the ankle forcefully inverts, which is called an ankle sprain (Figure 4.3). An ankle sprain results in physical damage to the lateral ankle ligaments, and is usually classified by the number of ligaments that are injured. With the foot in plantar flexed inversion, the biggest strain is on the anterior talofibular ligament. It may not be

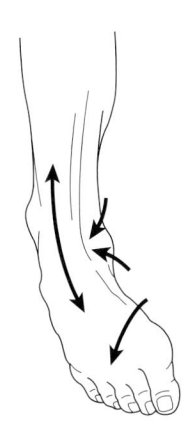

Figure 4.3. Ankle movement leading to an ankle sprain: whilst the foot is plantar flexed and slightly inverted, the foot is easily further inverted and/or rolled inwards leading to an excessive strain on the lateral ankle ligaments

surprising that this is the first ligament to tear during an ankle sprain. With increasing forces, the next ligament to tear is the calcaneofibular ligament, and in rare cases the posterior ligament is also injured.

Based on the mechanism described earlier, it is not surprising that most sports-related ankle sprains are a result of landing on other athletes, objects, or uneven surfaces. Even so, this explains (at least in part) the increased risk after an earlier ankle sprain. As said, a previous ankle sprain results in partial deafferentation that can compromise neuromuscular control of the ankle, a proprioceptive deficit. Ankle proprioception is an important regulatory system keeping the ankle in the safe "neutral" position. When one is unable to accurately detect the position of the ankle, its position will easily deviate from the "neutral" position. Additionally, the protective reflexes reacting to a sudden inversion of the ankle won't be able to detect changes in range of motion to such an extent that a proper reaction is possible. The term "feel" should be put into context here, since the proprioceptive system is regulated peripherally. In short it is the whole system consisting of muscle spindles, nerves, reflexes, etc. that subconsciously control ankle movement and position.

Examples from specific sports

One of the sports in which the events leading to an ankle sprain has been well documented, is volleyball. Nearly all volleyball-related ankle sprains result from player-to-player contact. Ankle sprains occur most frequently at the net, as the result of contact between the attacker and the opposing blocker(s) across the centerline (Verhagen et al., 2004a). It is well known from several studies that approximately half of all ankle sprains occur when a blocker lands on the foot of an opposing attacker who has legally crossed the centerline. It happens frequently that an attacker getting ready for a spike has to adjust his jump for a set that is too low and too close to the net. The resulting momentum and jump trajectory takes him under the net. As long as part of the attacker's foot touches the centerline this is allowed within the rules of volleyball. Unfortunately, for tactical reasons the blocker jumps later than the attacker, and may land on the attacker's foot within this "conflict zone" under the net. This situation accounts for about half of the ankle sprains in volleyball. Additionally, approximately one quarter of all ankle sprains occur when a blocker lands on a teammate's foot when participating in a multi-person block. Consequently, middle blockers and outside attackers are at greatest risk for ankle sprain (net positions), whereas setters and defensive specialists are at comparatively lower risk (back court positions).

Although in volleyball ankle sprain risk seems to be position specific, in sports such as basketball, soccer, and handball which also involve jumping, planting, and cutting, the risk of ankle ligament injury appears to be similar between positions. In these sports the different skills and tasks between positions do not vary as greatly as in volleyball. More importantly, players are not divided by a net and physical contact and jumping within close range of each other is not uncommon.

In soccer, it has been found that ankle sprains occur when the players gets hit in a late, sliding tackle, while the foot is being planted on the surface (Figure 4.4). A laterally directed hit on the medial side of the ankle or lower leg will put the ankle in a vulnerable, supinated position, and when the player puts weight on the ankle, this leads to an inversion sprain. In other words, it is not the tackle that ruptures the ligament, but the fact that the tackle causes the player to land in a vulnerable position.

In the end a vast amount of sports- and situation-specific examples of situations in which ankle sprains occur can be given. However, it is important to note that every ankle sprain has a single common underlying cause, that is, the

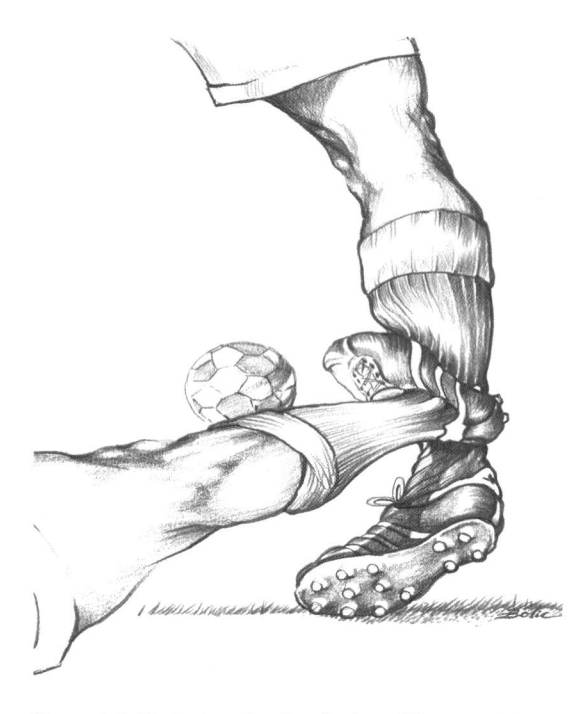

Figure 4.4. Typical mechanism for lateral ligament injury in football: opponent contact to the medial side of the leg, causing the player to put weight on an inverted ankle. Illustration reproduced with permission. ©Oslo Sports Trauma Research Center/T. Bolic

athlete's ankle is forced into a position of plantar flexed inversion after contact with another player, object, or surface.

Identifying risks in the training and competition program

Little is known about possible seasonal influences on the risk of sustaining an ankle sprain, and the meager evidence shows no strong relationships. This is not completely surprising, while ankle sprains occur most frequently in indoor sports with a high jump rate like volleyball or basketball. For that reason most research focuses on these sports in which weather conditions have no impact on ankle sprain risk whatsoever. However, by using common sense one can think of a number of reasons why during autumn and winter ankle sprain risk could be influenced by weather conditions. The fact that these relational influences have never been described is probably associated with rules prohibiting play on dangerous pitch conditions or athletes being aware of these risks.

Although seasonal influence may lack a scientific basis, in male amateur soccer players it has been shown that most ankle sprains occur during the first 2 months of the season (Kofotolis et al., 2007). This is in line with findings that in males low running speeds and low cardiorespiratory fitness are associated with ankle sprains (Willems et al., 2005b). After the summer break athletes will be less "fit," and the level of fitness will be regained during the course of the season. Therefore, it is advised to pay special attention to ankle sprains at the start of a new season. This can be done for instance by eliminating all external risk factors, by advocating preventive measure use to all players, or by planning training session aimed more at increasing fitness than skill.

Preventive measures

Based on the scientific evidence on etiology of ankle sprains and the injury mechanisms described earlier in this chapter, a matrix illustrating potential methods to prevent ankle sprains can be created (Table 4.3). It should be said that although for a number of potential ankle sprain risk factors there is (shallow) scientific evidence, most risk factors can be established by using common sense. Balls may wander around the pitch during training, during the winter time the field is harder and other cleats are required, a wet cross-country running track is slippery, three players jumping for a rebound under the basket, etc. Although general preventive guidelines based on proven risk factors can be given, each situation is different. Therefore, it is recommended to keep track of the ankle sprain causes in an injury log and perform a subsequent risk analysis on the acquired data. In this way recurring risks can be ascertained and dealt with accordingly.

Rule changes

In volleyball most ankle sprains occur under the net when a player lands on the foot of a teammate or an opponent after jumping for a spike or block.

Table 4.3 Injury prevention matrix for ankle sprains: potential measures to prevent injuries.

	Pre-crash	Crash	Post-crash
Athlete	Skill Neuromuscular function		Neuromuscular function
Rules	Rule changes		
Material		External ankle support	

It has been postulated that changing the net-line rule will avoid these collisions under the net. The current net-line rule allows a player to cross the line under the net as long as part the foot stays in contact with the line. Changing this rule to a state where a player may not cross or touch the net-line, will avoid the possibility to land on an opponent's foot. Thereby, an important cause of ankle sprains in volleyball will be eliminated. In a pilot study where this suggested rule was applied, it was found that too many rallies were stopped due to violations of this new rule, and the proposed rule change was discarded. Nevertheless, the rule could be applied during practice – both to reduce risk and to teach players techniques to win the ball without entering the potential conflict zone under the net.

Another example of a rule change intended to prevent ankle injuries is from soccer, where tackles from behind result in an automatic red card and expulsion from the game. Recent data suggest that red cards should also be considered for late sliding tackles against the lower leg.

It is obviously not always possible to develop effective rule changes that reduce injury risk. However, when keeping track of ankle sprain causes in an injury log one may identify situations where ankle injuries occur more frequently. One may conclude for instance that ankle sprains occur mostly on a wet and uneven surface in cross-country running, or in the goal area after a corner kick in soccer. Formal rule changes to avoid risky situations may not possible, because they change the nature of the game as in the previous volleyball example. Still, once established, players can be taught to recognize and avoid risky situations during training. Adjusted rules can be applied during training, one can avoid drills involving risky situations or even design drills to teach avoidance strategies in high-risk situations (provided the drills are done in a safe way, of course). Following the examples giving earlier, after heavy rain cross-country runners should avoid uneven and slippery surfaces during training. During practice soccer players may be instructed to restrict their dueling on corner kicks. Such measures can drastically decrease overall ankle sprain risk. One can only get injured while participating in sports, and training accounts for the highest exposure. A safe training environment will therefore have a great impact on injury risk.

Nonetheless, from a coaching perspective it is undesirable to avoid or modify all "risky" situations during training. The avoided or modified situations will most surely come up in an unmodified version in a competitive setting (e.g., there will be tough air duels after corner kicks). For that reason, it is also important to prepare the athlete for the risk situations encountered during competition. It is the challenge of the coach to find a balance between the safety of training drills and the true situations encountered in a competitive setting.

Improving player skills

With regard to high-risk situations in volleyball, a preventive program that included improvement of volleyball skills was evaluated (Bahr et al., 1997). Players were taught specific jumping and landing techniques that prevented them to land in the "conflict zone" under the net. Two seasons later there was a twofold reduction in the incidence of ankle sprains. In addition it was shown that the number of ankle sprains due to player contact in the "conflict zone" was decreased significantly. Although this example stems from volleyball, this shows that the overall idea to teach players (on how) to avoid risky situations is potentially very effective. Again an injury log may provide the information needed to develop skill training for specific sports and specific situations.

It should be noted that a difference in approach is needed between older (experienced) and younger athletes. Experienced athletes have been participating in sports for a relatively long time, and learning new "safer" skills requires an alteration of previously gained skills that are executed, by a large part, automatically. Younger athletes have not acquired sports specific skills to such an extent. Thereby, it is easier to teach younger players safe skills and to ensure they employ these skills in true sports situations.

Taping

Probably the most well known and already widely preventive measures against ankle sprains are tape and braces. Review of the prospective studies of the effect of taping and bracing on reduction of ankle sprains reveal a consistent finding; athletes with a history of ankle sprains, who regularly use a brace or tape experience a lower incidence of ankle sprains (Quinn et al., 2000).

Taping is a form of strapping that attaches tape to the skin in order to physically maintain a certain joint position. Taping of the ankle is the earliest prophylactic measure used to prevent ankle sprains. What one also does is stimulate additional nerve receptors on the ankle surface and to avoid any excessive ankle movements leading to an ankle sprain.

Over time a large variety of taping methods has been developed. Additionally, many different types of athletic tapes are manufactured, which can be divided into a non-elastic and elastic variant. For standard ankle application, the choice of tape is 3.8 or 5.1 cm white porous athletic non-elastic tape.

The two most commonly used and widely accepted methods are the so-called basketweave method and the figure-eight method (Box 4.1). Other taping methods are also available, as well as variations on the methods explained here. Applying tape can be difficult and, more importantly, frustrating at first. With a bit of practice one will be able to properly tape an ankle within a few minutes.

One of the greatest benefits of taping is that one can adjust the method of taping to the needs of the athlete. This starts with the preparation of the skin. The most common preparation is to clean and dry the lower leg, ankle, and foot. A layer of pre-wrap is applied to the ankle. Some athletes prefer to shave the hair around the ankle, and to have the tape applied directly to the skin. Whatever the wishes of the athlete, a quick drying adherent is recommended and may be sprayed onto the skin to allow for better tape adhesion. If wanted, heel and lace pads can be applied to areas of high friction (e.g., the dorsum of the ankle and the distal Achilles tendon) to prevent blisters.

Braces

The concept of ankle bracing evolved from ankle taping. Braces are currently being used instead of traditional taping by many athletes at all levels of competition. They offer several advantages in that they are self-applied, reusable, and readjustable. In the long run, they are also more cost-effective than taping. A brace will be a one time expense lasting a couple of seasons. Tape is not reusable, and every time new rolls of tape must be purchased. Although braces are considered to have important advantages over tape, many athletes do not feel as comfortable or as stable wearing braces, which can be a disadvantage to treatment. Braces also can become torn or lost and require replacement. Additionally, there is a common belief that braces affect performance by restricting too much ankle movement. Although this has never been shown in scientific studies, it is for instance likely that the use of an ankle brace alters the (feeling of) ball contact in soccer. Thereby, the advocation of braces in soccer may result in non-compliance, and it would be better to recommend the use of ankle tape.

Braces come in three different basic varieties (Box 4.2). These varieties may go by different names, but in general one can speak of the following:

1. *Ankle sleeves*: These provide no stability but provide compression and can be used for prevention due to their positive proprioceptive (balance and positioning) effect. These braces do not limit normal ranges of motion of the foot and ankle.

2. *Non-rigid ankle braces*: These come in two basic types (a) with an elastic sleeve with "wrap-around" straps, and (b) nylon, canvas, or neoprene lace-up brace with elastic wrap around straps. Both provide minimal stabilizing effect but assist with proprioception. Many of these braces can be uncomfortable. Fortunately, there is an abundance of various types and fits available, making it possible for each athlete to find a comfortable model.

Preventing ankle injuries 41

Box 4.1 Common methods for taping the ankle

General guidelines
1. Hold the tape between the thumb and the index finger of each hand with little to no gap between the thumbs. Quickly pull the hands in opposite directions to tear off a piece of tape.
2. Avoid wrinkles in the tape, these can lead to blisters and discomfort. Once applied the tape will be stuck solid, therefore one must smooth the tape while it is being applied.
3. Learn to use the angles naturally supplied by the ankle. When forcing tape in a specific direction it does not want to go will create wrinkles and results in a less effective application.
4. In general, tape strips should overlay each other by about one-half the width of the tape. Each area should be covered by two layers of tape. Uncovered areas within the taped ankle lead to blisters.
5. Do not use excessive force when applying tape. Constriction of blood flow is possible when tape is applied too tightly.

The basketweave method
Step 1: Wrap one piece of athletic tape under the heel of the foot and bring both ends up the ankle to either side of the leg. The tape should form a "U," like the stirrup on a horse's saddle.

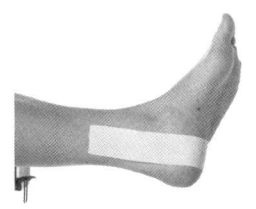

Step 2: Affix the tape to the skin just behind the knobby bone that juts out on either side of the ankle, pressing the tape firmly along the little groove behind the bone.

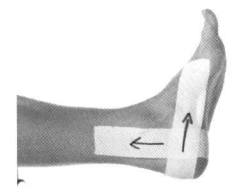

Step 3: Wrap a second piece of tape around the base of the heel, bringing the ends of the tape along either side of the foot, heading for the toes. It should form a 90° angle with the first piece of tape.

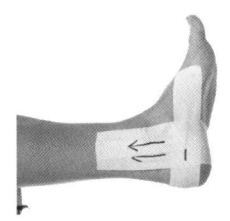

Step 4: Wrap a third piece of tape under the heel and up either side of the foot and ankle in the same manner as you wrapped the first piece of tape. Position the tape so that it runs adjacent to the first piece of tape—it should fall right over the knobby anklebone that juts out.

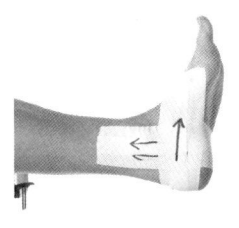

Step 5: Wrap a fourth piece of tape around the heel, running just above and adjacent to the second piece of tape, with the ends again heading for the toes along both sides of the foot. You now have the basic structure for the "basket weave"—overlapping pieces of tape that wrap around the heel, extend to the toe, wrap under the heel, and climb up to the ankle.

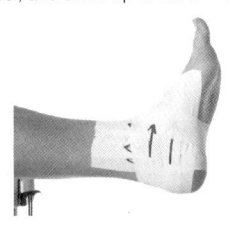

Step 6: Apply about eight more pieces of tape in this manner—four adjacent strips of tape that wrap around the heel pointing toward the toes, and four adjacent strips that wrap under the heel and head up the ankle. Alternating between strips that run along the foot and strips that run up the ankle will give you a weave that limits mobility and supports the entire ankle.

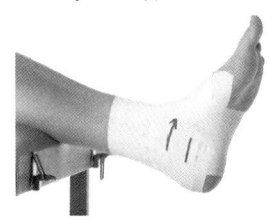

Figure-eight method with heel lock
Step 1: Place foot in the dorsiflexion position.
Apply pre-wrap from mid-foot to the base of the gastrocnemius/Achilles tendon junction.
Maintain foot in dorsiflexion.

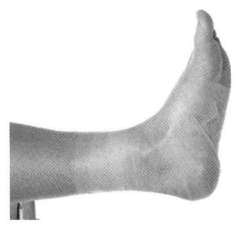

Step 2: Apply two anchor strips at the junction of the gastrocnemius/Achilles tendon, over-lapping one-half to a one-third. Angle tape down and back slightly to avoid gapping. Apply one anchor at the mid-foot, making sure to place distal to

(Continued)

Box 4.1 (Continued)

the head of the fifth metatarsal. *Placing directly over the head of the fifth metatarsal can cause discomfort.

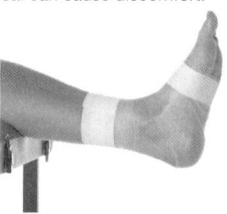

Step 3: Apply stirrups starting on the medial aspect of the upper anchor, place posterior to the medial malleolus, ending on the upper anchor on the lateral side. Always apply stirrups with a medial to lateral pull, as 90% of ankle sprains are inversion (outside part of ankle) in nature. Apply horseshoe, beginning on the medial aspect of the mid-foot anchor and proceed behind the calcaneous and ending on the lateral aspect of the mid-foot anchor.

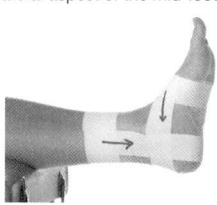

Step 4: Apply second stirrup in a similar fashion. Overlap one-half to a one-third of the previous stirrup, it should lie directly over the malleoli. Apply second horseshoe in a similar fashion proceeding up, overlapping one-half to a one-third of the previous, crossing behind the ankle and over the Achilles tendon.

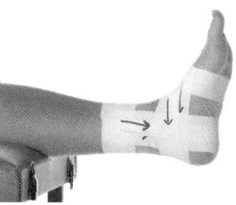

Step 5: Apply third stirrup and horseshoe, repeating the above process. The third (3rd) stirrup should lie anterior to the medial malleolus.

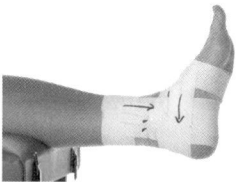

Step 6: Continue horseshoe strips until you have covered the ankle to the upper anchor.

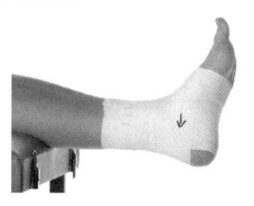

Step 7: Begin to apply the "figure eight." Starting on the dorsal aspect of the foot, move medially down the inside of the foot, across the plantar surface, pulling up on the outside of the foot. Continue by proceeding medially around the ankle, crossing the Achilles tendon, and returning to the starting point.

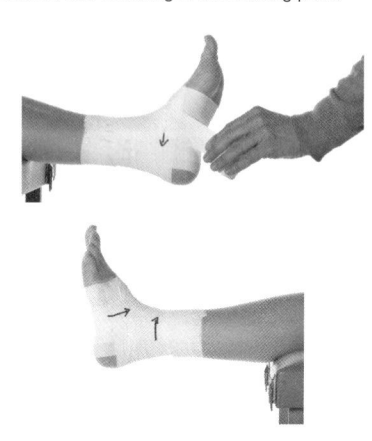

Step 8: Application of medial and lateral heel lock. Begin on the dorsum of the foot, as in the figure eight. Move medially down the inside of the ankle over the plantar surface of the foot. Pulling up on the outside of the foot.

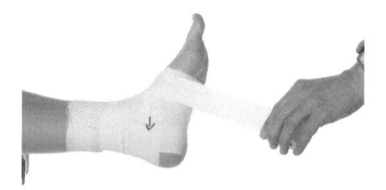

Step 9: Cross over front of ankle, crossing the medial malleolus, across the Achilles tendon, angling tape behind and below lateral malleolus. Angle tape underneath the foot and move back up to the dorsum of the foot.

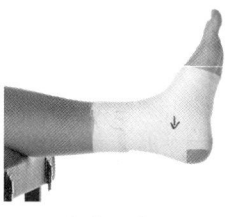

Step 10: Continue across the lateral malleolus, across the Achilles tendon, angling tape behind and below the medial malleolus. Continue tape around plantar aspect of the foot, ending on the dorsum of the foot.

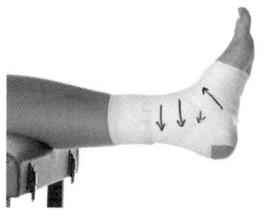

(Continued)

Box 4.2 Examples of various types of ankle braces

Ankle sleeves

Silipos Malleolar Ankle Sleeve
Provides mild compression to help reduce swelling in and around the ankle. Can be used to provide an additional protective layer to help prevent injuries. Two soft polymer gel pads are molded into the elastic sleeve.

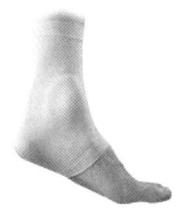

Banyan Healthcare Slip-on Ankle Compression
Provides even compression for ankle support and helps reinforce strained muscles. Constructed of knitted elastic and soft material for added comfort.

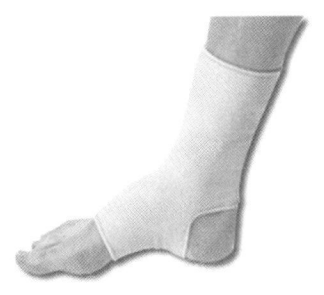

Non-rigid braces

Swede-O lace-up ankle brace
Provides good stability and can easily by retightened. Full elastic back ensures complete unrestricted blood flow to the Achilles' tendon. Internal U-shaped spiral stays provide extra support and further minimize the chance for ankle injury.

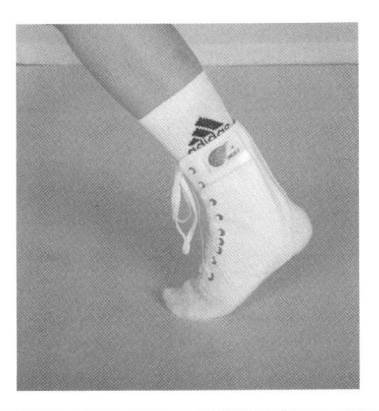

Captain Sports Adjustable Ankle Support with Spandex Wrap
Ankle sleeve with separate spandex wrap that provides additional support and stability to help prevent rolling of the ankle and limit joint stress.

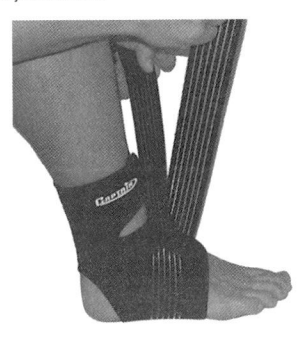

DonJoy Stabilizing Ankle Brace
Non-stretching adjustable nylon figure-eight straps which lock the calcaneus into place to help control abnormal eversion and inversion.

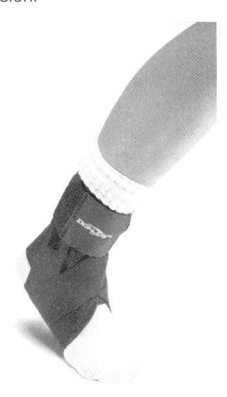

Core Deluxe Canvas Lace-up Ankle Strapping Support
Shares a close resemblance with semi-rigid braces using spandex wraps, but uses a lacing system. Offset eyelets and vinyl side supports help position the heel and stabilize the ankle. Can be easily retightened.

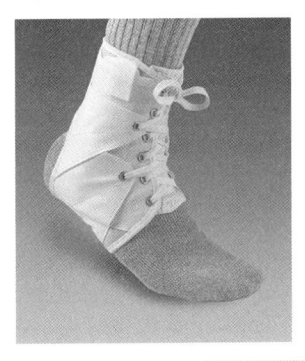

(Continued)

> **Box 4.2 (Continued)**
>
> **Semi-rigid braces**
> **Bauerfeind CaligaLoc Stabilizing Ankle Brace**
> Stabilizes the entire ankle giving both medial and lateral support, and by counteracting supination. Heat moldable and can be reshaped if necessary for an individual customized fit. 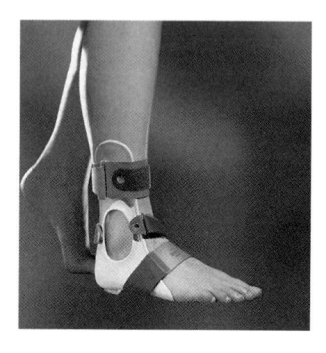 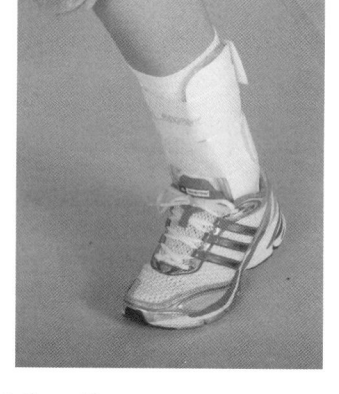
>
> **Rehband - Active ankle**
> Stable and easy to apply.
>
> **Aircast AirSport™ Ankle Brace**
> Low profile ankle brace specifically designed for professional athletes or chronic sufferers of ankle sprains. This support is beyond comparing to supports purchased over the counter because it is more often dispensed by orthopedic clinics or professional athletic trainers on the field. The only ankle brace to have been proven effective in preventing injuries in large trials.
>
> Incorporates features, such as, semi-rigid shells and foam filled aircells to provide both support and comfort. Additional compression and stabilization are provided by an anterior talofibular ligament cross-strap and by integrated forefoot and shin wraps.

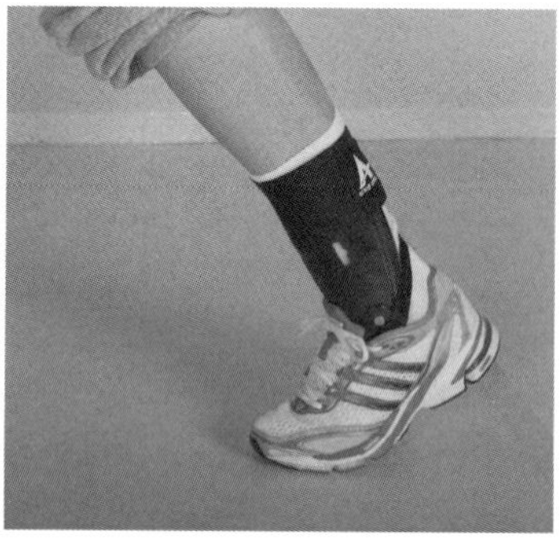

3. *Semi-rigid braces*: The construction of these braces is similar to the non-rigid versions, but with the added feature of molded plastic struts or air cushions. These are incorporated into the medial and lateral sides of the brace, similar in orientation to the stirrups used in ankle taping. These braces are effective at stabilizing the ankle in inversion (rolling out) and eversion (rolling in) but less effective when the athlete is in a dorsiflexed position (the most common mechanism of ankle sprain), provide more stability and often are chosen during the rehabilitation and return to play phases of ankle injury.

Braces versus tape

Many studies have been completed comparing taping versus bracing of the ankle to try and determine which is the better method. The general idea behind braces and tape is that both measures prevent excessive plantar flexed inversion when needed. It is known from previous research that in comparison to tape, braces have the best mechanical capabilities in terms of a reduction of ankle range of motion. Although tape appears to have an equal restricting effect directly after application, the mechanical support is already gone after short bouts of exercise. Braces do not show such loosening, and can be easily tightened, even during the match. Given

> **Box 4.3 Basic proprioceptive program for the ankle (originally described by Tropp (1985))**
>
> **Basic position**
> The athlete stands on one (straight) leg while the other leg is lifted in the air with the knee bent at 90°. The arms are crossed in front of the chest.
>
> **Exercise**
> The goal of the exercise is to attempt to make all balance correction using the ankle joint only, while using the arms, hips, and knees as little as possible.
>
> **Program**
> The program follows a "10–5–10" rule (i.e., 10 min, 5 times a week, for 10 weeks).
>
> **Level of difficulty**
> At first balancing on the floor may represent an adequate challenge. Exercise difficulty can be gradually increased during the program in the following order (1) perform exercises on a wobble board on a soft surface, (2) perform exercises on a wobble board on a hard surface, and (3) close the eyes.
>
> *Source:* Originally described by Tropp (1985)

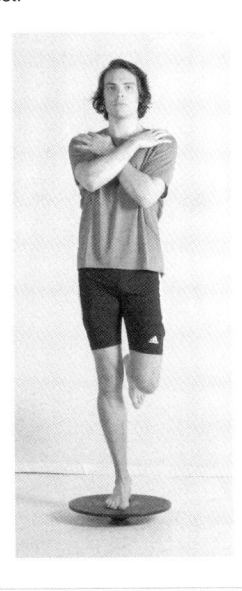

the etiology of ankle sprains, a forced plantar flexed inversion of the foot exceeding the anatomical range of motion it can then be argued that braces are the best crash measure against ankle sprains.

However, the superior restricting effect of braces does not translate to a superior preventive effect. Both tape and braces seem equally effective for the prevention of recurrent ankle sprains. Both measures have the effect to prevent ankle sprain recurrences and have less effect in "healthy" subjects, and in "healthy athletes" ankle sprains cannot be prevented using braces or tape.

The preventive effect of these measures does not result from a restriction in ankle range of motion only. A common belief is that external ankles supports prevent ankle sprains by affecting (or supporting) ankle proprioception instead of by restricting ankle inversion, or simply help guide the foot during landing to avoid landing in a vulnerable, inverted position. This also explains the inability to help players without previous ankle sprains, since healthy ankles have normal proprioception and do not have a tendency to land in an awkward foot position.

Balance training

One measure that has been studied extensively in the recent years is improvement of neuromuscular function, and more specifically balance board (proprioceptive) training. Trauma to mechanoreceptors of the ankle ligaments after an ankle sprain can produce a proprioceptive impairment in the ankle. This might explain the increased risk of re-injury within 1 year after an ankle sprain. Neuromuscular training is designed for the rehabilitation after an ankle sprain and is thought to improve proprioception by re-establishing and strengthening the protective reflexes of the ankle. Thereby, neuromuscular training of the ankle is a potentially very effective measure to reduce the risk of injury recurrences. This potential effect has been shown in studies in a variety of different sports, all showing an injury risk reduction for players with previous ankle sprains (Tropp et al., 1985; Verhagen et al., 2004b).

A basic proprioceptive training program is described in Box 4.3. Although such program is effective in preventing ankle sprain recurrences,

46 Chapter 4

Box 4.4 Volleyball-specific comprehensive balance training program developed by Verhagen et al. (2004b)

General information on the program

The training program consists of 14 basic exercises on and off the balance board, with variations on each exercise. Exercises are divided into four subcategories: (1) exercises without any material; (2) exercises with a ball only; (3) exercises with a balance board only; and (4) exercises with a ball and a balance board. The higher the exercise number the more difficult the exercise, where variations make the basic exercises more challenging.

Exercises should *not* lead to physical complaints. Once an athlete suffers pain in the ankle region after using this program, reduce the number of exercise bouts and/or choose easier exercises.

How to use the program

– During the execution of exercises the ankle may not be supported by brace or tape
– Exercises should be incorporated in the usual warm-up routine, and during each warm-up one exercise should be carried out lasting no more than 5 min.
– Each week one exercise from each subcategory should be carried out, and once an exercise has been carried out the same exercise cannot be chosen again during that week.
– During the season make exercises more challenging by choosing higher exercise numbers and variations on basic exercises.

Basic exercises
No material
Exercise 1
One legged stance with the knee flexed. Step-out on the other leg with the knee flexed and keep balance for 5 s. Repeat 10 times for both legs.
Variations 1 2 3 4

Exercise 2
One legged stance with the hip and the knee flexed. Step-out on the other leg with the hip and knee flexed, and keep balance for 5 s. Repeat 10 times for both legs.
Variations 1 2 3 4

Ball
Exercise 3
Make pairs. Stand both in one legged stance with the knee flexed. Keep a distance of 5 m. Throw and/or catch a ball 5 times while maintaining balance. Repeat 10 times for both legs.
Variations 1 2

Exercise 4
Make pairs. Stand both in one legged stance with the hip and knee flexed. Keep a distance of 5 m. Throw and/or catch a ball 5 times while maintaining balance. Repeat 10 times for both legs.
Variations 1 2

Balance board
Exercise 5
One legged stance on the balance board with the knee flexed. Maintain balance for 30 s and change stance leg. Repeat twice for both legs.
Variations 1 2 3 4

Exercise 6
One legged stance on the balance board with the hip and knee flexed. Maintain balance for 30 s and change stance leg. Repeat twice for both legs.
Variations 1 2 3 4

Exercise 10
Step slowly over the balance board with one foot on the balance board. Maintain the balance board in a horizontal position while stepping over. Repeat 10 times for both legs.

Exercise 11
Stand with both feet on the balance board. Make 10 knee flexions while maintaining balance.

Exercise 12
One legged stance on the balance board with the knee flexed. Make 10 knee flexions while maintaining balance. Repeat twice for both legs.

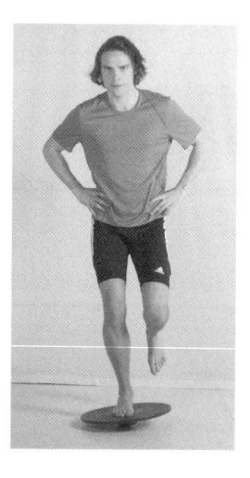

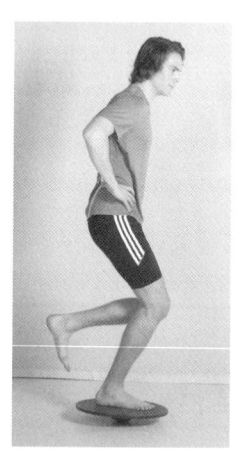

Ball and balance board
Exercise 7
Make pairs. One stands with both feet on the balance board. Throw and/or catch a ball 10 times with one hand while maintaining balance. Repeat twice for both players on the balance board.

Exercise 8
Make pairs. One stands in one legged stance with the knee flexed on the balance board, the other has the same position on

(Continued)

Box 4.4 (Continued)

the floor. Throw and/or catch a ball 10 times with one hand while maintaining balance. Repeat twice for both legs and for both players on the balance board.
Variations 1 2

Exercise 9
Make pairs. One stands in one legged stance with the hip and knee flexed on the balance board, the other has the same position on the floor. Throw and/or catch a ball 10 times with one hand while maintaining balance. Repeat twice for both legs and for both players on the balance board.
Variations 1 2

Exercise 13
Make pairs. One stands with both feet on the balance board. Play the ball with an upper hand technique 10 times while maintaining balance. Repeat twice for both legs and for both players on the balance board.
Variations 5 6 7 8

Exercise 14
Make pairs. One stands in one legged stance with the knee flexed on the balance board, the other has the same position on the floor. Play the ball with an upper hand technique 10 times while maintaining balance. Repeat twice for both legs and for both players on the balance board.
Variations 5 6 7 8

Variations on basic exercises
1. The standing leg is stretched.
2. The standing leg is bent.
3. The standing is stretched and the yes are closed.
4. The standing leg is bent and the eyes are closed.
5. The standing leg is stretched and upper hand technique.
6. The standing leg is bent and upper hand technique.
7. The standing leg is stretched and lower hand technique.
8. The standing leg is bent and lower hand technique.

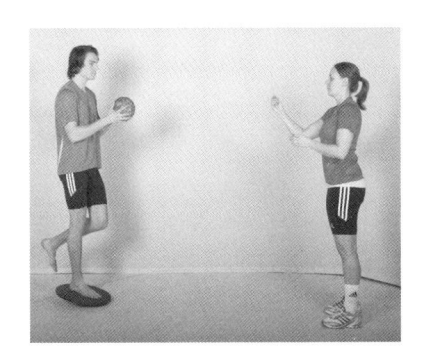

an athlete's motivation to comply with the program may diminish during the 10-week time span. Additionally, this basic program consists of one static exercise, while most ankle sprains occur during dynamic situations. Thereby, based on this basic proprioceptive program, more elaborate dynamic, and sports-specific programs may be developed to keep athletes motivated and to introduce dynamic exercises. As an example, Box 4.4 shows a more elaborate volleyball-specific proprioceptive program which has been proven effective in a large trial (Verhagen et al., 2004b). Similar programs may be developed for other sports.

Take-home message

Preventive measures should be advocated to all athletes, especially the subgroup with a history of previous sprains or instability episodes. In this subgroup, subsequent re-injury risk is highly dependent on the type of rehabilitation done, whether or not the subject complied with the rehabilitation program, and the quality of recovery that was achieved. From this perspective, structured rehabilitation programs that include restoration of normal ankle motion, strengthening, and restoration of neuromuscular control and proprioception of the ankle complex should be advocated to all injured athletes. Until function is completely normal, athletes should be urged to make use of either a tape or a brace.

References

Bahr, R., Lian, O., Bahr, I.A. (1997) A twofold reduction in the incidence of acute ankle sprains in volleyball after the introduction of an injury prevention program: a prospective cohort study. *Scandinavian Journal of Medicine and Science in Sports* **7**, 172–177.

de Noronha, M., Refshauge, K.M., Herbert, R.D., Kilbreath, S.L., Hertel, J. (2006) Do voluntary strength, proprioception, range of motion, or postural sway predict occurrence of lateral ankle sprain? *British Journal of Sports Medicine* **40**, 824–828.

Hertel, J. (2000) Functional instability following lateral ankle sprain. *Sports Medicine* **29**, 361–371.

Kofotolis, N.D., Kellis, E., Vlachopoulos, S.P. (2007) Ankle sprain injuries and risk factors in amateur soccer players during a 2-year period. *American Journal of Sports Medicine* **35**, 458–466.

Morrison, K.E., Kaminski, T.W. (2007) Foot characteristics in association with inversion ankle injury. *Journal of Athletic Training* **42**, 135–142.

Quinn, K., Parker, P., de Bie, R., Rowe, B., Handoll, H. (2000) Interventions for preventing ankle ligament injuries. *Cochrane Database of Systematic Reviews (Online)* **2**, CD000018.

Tik-Pui Fong, D., Hong, Y., Chan, L., Shu-Hang Yung, P., Chan, K. (2007) A systematic review on ankle injury and ankle sprain in sports. *Sports Medicine* **37**, 73–94.

Tropp, H., Askling, C., Gillquist, J. (1985). Prevention of ankle sprains. *American Journal of Sports Medicine* **13**, 259–262.

Willems, T.M., Witvrouw, E., Delbaere, K., Philippaerts, R., De Bourdeaudhuij, I., De Clercq, D. (2005a) Intrinsic risk factors for inversion ankle sprains in females—a prospective study *Scandinavian Journal of Medicine and Science in Sports* **15**, 336–345.

Willems, T.M., Witvrouw, E., Delbaere, K., Mahieu, N., De Bourdeaudhuij, I., De Clercq, D. (2005b) Intrinsic risk factors for inversion ankle sprains in male subjects: a prospective study. *American Journal of Sports Medicine* **33**, 415–423.

Verhagen, E., van der Beek, A., Bouter, L., Bahr, R., van Mechelen, W. (2004a) A one season prospective cohort study of volleyball injuries. *British Journal of Sports Medicine* **38**, 477–481.

Verhagen, E., van der Beek, A.J., Twisk, J.W.R., Bahr, R., Bouter, L.M., Van Mechelen, W. (2004b). The effect of a proprioceptive balance board training program for the prevention of ankle sprains, a prospective controlled trial. *American Journal of Sports Medicine* **32**, 1385–1393.

Further reading

Bahr, R. (2004a) Acute ankle injuries. In R. Bahr & S. Maehlum (eds) *Clinical Guide to Sports Injuries*, pp. 393–407. Human Kinetics, Champaign.

Bahr, R. (2004b) Pain in the ankle region. In R. Bahr & S. Maehlum (eds) *Clinical Guide to Sports Injuries*, pp. 408–418. Human Kinetics, Champaign.

Bahr, R. (2007) Can we prevent ankle sprains? In D. MacAuley & T. Best (eds) *Evidence-Based Sports Medicine*. Blackwell BMJ Books, London.

Hansen, K.J., Bahr, R. (2004) Rehabilitation of ankle injuries. In R. Bahr & S. Maehlum (eds) *Clinical Guide to Sports Injuries*, pp. 419–422. Human Kinetics, Champaign.

Chapter 5
Preventing knee injuries

Timothy E. Hewett[1], Bruce D. Beynnon[2], Tron Krosshaug[3] and Grethe Myklebust[3]

[1]Cincinnati Children's Hospital Medical Center, University of Cincinnati College of Medicine, Cincinnati, Ohio, USA
[2]Department of Orthopaedics and Rehabilitation, McClure Musculoskeletal Research Center, The University of Vermont, VT, USA
[3]Oslo Sports Trauma Research Center, Norwegian School of Sport Sciences, Oslo, Norway

Epidemiology of knee injuries in sports

This chapter will not focus on the prevention of knee injuries in general. Instead, it will review the epidemiology of one of the most serious knee injuries experienced during participation in Olympic Sports; disruption of the anterior cruciate ligament (ACL). This injury is not the most common ligament injury experienced in sports. However, as described below it is one of the most serious in terms of absence from sport, pain, disability, and an increased risk of development of osteoarthritis about the knee joint. In Olympic summer sports, the highest ACL injury incidences occur during participation in basketball, soccer, and team handball. The highest injury risk is among top level female athletes who compete in team handball and soccer (Table 5.1).

A gender difference is very apparent in ball sports, where female athletes suffer ACL injuries 4–6 times more often than their male counterparts taking part in the same sports at the same level of competition (Table 5.1). The injury mechanism is frequently the "non-contact" type which means that there is limited contact between the opponent and the athlete about the lower extremity immediately before and during the injury. In many situations, athletes are perturbed just before the injury occurs, and the injury is often incited by a push from an opponent. The inciting moment of the injury often surprises the players since they are performing movements that they have done many times in the past.

Among the Olympic winter sports, ACL injuries are most the common in the sport of alpine skiing. Alpine ski injuries are typically reported as the number of ACL injuries per 100,000 skier days (Table 5.1) and, therefore, a comparison of these data with that from other sports cannot be made in a direct manner. The injury often occurs during high speed situations with considerable magnitudes of forces and torques produced across the athlete's knee. The new Olympic sport of snowboarding includes the different disciplines of "big air," "snowboard cross," "half pipe," and "slalom." Most consider these sports to be associated with high numbers of knee injuries; however, precise injury data are currently not available. This is a sport that is under development and therefore we must follow it closely and carry out prospective studies to record the incidence rates of knee and ACL injuries.

There is no consistent data regarding sex differences in recreational alpine skiers; however, female competitive alpine skiers have twice the incidence rate of ACL injuries in comparison to male competitive alpine ski racers. In the sport of ice hockey the incidence of ACL injuries is low; however, a greater number of medial collateral ligament (MCL) injuries are seen as a result of a direct blow to the lateral aspects of the knee by an opponent. MCL injuries are also common in soccer, often with the same injury mechanism as in ice hockey.

Sports Injury Prevention, 1st edition. Edited by R. Bahr and L. Engebretsen Published 2009 by Blackwell Publishing
ISBN: 9781405162449

Table 5.1 Risk of ACL injury in different sports. The numbers reported are average estimates based on the studies available.

Sport	Competition incidence[1]	Training incidence[1]	Rank[2]	Comments
Team sports				
Basketball	0.28–0.40 ♀	*0.14 ♀	15–17	NBA & WNBA
	0.08–0.16* ♂	*0.04 ♂		*NCAA data 2006
Soccer	0.33–2.2 ♀	*0.10 ♀	15-Sep	*NCAA data 2006
	0.12 ♂	*0.04 ♂		
Team handball	1.3–2.8 ♀	0.03 ♀	10-Aug	Elite level
	0.23 ♂			
Volleyball	0.19 ♀	0.05 ♀	NA	NCAA data 2006
Field hockey	0.15 ♀	0.05 ♀	NA	NCAA data 2006
Ice hockey	0.14 ♀		NA	NCAA data 2006
	0.21 ♂	0.02 ♂		
Individual sports				
Alpine skiing	4.4 ♀**		NA	♀ twice of ♂ in some studies
	4.0 ♂**			
Gymnastics	0.33 ♀*		15-Dec	
Wrestling	0.70 ♂	0.06 ♂	NA	NCAA data 2006

[1]Incidence is reported for adult, competitive athletes as the number of injuries per 1000 hours of training and competition (*per 1000 athletic exposures) or **per 100,000 skiing days in alpine skiing.
[2]Rank indicated the relative rank of ACL injuries within the sport in question.
NA: Not available.

The incidence of ACL injuries appears to be significantly greater during competition than during training (Table 5.1), and this finding is consistent in sports. Studies of European team handball athletes have shown that the relative risk of sustaining an ACL injury is approximately 30 times greater during competition than during training. This difference is expected, since the intensity and corresponding loads transmitted to the knee and ACL are higher during competition when compared to training sessions. In most sports, training sessions include warm-up exercises and technical drills, which are associated with a lower risk of injury.

ACL injury has received great attention even though it is not the most frequent injury suffered during participation in sports. The primary reason for this is the severity of the injury: For most athletes involved with Olympic sports, surgery is necessary to return them to their sport at the same level of competition they were capable of prior to injury and rehabilitation and recovery requires a long absence from sport. A recovery time that ranges between 6 and 12 months is not unusual. Studies have shown that the long-term risk of suffering premature osteoarthritis is considerably greater among ACL injured athletes in comparison with athletes who do not suffer these severe injuries. This results in substantial direct and indirect treatment costs in relation to medical disability. Osteoarthritis occurs, at a rate that is 10 times greater, for athletes who suffer an ACL injury regardless of whether they choose reconstructive surgery or non-operative treatment. The cost of this injury is estimated to be 17,000 dollars including surgical and rehabilitation costs, and these costs can be considerably higher over the athlete's life span with a long-term disability, sick leave, and the possibility of additional surgical procedures.

Key risk factors: how to identify athletes at risk

A large number of studies have investigated the potential risk factors for severe knee injuries and a majority of this work has focused on ACL injuries. However, there remains a significant knowledge gap concerning the risk factors for serious knee injuries such as an ACL disruption. This is because only a few well-designed prospective studies are available and most studies have assessed only one factor in isolation. Considering that the risk factors for ACL injury are multifactorial (e.g., multiple risk factors act in combination to increase an athlete's risk of suffering an ACL injury), this approach is not appropriate to assess how risk factors act in combination to increase an individual's risk of suffering a severe knee ligament injury. Further, the majority of these studies have identified sex differences in anatomy as well as hormonal and neuromuscular function; however, they fail to relate these differences to the risk of suffering a severe knee ligament injury (Table 5.2).

External risk factors: shoe–surface interaction

The shoe–surface interaction has been studied as an ACL injury risk factor in different sports. A study of Australian football athletes has reported that the risk of sustaining non-contact ACL injuries increased during high-evaporation and low-rainfall periods. Studies of soccer athletes reported that competing on artificial turf does not increase the risk of knee injuries compared with natural grass. In contrast, recent studies of professional American football athletes suggest that the incidence of ACL injuries may be greater on the new artificial turf designs in comparison with the older turf designs. In the sport of European team handball, it was shown that the risk of ACL injury was 2.4 times greater when competing on artificial floors (with an increased coefficient of friction) compared with wooden floors. Earlier studies of American football athletes have shown that the use of longer cleat lengths and an associated higher torsional resistance at the foot–turf interface places these athletes at an increased risk of suffering knee injuries. There is little doubt that the shoe–playing surface interface is important to consider when developing intervention strategies to reduce the incidence rate of serious knee injuries.

Internal risk factors: previous knee injury

Recent studies have suggested that having a previous injury may be a risk factor for subsequent injury—either a rupture of the ACL graft, an ACL rupture to the contralateral knee, or another type of acute or overuse knee injury. One study also showed that females experience ACL re-rupture at a rate twice that of men.

Age

Although there appears to be a consensus that the risk of suffering an ACL injury increases for female athletes during their growth spurt, there are no investigations that have included age as a potential risk factor in analysis of serious knee injuries in skeletally mature athletes. Similarly, no investigations of the effect of age on the likelihood of suffering a knee injury in skeletally immature athletes exist.

Body composition

An increased body mass index (BMI) has been found to be associated with an increased risk of suffering ACL injuries in female cadets attending the US Military academy. However, other studies have not found such a relationship. The data on BMI appear to be inconsistent, making it difficult to establish reliable conclusions.

Familial tendency and ethnicity

Two case-control studies reported that familial tendency is a risk factor for ACL injury. Athletes who suffer an ACL tear are twice as likely to have a relative with an ACL tear compared with age, sex, and sport-matched controls.

In a recent 4-year cohort study, it was found that white European American athletes were 6.6 times more likely to suffer an ACL tear compared with other ethnic groups.

Anatomical factors

The Q-angle of the knee (Figure 5.1) has been studied as a possible explanation for the gender difference

Table 5.2 Internal and external factors for knee ligament sprains in different sports. The numbers reported are average estimates based on the studies available.

Risk factor	Relative risk[1]	Evidence[2]	Comments
External risk factors			
Surface	2–2.4×*	+	Few studies. Greater risk of injury when competing on artificial floors relative to natural wood floors, but only for women.
Meteorological conditions	1.9–2.8×	+	Only one study. Non-contact ACL injuries more frequent during high evaporation and low-rainfall periods.
Footwear	NA	+	Only two studies. Shoes with longer cleats produced significantly greater ACL injury rates.
Game versus practice	29.9×	+ (+)	Higher ACL injury rate during competition.
Internal risk factors			
Gender	2–8×	+ +	Risk of ACL injury is greater in women compared to men when participating in the same sport at the same level of competition.
Previous injury	3.1–11.3×	+	Risk for new knee injuries in general as well as new ACL injuries, both in the reconstructed and the contralateral knee.
Age	NA	0	No studies were found that included age as a potential risk factor for ACL injury.
BMI	3.5×	+	Few studies. Higher risk of ACL injury for women with high BMI. Conflicting results.
Familial tendency	2.0×*	+	Only two studies. Athletes with an ACL tear are two times more likely to have a relative with an ACL tear.
Race	6.6×*	+	Only one study. White European American players more susceptible to ACL tears compared with other ethnic groups.
Q-angle	NA	+	Higher Q-angle in females. Conflicting results.
Leg length	NA	+	Long femur relative to tibia may be a risk factor in skiers. Wide pelvis relative to femur predicts dynamic valgus in one-legged squats.
Intercondylar notch width index	3.7–6.0×	+	Small notch width index may lead to increased risk of suffering an ACL injury. Several positive studies, but also some studies with conflicting results.
(Ligament cross-sectional area)	NA	0	No risk factor studies. Relative larger cross-sectional area in males after adjusting for body weight.
(Ligament material properties)	NA	0	No risk factor studies. Female ligaments have lower strain and strain energy density at failure, as well as lower modulus of elasticity compared to males.
Anterior knee laxity	2.7×	+	Only two studies. The larger, prospective study found a 2.7-fold increased risk for ACL injury in females with A-P knee laxity values greater than 1 SD of the mean. A-P knee laxity had no effect on risk of ACL injury in males.
General joint laxity	2.8×	+	Few studies. Females exhibit greater joint laxity than males. Skiers with increased hyperextension of the knee are in significantly increased risk of suffering ACL injury.
Patella tendon-tibia shaft angle (PTTSA)	NA	0	No risk factor studies. PTTSA is greater in females compared to males.
Foot pronation/navicular drop	NA	+	Three studies found a relationship, whereas one study found no relationship.
Phase of menstrual cycle	3.2 ×*	+	Studies that have accurately measured phase of cycle with serum- or urine-based assays of estradiol and progesterone have observed a greater proportion of ACL injuries in the pre-ovulatory phase of the menstrual cycle in comparison with the post-ovulatory phase. One study of recreational alpine skiers found the odds ratio of suffering an ACL disruption was 3.2 times greater during the pre-ovulatory phase compared to the post-ovulatory phase of the menstrual cycle in recreational alpine skiers.
Knee flexion during landing	NA	0	Only one risk factor study that showed no relationship. Conflicting results among studies looking at gender differences.
Valgus motion and valgus moment during landing	NA	+	Only one risk factor study. Valgus moments have a sensitivity of 78% and a specificity of 73% for predicting ACL injury status.

(Continued)

Table 5.2 (Continued)

Risk factor	Relative risk[1]	Evidence[2]	Comments
Leg dominance during landing	NA	0	Only one risk factor study, but no significant effect of this variable on ACL injury risk. Females have greater side-to-side (leg dominance) differences in knee loads.
Quadriceps dominance	NA	0	No risk factor studies. Females exhibit greater quadriceps dominance than males.
Muscle stiffness	NA	0	No risk factor studies. Females have lower muscle stiffness than males.
Muscle strength	NA	0	No risk factor studies. Females have lower muscle strength than males.
Muscle reaction time	NA	0	No risk factor studies.
Time to peak force	NA	0	No risk factor studies.
Fatigue	NA	0	No risk factor studies. No gender differences. Fatigue may alter the neuromuscular control of knee biomechanics.

[1]Relative risk indicates the increased risk of injury to an individual with this risk factor relative to an individual who does not have this characteristic. A relative risk of 1.2× means that the risk of injury is 20% higher for an individual with this characteristic.
[2]Evidence indicates the level of scientific evidence for this factor being a risk factor for ligament sprains: ++—Convincing evidence from high-quality studies with consistent results; +—evidence from lesser quality studies or mixed results; 0—expert opinion or hypothesis without scientific evidence.
*Odds ratio and not relative risk.
NA: Not available.

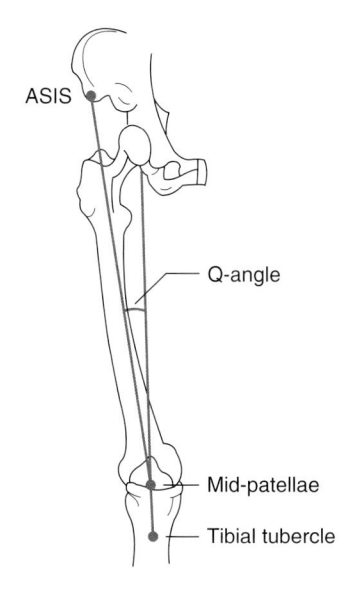

Figure 5.1. The Q-angle is formed in the frontal plane by two lines: (1) the line between the tibial tubercle to the middle of the patella and (2) the line from the middle of the patella to the anterior superior iliac spine

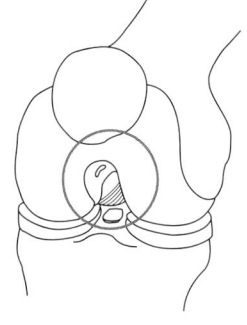

Figure 5.2. A narrow intercondylar notch width has been proposed as a risk factor for ACL injuries

in ACL injury rates, with the rationale that high Q-angles may be associated with an excessive valgus loading of the knee. These studies consistently report higher Q-angles in females. In a recent case-control study, it was reported that the mean Q-angles of athletes sustaining knee injuries were significantly larger than the mean Q-angles for athletes who were not injured (14° versus 10°). In contrast, others have reported that the risk of suffering a knee injury was not related to anatomical alignment differences such as Q-angles. One study reported that pelvic width to thigh length ratio, and not Q-angle, predicts dynamic valgus angulation of the knee during the single leg squat. It has also been shown that a long thigh to shank ratio may be a risk factor for ACL injuries in competitive alpine skiers.

One of the most studied factors in relation to ACL injury is the femoral intercondylar notch width (Figure 5.2). Several investigators have hypothesized that a narrow intercondylar notch or notch width index (e.g., the ratio of the width of the femoral notch to the width of femoral condyles when observed through X-ray in a coronal plane view) may predispose athletes to an increased risk of ACL injury. One cause could be that a narrower femoral notch is associated with a smaller, weaker ACL. This hypothesis has been challenged by recent studies that used MRI to correlate the size of the ACL with the size of the intercondylar notch. These studies suggest that the size of the ACL cannot be predicted by the size of the femoral intercondylar notch. Another possibility is that impingement of the ACL against the femoral intercondylar notch may be more predominant when the notch is narrow and this may induce microtears of the ligament during participation in athletics that subsequently progress to macrotears that weaken the ligament and predispose it to an increased risk of a complete tear. Research is needed to delineate the role of notch impingement as an ACL injury risk factor. Three prospective cohort studies, as well as several other lesser quality studies, have found that athletes with a decreased femoral notch width are at an increased risk of suffering an ACL injury. There are, however, several studies that do not show such an association and as a consequence it remains unclear how notch width geometry, or notch width index, is related to increased risk of suffering an ACL injury.

Ligament material properties and joint laxity

The size and material properties of the ACL are factors that may influence the risk of this ligament tearing. It has been shown that ACLs in females are smaller than in males when normalized for body weight. In addition, it has been reported that female ligaments have lower strain and strain energy density at failure as well as 22.5% lower modulus of elasticity. However, at the curren point in time, no risk factor studies have considered these variables. On the other hand, there are studies that have established increased anterior knee laxity as a risk factor for females, and this may be a result of differences in the size and material properties of the ACL. It is important for us to point out that these studies are relatively small and such factors can only explain a relatively small proportion of the variance in ACL injury risk. Generalized joint and ligament laxity have also been proposed as risk factors for knee ligament injuries; however, most of these studies have evaluated the effect of these variables on all lower extremity injuries as a group and not knee ligament injuries in isolation. A few exceptions exist and these studies suggest that increased generalized joint laxity and increased hyperextension of the knee may be associated with increased risk of suffering an ACL injury.

Foot pronation

It has been suggested that foot pronation may lead to anterior tibial translation, and subsequently strain the ACL; however, the results are conflicting. Three case-control studies found a relationship between foot pronation/navicular drop and ACL injuries whereas one found no such relationship.

Hormonal factors

To determine how different phases of the menstrual cycle affect ACL injury risk, it appears necessary to accurately describe the hormone milieu with serum- or urine-based measures of hormone concentrations and then use these data to accurately identify the phase of the cycle when injury occurs. The use of an athlete's self-report of menstrual history is inadequate to determine the phase of cycle at the time of injury. Review of studies that have used serum- and urine-based measures of hormone concentrations reveal that the risk of suffering a non-contact ACL injury can be threefold greater during the pre-ovulatory phase of the menstrual cycle in comparison to the post-ovulatory phase.

Patella tendon-tibia shaft angle and tibial plateau slope

One of the most investigated hypotheses in recent years is whether a quadriceps contraction performed with the knee near extension can create a force of sufficient magnitude on the patellar tendon such that it produces an anterior translation of the tibia relative to the femur and ruptures the ACL (see also description of Injury mechanisms later for further explanation). The patella tendon-tibia shaft angle (PTTSA) is the sagittal plane angle between the tibia (ankle to knee joint) and the line of action of the patellar tendon. When the knee is near extension, an increased PTTSA produces a larger magnitude of anterior-directed force on the tibia and increases the loads transmitted to the ACL. It has been showed that females have greater PTTSA throughout the range of knee flexion compared to males, and that this angle is greater when the knee is close to full knee extension. However, no risk factor studies have included PTTSA in the analyses. The same is true for the slope of the tibial plateau in the sagittal plane. An increased slope of the plateau will generate an increased anterior-directed force on the tibia when compression forces, such as that produced during landing or plant and cut maneuvers, are produced across the knee.

Movement patterns

Another explanation for the gender difference in ACL injury rate is that females may perform a certain movement different from males. Landing with straighter knees implies higher PTTSA and thereby an increased anterior-directed shear force component on the tibia. Although several studies have investigated if females land with straighter knees compared with males, there is no consensus in the literature. Furthermore, in a recent prospective risk factor study of 205 female athletes who participated in soccer, basketball, or volleyball, where knee flexion angles produced during jump landings were assessed, no significant differences were found between injured and un-injured subjects. The same study showed that the valgus motion and valgus moments that were produced when landing from a jump predicted ACL injuries with a sensitivity of 78% and a specificity of 73%. Also, leg dominance was studied, but this factor was not found to be associated with risk of suffering an ACL injury. It should be mentioned that only nine ACL injuries were included in this study, so the results should be interpreted with caution until confirmed in other studies. For more information on how movement patterns can contribute to ACL injuries, see section on Injury mechanisms later.

Other neuromuscular measures

Several neuromuscular measures have been proposed as possible risk factors for ACL injury. Quadriceps dominance, muscle reaction time, time to peak force, muscle stiffness, and muscle strength and fatigue are all factors that may have an influence on an athlete's risk of suffering an ACL injury. It has been shown that females exhibit greater quadriceps dominance and that they have less muscle stiffness and muscle strength compared to males. However, none of these factors have been studied as ACL injury risk factors and consequently it is not possible to determine the relative importance of these factors at this point in time.

Take-home message

It appears that the risk factors for serious knee ligament injuries are likely multifactorial in nature. It has been shown that the combination of risk factors such as a small femoral notch width and large body mass results in a dramatic increase in the risk of ACL injury (relative risk 26.2) compared to having only one of the two factors in isolation (relative risks of 3.5 and 4.0, respectively). However, as is apparent from this chapter, our current knowledge on the many potential risk factors for serious knee injuries is limited.

Perhaps, the most important from the athlete's point of view is the finding that a suboptimal movement pattern will increase the risk of such injuries. This finding also agrees well with numerous studies that have shown beneficial effects of neuromuscular training programs focusing on strength, balance, and maintaining the "knee-over-toe" position during dynamic movements. Drop-jumps and one-legged squats are simple tests that can be used to screen athletes with poor strength, balance, and "knee-over-toe" control. Furthermore, one should avoid excessive shoe–floor friction by making sure to wear shoes that "fit" the playing surface.

It should be noted that other factors such as anatomic alignment and ligament properties are not easily modifiable, and therefore, direct intervention on such factors may be difficult. Nevertheless, if we can identify individuals at increased risk (e.g., athletes that are at increased risk of suffering ACL injury based on poor anatomic alignment), it may be possible to initiate individualized injury prevention measures on these individuals and reduce their risk of injury by enhancing their neuromuscular control.

Injury mechanisms

A simple description of non-contact ACL injury situations in ball/team sports

During most Olympic sports, ACL injuries are commonly non-contact in nature and can occur during plant and cut maneuvers (Figure 5.3), but a high proportion of these injuries also occur during landings (Figure 5.4). In basketball, landings are the most frequently reported mechanism for ACL injuries.

It is important to realize that while an athlete may appear to land on both feet with body weight equally distributed between legs, at the point of impact the entire ground reaction force may be supported by the leg that suffers an injury. Previous studies have suggested that the knee is near extension at the time of ligament injury (i.e., less than 30°); however, recent studies that have used more sophisticated video analysis with multiple camera angles indicate that the knee is injured when it is in a position of greater flexion. Although the majority of ACL injuries that occur in Olympic sports are non-contact by definition, the movement patterns often involve perturbation by an opponent (e.g., body contact before the injury). However, even if a few details are known, we still lack vital knowledge about the injury mechanisms. A complete biomechanical description should quantify entire body and knee kinematics, loading directions and magnitudes, and the rate of application of external and internal forces about the lower extremity.

Knee ligament injury mechanisms in alpine skiing

Knee ligament injury mechanisms that occur during traditional alpine skiing have been investigated for some time, and various injury mechanisms have been proposed, both for ACL injuries and other ligament injuries. Some knee injury mechanisms are equipment related, such as when the back portion of the ski boot acts to produce a "boot-induced anterior drawer" (e.g., an anterior directed force on the tibia that tears the ACL), or when the edge of the ski is caught in the snow.

Some injury mechanisms are associated with certain circumstances, such as a backward fall, with the weight of the skier on the inner edge of the tail of the ski resulting in a sharp uncontrolled inward twist of the lower leg (Figure 5.5). This scenario is termed as the "phantom foot mechanism" and is considered the most common ACL injury mechanism in alpine skiing.

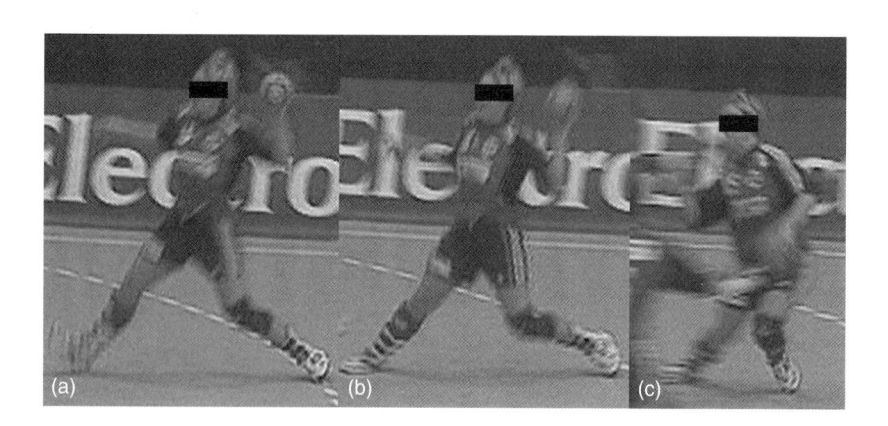

Figure 5.3. Frame sequence of a plant and cut ACL injury showing the team handball athlete (a) at initial ground contact, (b) at 40 ms, and (c) at 100 ms, respectively. Reproduced with permission from the *Scandinavian Journal of Medicine and Science in Sports*

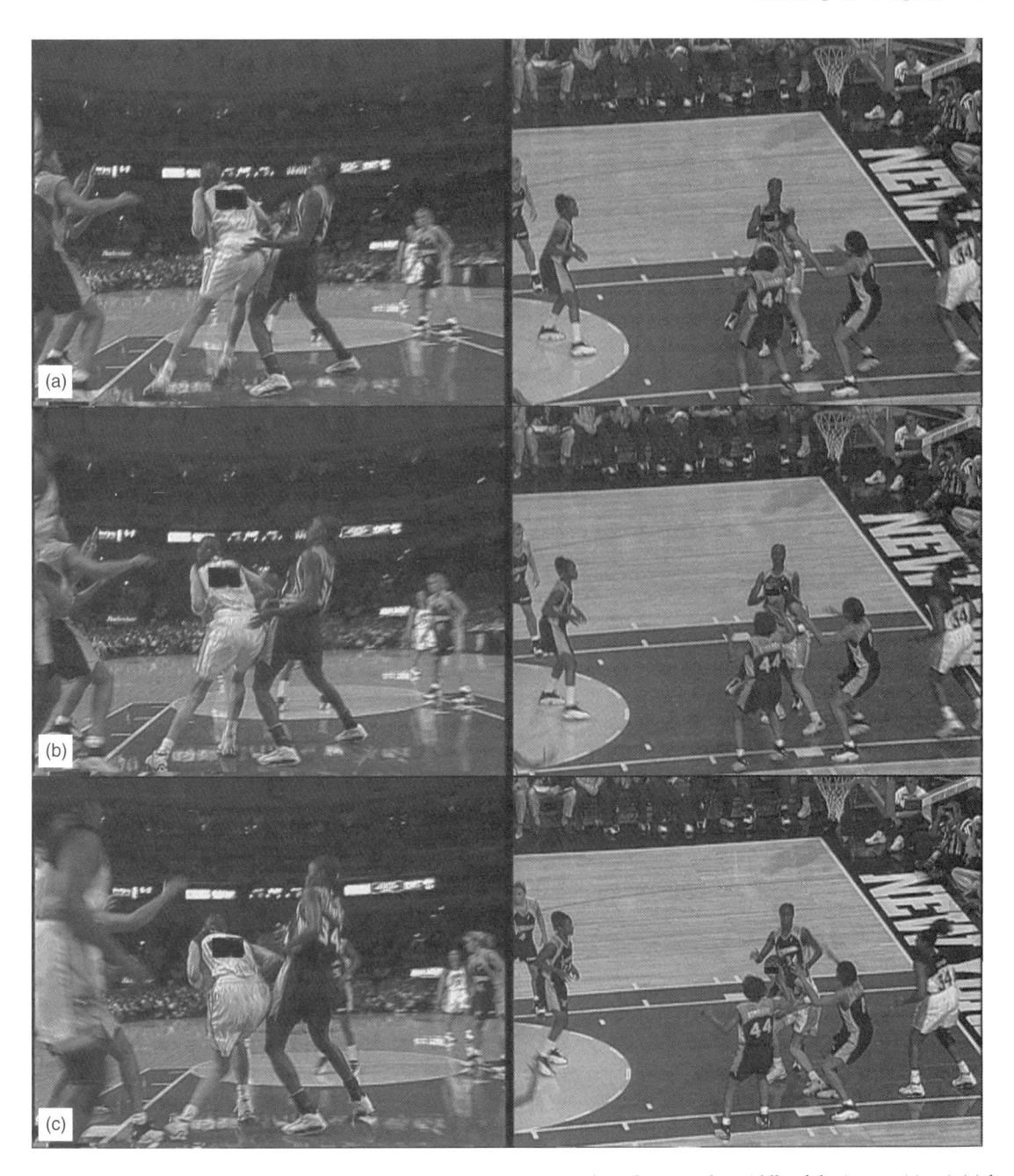

Figure 5.4. Landing injury in basketball. The injured player is seen in white shorts in the middle of the images (a) at initial ground contact, (b) 33 ms after initial contact, corresponding to the approximate estimated time of rupture, and (c) 133 ms after initial contact. Reproduced with permission from the *American Journal of Sports Medicine*

However, previous studies on knee ligament injury mechanisms produced during alpine skiing have mainly used approaches such as athlete interview and visual inspection of injuries captured on video. These approaches have methodological limitations, and there is a need for the improvement of the existing injury mechanism descriptions.

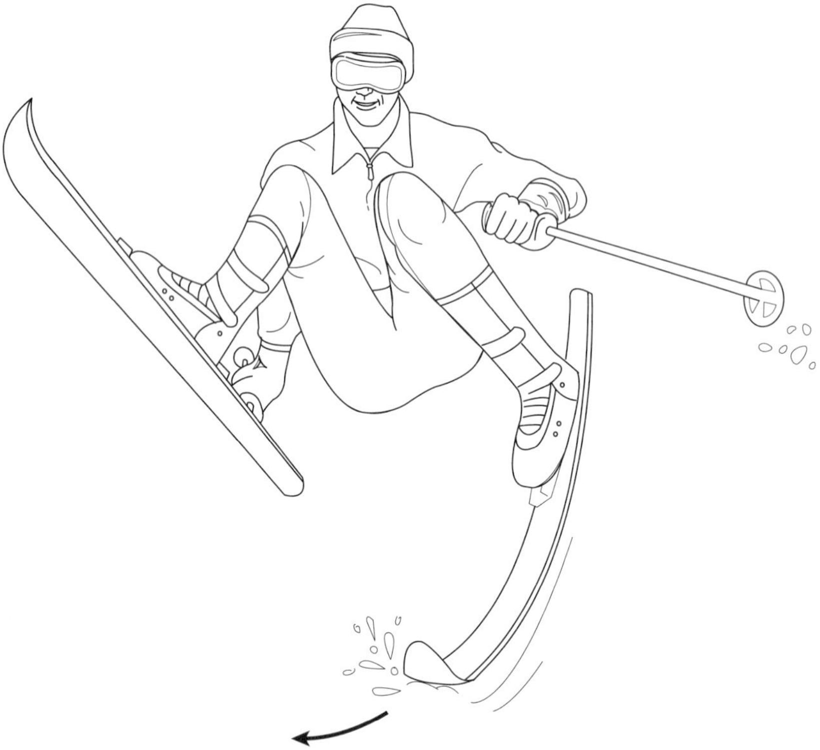

Figure 5.5. Drawing of the body position in the "phantom foot" injury mechanism. The weight of the skier is on the inner edge of the tail of the ski resulting in a sharp uncontrolled inward twist of the lower leg. Copyright: ACL awareness training—Phase II, Vermont Safety Research, 1994. Illustration is copyrighted by William Hamilton, 1988 and is adapted with permission

Non-contact ACL injury mechanisms in ball/team sports: different hypotheses

Although gross biomechanical information about serious knee injuries exists, detailed biomechanical information (i.e., joint loading) is not known. For injuries that are caused by a direct blow to the knee, which is the case for many MCL injuries, the loading patterns are more obvious. However, for non-contact ACL injuries, different hypotheses are heavily debated in the scientific community.

Valgus loading

Studies have shown that external tibial rotation combined with valgus rotation with the knee in an extended or partially flexed position initiates ACL strain, as the ligament contacts and then impinges against the medial aspect of the lateral femoral condyle (Figure 5.6).

The ligament impingement theory has also been suggested in video analysis studies. Although it remains unknown how the ligament impinges against the medial aspect of the lateral femoral condyle and strains the ACL, there is evidence that valgus loading of the tibia relative to the femur is an important aspect of the loads applied to the knee during an ACL injury. A recent prospective risk factor study showed that increased valgus loading when landing from a jump was associated with increased risk of suffering an ACL injury amongst soccer, basketball, and volleyball athletes. Several studies also report that MCL injuries are frequently seen in combination with non-contact ACL injuries, indicating that valgus loading was present. Interestingly, laboratory-based motion analysis studies have demonstrated that females develop larger magnitudes of valgus and external torques about the knee when landing from a jump in comparison to males, suggesting that knee valgus loading may explain, at least in part, the larger incidence rate of ACL injuries seen in females compared to males taking part in the same sport at the same level of competition. A recent video-based analysis study of actual ACL injury situations reported a large number of valgus collapses about the knee for female athletes.

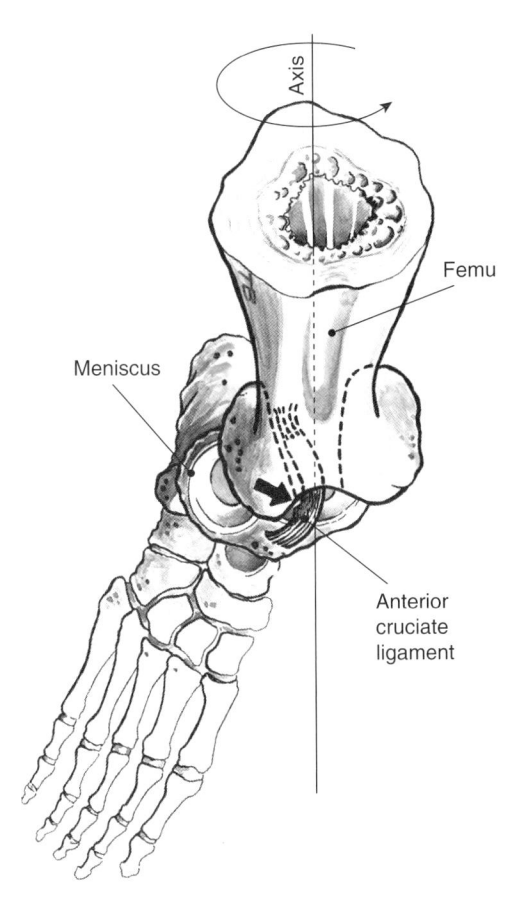

Figure 5.6. A sidestep cutting maneuver may lead to valgus and external tibial rotation. The solid arrow indicates a possible impingement of the ACL against the intercondylar notch. Reproduced with permission from Gazette Bok

This evidence suggests that valgus loading plays an important role in many of the non-contact ACL injury situations, at least amongst female athletes. However, there are likely to be other forces and torques applied to the knee during injury, since it has been shown that pure valgus loading will rupture the MCL first, then the ACL secondly—only a limited number of MCL ruptures are found in conjunction with non-contact injury of ACL injuries.

Quadriceps-induced anterior tibial drawer

Several cadaver studies have shown that quadriceps loading strains the ACL when the knee is near extension. It has been hypothesized that a vigorous quadriceps contraction when landing on an extended knee can produce high ACL strain values. In this theory, contraction of the quadriceps muscle group and subsequent engagement of the patellofemoral joint produces a load on the patella tendon which has an anterior-directed angulation relative to the tibia when the knee is near extension, and this generates an anterior-directed force component on the tibia. As the knee is moved from an extended to a flexed position, the orientation of the patellar tendon relative to the tibia moves from an anterior to a posterior direction as does the corresponding direction of the force produced by the quadriceps extensor mechanism. Understanding this biomechanical relationship, studies have investigated if the gender difference in ACL injury incidence can be explained by the fact that females appear to land with their knee and hip in a more extended position. The findings from these studies conflict. In actual injury situations, females are found to be at significantly greater knee and hip flexion angles at initial contact with the playing surface and at the assumed point of injury in comparison to males. This finding suggests that landing on straighter knees may not be an important explanation for the observed difference in ACL injury incidence rates between males and females. Although a novel cadaver study demonstrated that the quadriceps-induced anterior drawer mechanism is capable of producing ACL rupture, this approach was criticized for not including ground reaction forces, which may act posteriorly on the tibia and help restrain anterior translation of the tibia. Three mathematical model simulation studies of landing and plant and cut maneuvers, which included the effect of ground reaction and hamstrings forces, all concluded that the anterior-directed shear force that acts on the tibia cannot generate sufficient magnitude to rupture the ACL, even in extreme cases where hamstrings forces are non-existent. Still, the results of these studies were quite different, possibly due to the fact that realistic modeling and simulation of the knee joint is challenging. In contrast to the findings from mathematical modeling studies, a recently published cadaver study demonstrated that anterior tibial translation and ACL strain proportional to the applied quadriceps force were generated when the ground contact forces were also included. However, since the loading was far from injury levels, it is not possible to make firm conclusions regarding the quadriceps-induced anterior drawer mechanism from this study. Further investigations are required to delineate the role of quadriceps-induced anterior drawer loading of the tibia in producing ACL injuries.

Internal tibial rotation

There are several factors that suggest internal rotation of the tibia relative to the femur on a relatively extended knee could be a potential mechanism of non-contact ACL injuries. First, cadaver and human studies have shown that the ACL is strained when torques are applied to internally rotate the tibia relative to the femur. Second, internal rotation is frequently reported to be the mechanism of injury in athlete interview studies, in video analysis, as well as suggested from the associated clinical findings. Motion analysis studies of sidestep cutting maneuvers usually show a dominance of internal tibial rotation during the stance phase. However, males are reported to exhibit this pattern to a larger degree than females indicating that other loading scenarios are likely to be associated with many female non-contact ACL injuries. Hyperextension has also been proposed as a possible mechanism, but this seems unlikely considering that such injuries have not been reported in any video analysis studies.

Take-home message

Currently, little is known about the specific knee loads that cause non-contact ACL injuries. What seems clear is that valgus loading is an important factor in many cases; implying that avoiding valgus knee motion (or "kissing knees") is important.

Identifying risks in the training and competition program

The risk of suffering a serious knee injury may increase during championships or playoff situations, when the best players are exposed to an abnormally high number of matches during a short-time period. In planning championships and Olympic Games, it is important to allow an adequate number of days for the athlete to recover. For young athletes who participate in sports at a high level, there is a clear tendency for participation on many teams and to compete at different age levels. This increases the number of matches/competition and reduces the time they have, available for rest and training. Every sports federation should be aware of this and try to protect the young athletes from over participation in sports.

Another aspect that must be considered for pivoting sports that are performed on courts and turf is the friction between the floor and the shoes. Playing surfaces with a low coefficient of friction can prevent ACL injuries. Athletic shoes should be designed to provide sufficient friction and mechanical interlock with the playing surface to allow optimal performance, not making pivoting difficult, yet not producing injury. Athletes who take part in sports that are performed on surfaces with different friction levels should consider the use of different types of shoes. For example, one for high- and another for low-friction playing surfaces. This is an important factor in relation to prevent an ACL injury. We must also keep in mind that proper cleaning and maintenance of the playing surfaces influences the friction at the shoe–surface interface for both indoor floors and turfs.

In relation to ACL injuries among the different skiing disciplines, there are several risk situations that are important. Among alpine skiers, it is extremely important that the athletes use equipment and bindings adjusted by trained and certified technicians. Alpine resorts must take precautions to prevent over-crowding in an effort to avoid collisions, and obstacles must be sufficiently padded and marked.

Snowboard facilities should be properly maintained and appropriate construction of the half-pipe and jumps are important to reduce the risk of suffering injury.

Preventive measures

Neuromuscular training appears to be effective at reducing ACL injury risk, particularly for female athletes in sports performed on courts and turf. For the optimal design of ACL intervention programs, we can learn much from a systematic analysis of the common components of the published interventions, successful and unsuccessful, designed to reduce ACL injury risk in athletes. Analyzing the common components of the most effective and least effective programs is useful for the development of effective intervention protocols. Hewett et al., (2006a) performed a systematic review of intervention studies designed to reduce ACL injury risk in female athletes and revealed that several programs appear to reduce ACL injury risk. In contrast, other studies have failed to show an effect of neuromuscular training on the reduction of ACL injury rates or establish that they can alter lower extremity biomechanics. Most of what is known has come from studies of female athletes, as they are at increased risk of ACL injury. As described earlier, the mechanism of ACL injury may differ between females and males, particularly with respect to the dynamic positioning and control of the knee, as females demonstrate greater valgus collapse of the lower extremity, primarily in the coronal plane. However, female athletes may serve as a working model for any athlete at increased risk of suffering an ACL injury. In this section, we will describe many of the prevention methods and neuromuscular training programs and provide broad instructions and guidelines for the exercises. In addition, we will review as many components of the successful, and unsuccessful, programs as possible within the specific purview of ACL injury prevention in athletes.

There appears to be a measurable effect of neuromuscular training interventions on the reduction of severe knee and ACL injuries. A comprehensive review of the literature revealed that five of the six studies demonstrated neuromuscular training reduced lower extremity injury risk, four of the six studies found neuromuscular training reduced serious knee injury risk and three of the six reported decreased ACL injury risk (Hewett et al., 2006c). The components of the most successful programs are summarized later. In sum, plyometric training and biomechanical analysis of landing, cutting, and jumping technique were common components of the studies that were effective at reducing the risk of ACL injury in athletes.

Safety equipment

Two investigations have studied the effect of prophylactic knee bracing on American football athletes (Sitler et al., 1990; Albright et al., 1994). The first study found significantly fewer MCL injuries occurred in athletes who used prophylactic bracing in comparison to those who did not use braces; however, the effect of prophylactic bracing on ACL injures could not be determined because of the small sample size (Sitler et al., 1990). In contrast, the second study did not find statistically significant differences between braced and unbraced athletes in terms of the risk of sustaining MCL injuries (Albright et al., 1994). Additional research is needed in this area to establish the effect that prophylactic braces have on knee injuries.

Although alpine ski bindings have been developed to effectively protect skiers from tibia and ankle fractures, the present day alpine ski binding designs are inadequate for preventing ACL disruptions, even when the bindings function as designed and are properly adjusted. In a large prospective study of ACL-deficient professional alpine skiers, the risk of sustaining a subsequent knee injury (e.g., injury to other structures about the knee such as articular cartilage and the menisci) was 6.4 times greater for non-braced skiers in comparison to braced skiers (Kocherc et al., 2003).

Targeting participation in ACL injury interventions to individuals or teams

Athletes at the greatest risk of ACL injury should participate in neuromuscular training interventions to decrease the risk of injuring this important ligament. This approach is specific to the individual athlete. The neuromuscular training protocol should preferably be designed and instituted specifically for and with athletes selected for neuromuscular training based on identified neuromuscular deficiencies and imbalances (Table 5.3).

In order to correct ligament dominance in female athletes (Table 5.3), a neuromuscular training program must be designed to teach the athlete to control dynamic knee motion in the coronal (abduction and valgus) plane. The first concept that the athlete and coach are taught is the knee

Table 5.3 Injury prevention matrix applied to ACL injury prevention: potential measures to prevent injuries.

	Pre-injury	Injury	Post-injury
Athlete	Sex/gender Body Mass Index	Training status Falling techniques	Rehabilitation Restoration of neuromuscular function

	Neuromuscular imbalance
	1. Ligament dominance:
	   –Technique/biomechanics
	2. Quadriceps dominance:
	   –Hamstrings power
	3. Leg dominance: single leg balance/symmetry
		Safe technique and biomechanics	

	–"Core"/trunk instability –Trunk control training		
Surroundings	Floor friction Playing rules	Safety nets	Emergency medical coverage
Equipment	Shoe friction and torsional resistance with the playing surface	Knee brace Tape	First aid equipment Ambulance Ice

is a single-plane hinge, not a ball-and-socket joint. Reeducation of the female neuromuscular system away from multi-planar motion of the knee to dynamic control of knee motion in the sagittal plane only is achieved through a progression of single, then multi-planar exercises.

Quadriceps dominance (Table 5.3) can be corrected through the use of exercises that emphasize co-contraction of the knee flexor (hamstrings) and extensor (quadriceps) muscles. It is a challenging task to develop more appropriate firing patterns for the knee flexors, while utilizing exercises that also strongly activate the knee extensors. At angles greater than 45°, the quadriceps is an antagonist to the ACL. Therefore, it is important to use deep knee flexion angles to put the quadriceps into an ACL agonist position. By training the athlete with deep knee flexion jumps, she learns to increase the amount of knee flexion and decrease the amount of time in the more dangerous straight-legged position. At the same time the athlete can reprogram peak flexor/extensor firing patterns, increasing co-firing and quadriceps firing in deep flexion for greater protection of the ACL.

Dominant leg imbalance can be addressed in the female athlete via exercises that force the correction of dynamic contralateral imbalances (Table 5.3). These imbalances are addressed throughout the entire training protocol. Equal leg-to-leg strength, balance and foot placement are stressed through all the neuromuscular training exercises. In order to correct for leg dominance, the neuromuscular training must progressively emphasizes double then single movements through progressive training phases.

Finally, "core" or trunk/pelvis instability, as evidenced by increased trunk motion, must be corrected in those female athletes who demonstrate instability with the latest core stability training techniques. These include progressive neuromuscular training techniques that target the balanced and synchronized turn-on of the dynamic stabilizing musculature of the trunk, pelvis and hip. Unstable surfaces, single-leg balancing and perturbation training should be employed (Table 5.3).

The authors realize that the individualized approach may not be tenable for team athletes and their coaches. Though we do not know if the generalizations from our systematic review of the literature discussed earlier apply to all athletes or just those that participate in jumping, landing and cutting sports; we can assume that there will be positive effects of neuromuscular training programs designed around these basic commonalities in effective interventions. These broad generalizations for the athlete in cutting and landing sports, for "team training" from the studies discussed above should be effective if plyometrics and landing, cutting and jumping technique training are included in the intervention.

Plyometrics is an important component for reduction of ACL injury risk in athletes

The evidence for including a plyometric component as a portion of an ACL injury prevention program is relatively strong. A systematic review of the literature found that reduced ACL injury risk occurred in those interventions that included plyometrics as part of the training program, while those that did not include plyometrics did not reduce an ACL injury risk (Hewett et al., 2006c). The focus of plyometrics should be on proper landing, cutting, and jumping techniques and body mechanics during these movements. Training programs that incorporate plyometrics result in safe levels of varus or valgus stress about the knee, and may increase "muscle dominant" and reduce "ligament dominant" neuromuscular control patterns while correcting for these and other neuromuscular imbalances in athletes (Table 5.3).

Studies by Hewett et al. (1996, 1999, 2006a), Myklebust et al. (2003), and Mandelbaum et al. (2005) all incorporated high intensity plyometric movements into the design of their intervention programs (Boxes 5.1 and 5.2), but the studies by Heidt et al. (2000) and Söderman et al. (2000), which did not reduce ACL injury risk, did not. This can be explained, at least in part, by the fact that the studies by Söderman et al. (2000) and Heidt et al. (2000) had little chance of establishing if their intervention could reduce the risk of injury because the sample size was likely too small and from this perspective these should be considered preliminary studies. With this caveat, the studies that incorporated high intensity plyometrics reported reduced ACL injury risk, while the studies that did not incorporate high intensity plyometrics did not report reductions in ACL injury risk. Hence, the plyometric component of a pre-season intervention program appears to reduce serious ligamentous injuries, specifically ACL injuries.

Plyometrics may be used as combined analysis and training tools, with verbal or visual feedback, for control of body motion, both during deceleration and acceleration, and knee loading, especially with respect to the reduction of abduction (or "valgus") torque about the knee. For example, Hewett et al. (1996, 1999, 2006a) have shown that tuck jumps force control of knee abduction torque (Box 5.1). The other exercises that were included in the interventions that reported decreased ACL injury risk were lateral jumps over barriers (this forces trainees to stabilize their trunk in the coronal plane while moving both lower extremities side-to-side), landing and balancing on compliant surfaces and perturbed single-leg balancing and hop and holds for extended periods (Box 5.1).

Movement biomechanics, technique and education components: coronal plane is key

The evidence in support of including movement biomechanics, landing, cutting and jumping technique, and education components of the effective interventions is also relatively strong. Olsen et al. (2005) have reported that in sports performed on court and turf surfaces most ACL injuries occur by non-contact mechanisms during landing and lateral pivoting. The biomechanics of these landing and cutting movements can be improved with neuromuscular training. Neuromuscular training can increase coronal and sagittal plane control of the lower extremity. For example, during a squat jump (Box 5.1), a two-footed plyometric activity, post training results show that lower extremity valgus alignment can be reduced at the knee and hip. Conversely, during a single-leg tasks such as a hop and hold maneuver (Box 5.1), the most significant changes may occur in the sagittal plane of the knee.

There is strong evidence in support of landing, cutting and jumping technique training and its effect on reducing ACL injury risk. Hewett et al. (1996, 1999, 2006a) reported that technique and phase-oriented training that corrected jump and landing techniques in athletes reduced ACL injuries in a female intervention group compared to female controls and resulted in injury levels

Box 5.1 Dynamic neuromuscular analysis (DNA) training program

(Courtesy of Cincinnati Children's Hospital, www.cincinnatichildrens/sportsmed).

Athletic position
The athletic position is a functionally stable position with the knees comfortably flexed, shoulders back, eyes up, feet approximately shoulder-width apart, the body mass balanced over the balls of the feet. The knees should be over the balls of the feet and chest should be over the knees. This is the athlete-ready position and is the starting and finishing position for most of the training exercises. During some of the exercises the finishing position is exaggerated with deeper knee flexion in order to emphasize the correction of certain biomechanical deficiencies.

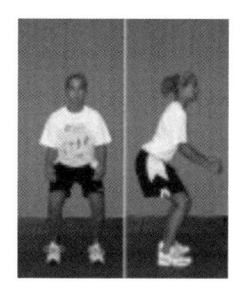

Wall jump
The athlete stands erect with her arms semi-extended overhead. This vertical jump requires minimal knee flexion. The gastrocnemius muscles should create the vertical height. The arms should extend fully at the top of the jump. Use this jump as a warm-up and coaching exercise as this relatively low-intensity movement can reveal abnormal knee motion in athletes with poor side-to-side knee control.

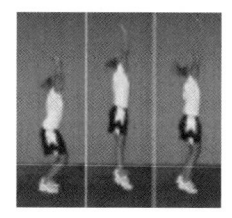

Tuck jump
The athlete starts in the athletic position with her feet shoulder-width apart. She initiates the jump with a slight crouch downward while she extends her arms behind her. She then swings her arms forward as she simultaneously jumps straight up and pulls her knees up as high as possible. At the highest point of the jump, the athlete is in the air with her thighs parallel to the ground. When landing the athlete should immediately begin the next tuck jump. Encourage the athlete to land softly, using a toe to mid-foot rocker landing. The athlete should not continue this jump if they cannot control the high landing force or if they utilize a knock-kneed landing.

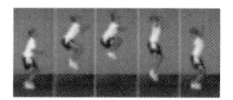

Broad jump and hold
The athlete prepares for this jump in the athletic position with her arms extended behind her at the shoulder. She begins by swinging her arms forward and jumping horizontally and vertically at approximately a 45° angle to achieve maximum horizontal distance. The athlete must stick the landing with her knees flexed to approximately 90° in an exaggerated athletic position. The athlete may not be able to stick the landing during a maximum effort jump in the early phases. In this situation, have the athlete perform a sub-maximal broad jump in which she can stick the landing with her toes straight ahead and no inward motion of her knees. As her technique improves, encourage her to add distance to her jumps, but not at the expense of perfect technique.

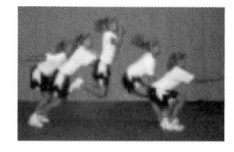

180-degree jump
The starting position for this jump is standing erect with feet shoulder width apart. She initiates this two-footed jump with a direct vertical motion combined with a 180° rotation in mid air, keeping her arms away from her sides to help maintain balance. When she lands she immediately reverses this jump into the opposite direction. She repeats until perfect technique fails. The goal of this jump is to achieve maximum height with a full 180° rotation. Encourage the athlete to maintain exact foot position on the floor, by jumping and landing in the same footprint.

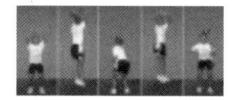

Squat jump
The athlete begins in the athletic position with her feet flat on the mat pointing straight ahead. The athlete drops into deep knee, hip and ankle flexion, touches the floor (or mat) as close to her heels as possible, then takes off into a maximum vertical jump. The athlete then jumps straight up vertically and reaches as high as possible. On landing she immediately returns to starting position and repeats the initial jump. Repeat for the allotted time or until her technique begins to deteriorate. Teach the athlete to jump straight up vertically, reaching as high overhead as possible. Encourage her to land in the same spot on the floor, and maintain upright posture when regaining the deep squat position. Do not allow the athlete to bend forward at the waist to reach the floor. The athlete should keep her eyes

(Continued)

Box 5.1 (Continued)

up, feet and knees pointed straight ahead, and have their arms to the outside of their legs.

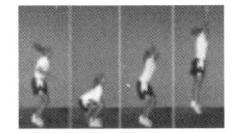

Broad Jump to Vertical Jump
The athlete performs three successive broad jumps, and immediately progresses into a maximum effort vertical jump. The three consecutive broad jumps should be performed as quickly as possible and attain maximal horizontal distance. The third broad jump should be used as a preparatory jump that will allow horizontal momentum to be quickly and efficiently transferred into vertical power. Encourage the athlete to provide minimal braking on the third and final broad jump to ensure that maximum energy is transferred to the vertical jump. Coach the athlete to go directly vertical on the fourth jump and not move horizontally. Utilize full arm extension to achieve maximum vertical height.

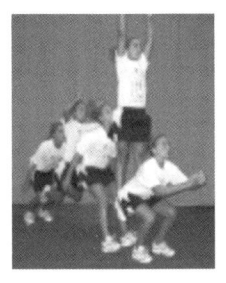

Hop and Hold
The starting position for this jump is a semi-crouched position on a single leg. Her arms should be fully extended behind her at the shoulder. She initiates the jump by swinging the arms forward while simultaneously extending at the hip and knee. The jump should carry the athlete up at an approximately 45° angle and attain maximum distance for a single-leg landing. Athletes are instructed to lands on the jumping leg with deep knee flexion (to 90°). The landing should be held for a minimum of 3 s. Coach this jump with care to protect the athlete from injury. Start her with a submaximal effort on the single leg broad jump so she can experience the level of difficulty. Continue to increase the distance of the broad hop as the athlete improves her ability to stick and hold the final landing. Have the athlete keep her visual focus away from her feet, to help prevent too much forward lean at the waist.

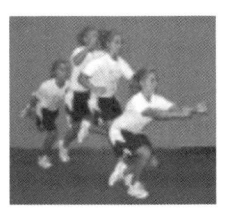

X-Hops
The athlete begins faces a quadrant pattern stands, on a single limb with their support knee slightly bent. She hops diagonally, lands in the opposite quadrant, maintains forward stance and holds the deep knee flexion landing for 3 s. She then hops laterally into the side quadrant and again holds the landing. Next she hops diagonally backward and holds the jump. Finally, she hops laterally into the initial quadrant and holds the landing. She repeats this pattern for the required number of sets. Encourage the athlete to maintain balance during each landing, keeping her eyes up and visual focus away from their feet.

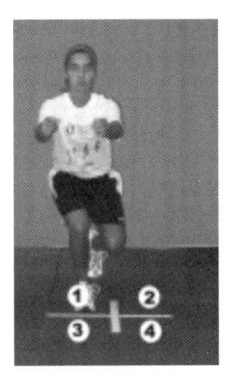

Single Leg Balance
The balance drills are performed on a balance device that provides an unstable surface. The athlete begins on the device with a two-leg stance with feet shoulder width apart, in athletic position. As the athlete improves the training drills can incorporate ball catches and single leg balance drills. Encourage the athlete to maintain deep knee flexion when performing all balance drills.

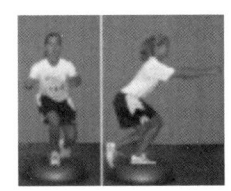

Bounding
The athlete begins this jump by bounding in place. Once she attains proper rhythm and form encourage her to maintain the vertical component of the bound while adding some horizontal distance to each jump. The progression of jumps progresses the athlete across the training area. When coaching this jump, encourage the athlete to maintain maximum bounding height.

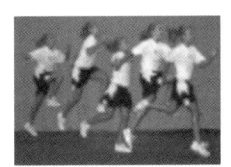

similar to a male control group. Myklebust and Bahr (2005) reported that the incidence of ACL injury in elite handball was reduced with training designed to improve awareness of lower extremity alignment and knee control during cutting and landing activities (Box 5.2). The studies by Hewett et al. (1996, 1999, 2006a), Mandelbaum et al. (2005), and Myklebust and Bahr (2005), which successfully reduced ACL injury risk, all incorporated landing technique analysis and feedback during training into their intervention programs. Of the non-effective studies, none incorporated landing/cutting technique and while only the Wedderkopp et al. (2003) study found a decrease in traumatic lower extremity injuries, none of these interventions reduced ACL injury risk. Methods for altering biomechanical technique include those of Hewett et al. (1996, 1999, 2006a) that utilized a trainer to provide feedback and awareness to an athlete during training, and Myklebust and Bahr (2005) that utilized partner training to provide the critical feedback regarding lower extremity alignment, particularly valgus (inward) positioning of the knee (Figure 5.7).

Johnson (2001) reported that education and public awareness of the high occurrence and mechanisms of ACL injury can decrease injuries in alpine skiers by

---

Box 5.2 ACL prevention program for team handball

(Courtesy of the Oslo Sports Trauma Research Center, www.ostrc.no).

Floor exercises

Week 1: Running and planting, partner running backward and giving feedback on the quality of the movement, change position after 20 s.

Week 2: Jumping exercise—right leg–right leg over to left leg–left leg and finishing with a two-foot landing with flexion in both hips and knees.

Week 3: Running and planting (as week 1), now doing a full plant and cut movement with the ball, focusing on knee position.

Week 4: Two and two players together two-leg jump forward and backwards, 180° turn and the same movement backward. Partner tries to push the player out of control but still focusing on landing technique.

Week 5: Expanding the movement from week 3 to a full plant and cut, then a jump shot with two-legged landing.

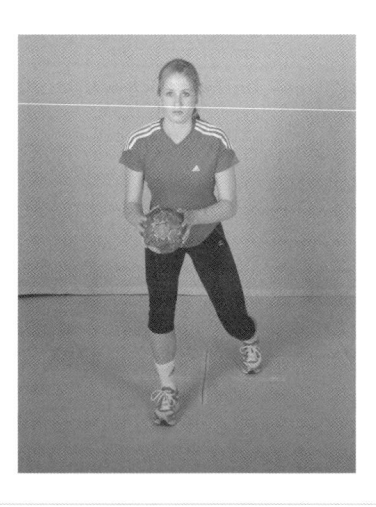

Mat exercises

Week 1: Two players standing on one leg on the mat throwing to each other.

Week 2: Jump shot from a box (30–40 cm high) with a two-foot landing with flexion in hip and knees.

Week 3: "Step" down from box with one-leg landing with flexion in hip and knee.

Week 4: Two players both standing on balance mats trying to push partner out of balance, first on two-legs, then on one leg.

Week 5: The players jump on a mat catching the ball, then take a 180° turn on the mat.

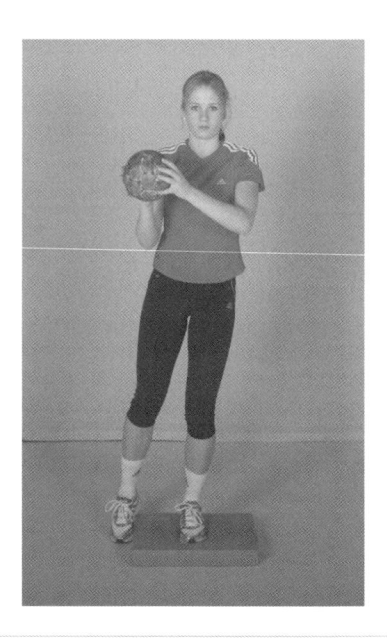

(Continued)

Box 5.2 (Continued)

Wobble board exercises

Week 1: Two players two-legged on the board throwing to each other.

Week 2: Squats on two legs, then on one leg.

Week 3: Two players throwing to each other, one foot on the board.

Week 4: One foot on the board, bouncing the ball with their eyes shut.

Week 5: Two players, both standing on balance boards trying to push partner out of balance, first on two legs, then on one leg.

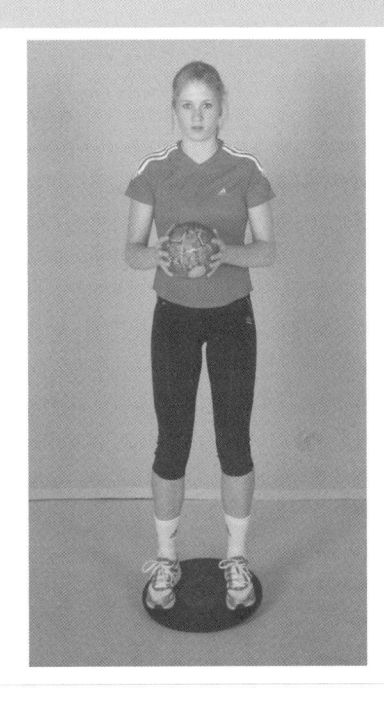

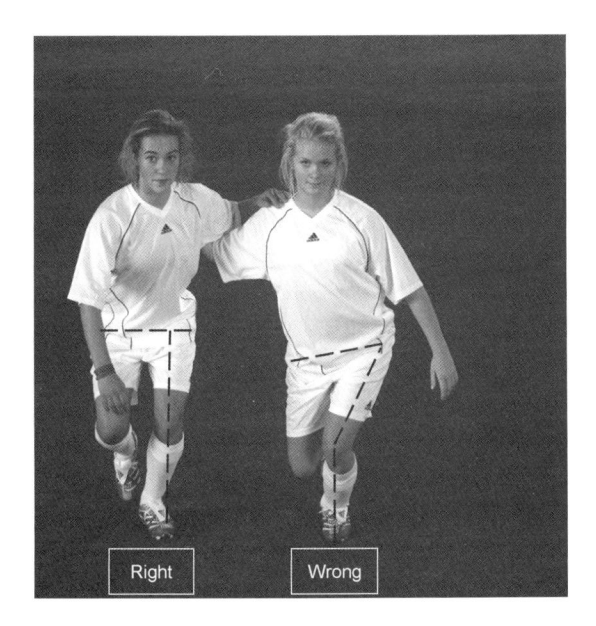

Figure 5.7. Hip and knee control. In single leg squats and balance training exercises the athlete should maintain a straight line through the hip, knee, and toe. She should keep a horizontal orientation of the hips and avoid a pelvic tilt during one legged squat, balance exercises, etc. Encourage the athlete to reach deep knee flexion when performing these drills

greater than 50%. A reduction of ACL injuries in ski instructors was achieved by using "guided learning" techniques that educated skiers to avoid "high risk" skiing positions, such as the skier positioned with a majority of the weight on the downhill ski and their hips below their knees. This approach is supported by findings that verbal or visual or bio-feedback regarding technique may decrease reaction forces at the knee and reduce ACL injuries.

Single leg balancing component and ACL injury risk

Though single leg balance training alone may not be effective for decreasing ACL injury rates in female athletes, as the small studies that incorporated single leg balancing alone did not report decreased ACL injury risk in female athletes, it may be an important component of neuromuscular training designed to decrease non-contact ACL injury. The studies by Hewett et al. (1996, 1999, 2006a) and Mandelbaum et al. (2005) incorporated single leg stability training, primarily utilizing hold positions from a decelerated landing. Single leg stability can be gained with balance training on unstable surfaces. Myklebust and

Bahr (2005) utilized partner training on Airex mats, wobble boards or the floor (Box 5.2). Again, however, the intervention programs that used balance training in isolation were not effective in reducing knee injuries in females. Wedderkopp et al. (2003) reported a reduction in all soccer-related injuries, though not knee or ACL injuries. Söderman et al. (2000) were not effective in reducing injuries in female soccer players. Wedderkopp et al. (2003) and Söderman et al. (2000) focused on balance training, primarily utilizing unstable wobble boards. Therefore, balance training alone may not be as effective for ACL injury prevention as when it is combined with other types of training. Interestingly, Caraffa et al. (1996) studied male soccer players and showed a significant effect of balance board exercises on reducing ACL injury and reported that balance training may be more effective in males than females.

A core component? Evidence for the effects of "core stability" training

There is not clear evidence whether "core stability" exercises should be incorporated into an intervention to reduce knee ligament injuries. It is not clearly defined what "core stability" exercises actually represent and what their effects are on the muscles that stabilize the trunk, hip, and pelvis. However, Zazulak et al. (2007) demonstrated that measures of "core" or trunk proprioception and displacement predicted risk of ACL injury in collegiate athletes with high sensitivity and specificity. Interestingly, this effect was observed in female, but not male, collegiate athletes. This may indicate the need for including trunk perturbation and strengthening in optimal interventional training programs. The findings support the integration of proprioceptive stability training in ACL injury interventions, at least for females. Krosshaug et al. (2007) suggested that preventive programs to enhance knee control should focus on avoiding valgus motion about this joint and include distractions resembling those seen in match situations.

Strength training effects on ACL injury risk

Resistance training alone has not been shown to reduce ACL injuries. However, inferential evidence suggests that resistance training may reduce injury based on beneficial adaptations that occur in bones, ligaments, and tendons after training. For example, Lehnhard et al. (1996) significantly reduced injury rates with a strength training regimen in men's soccer. The studies by Hewett et al. (1996), Kocher et al. (2003), Myklebust et al. (2003), and Mandelbaum et al. (2005) incorporated strength training in their intervention protocols. Myklebust and Bahr (2005), Heidt et al. (2000), and Söderman et al. (2000) did not include strength training in their interventions. The designs that incorporated strength training were among the most effective at decreasing ACL injury rates. But strength training in isolation may not be a pre-requisite for prevention, as the Myklebust and Bahr (2005) study was effective in reducing ACL injury risk and it did not incorporate strength training. In the final analysis, weight training alone has not been reported to be effective at decreasing ACL injury rates and may not need to be incorporated into a successful intervention. It is important for us to point out that this may apply only to those subjects who have adequate strength prior to entering an injury prevention program.

The proper "training dose:" How much and how often interventions should be performed

Neuromuscular power can increase within 6 weeks of training and may result in decreases in peak impact forces and knee abduction torques. The evidence from the literature indicates that training sessions should be performed more than one time per week, preferably at least two and up to five times per week. The total pre-season training duration of the intervention program should be a minimum of 6, preferably 8 or more, weeks in length. Pfeiffer et al. (2006) reported that 20 min of "in-season" exercise 2 days per week was not sufficient to decrease an ACL injury risk in high school age female basketball players. Gilchrist et al. (2008) also reported that an "in-season" program, with no "pre-season" component was only effective in the last half of the season.

The most effective programs are progressive in nature. Exercises should progress to techniques that initiate perturbations that force the athlete to decelerate and control the body in order to successfully perform the landing, cutting and jumping techniques. The intervention should preferably be phasic in nature. Three exercise phases, such as technique, power, and performance phases are often utilized to facilitate progressions designed to improve the athletes' ability to control body motion during dynamic activities. All exercises in each phase should be progressed to exercise techniques that incorporate perturbations that force the athlete to decelerate and control the body in multiple planes of motion, particularly the coronal plane, in order to successfully perform each technique with optimal form and safety level.

Several studies have highlighted the importance of the athlete's fitness with regard to prevention of injuries. In relation to ACL injuries we know that in addition to strength, endurance, and general fitness it is highly recommended to improve every athlete's sport specific skills. This includes more "ACL-friendly" movements in the different sports, such as a two footed landings after a jump and two- to three-step stop instead of a one-step stop and pivoting.

Finally, fair play is an important factor in our work for less serious injuries. In contact sports sometimes ACL injury is produced by brutal and unfair play. This is an educational and attitude challenge for coaches and officials.

Take-home message

There is good evidence that neuromuscular training decreases ACL injury incidence in female athletes. Plyometrics in combination with biomechanics and technique (e.g., jumping/landing) training appear to induce neuromuscular changes that reduce ACL injury risk. Increased lower extremity muscle recruitment and strength likely have a direct effect on the loading of the ACL during activities that involve cutting and landing. Though ACL injuries likely occur too quickly (less than 70 ms) for reflexive muscular activation (greater than 100 ms), athletes can adopt preparatory muscle recruitment and movement patterns that reduce the incidence of injuries caused by unexpected perturbations. The studies discussed earlier provide strong, but not unequivocal, evidence that neuromuscular intervention training and education programs are likely to be an effective solution to the problem of gender inequity in ACL injury. Selective combination of neuromuscular training components may provide additive effects, further reducing the risk of ACL injuries.

It appears that plyometric power and biomechanics technique training specific to landing, cutting and jumping activities can induce neuromuscular changes and prevent ACL injury, at least in female athletes. Balance, core stability, and strength training may be useful adjuncts. However, we do not yet know which of these components are most effective or whether their effects are combinatorial. Future research efforts will assess the relative efficacy of these interventions alone and in combination in order to achieve the optimal effect in the most efficient manner possible. Selective combination of neuromuscular training components may provide additive effects, further reducing the risk of ACL injuries in female athletes.

Neuromuscular training interventions designed to prevent injury should be based on the previously published literature. Final conclusions are that neuromuscular and educational training reduce ACL injury risk in females athletes if: plyometric exercises and biomechanical technique training are incorporated into the protocol, training sessions are performed more than 1 time per week and the duration of the training program is a minimum of 6 weeks in length. The studies by Hewett et al. (2006b), Myklebust and Bahr (2005), and Mandelbaum et al. (2005) all incorporated plyometrics and biomechanical movement analysis and feedback into their injury prevention programs and applied these basic rules of proper intervention "dose."

References

Albright, J.P., Powell, J.W., Smith, W., Martindale, A., Crowley, E., Monroe, J., Miller, R., Connolly, J., Hill, B.A., Miller, D. (1994) Medial collateral ligament knee sprains in college football. Effectiveness of preventive braces. *American Journal of Sports Medicine* **22**, 12–18.

Caraffa, A., Cerulli, G., Projetti, M., Aisa, G., Rizzo, A. (1996) Prevention of anterior cruciate ligament injuries in soccer. A prospective controlled study of proprioceptive training. *Knee Surgery Sports Traumatology and Arthroscopy* **4**, 19–21.

Heidt Jr., R.S., Sweeterman, L.M., Carlonas, R.L., Traub, J.A., Tekulve, F.X. (2000) Avoidance of soccer injuries with preseason conditioning. *American Journal of Sports Medicine* **28**, 659–662.

Hewett, T.E., Ford, K.R., Myer, G.D. (2006a) Anterior cruciate ligament injuries in female athletes: Part 2, A meta-analysis of neuromuscular interventions aimed at injury prevention. *American Journal of Sports Medicine* **34**, 490–498.

Hewett, T.E., Myer, G.D., Ford, K.R. (2006b) Anterior cruciate ligament injuries in female athletes: Part 1, Mechanisms and risk factors. *American Journal of Sports Medicine* **34**, 299–311.

Hewett, T.E., Myer, G.D., Ford, K.R., Slauterbeck, J.L. (2006c) Preparticipation physical exam using a box drop vertical jump test in young athletes: the effects of puberty and sex. *Clinical Journal of Sports Medicine* **16**, 298–304.

Hewett, T.E., Paterno, M.V., Noyes, F.R. (1999) Differences in single leg balance on an unstable platform between female and male normal, ACL-deficient and ACL-reconstructed knees. In S. Lephardt, F.H. Fu (eds.) *Proprioception and Neuromuscular Control in Joint Stability*, pp. 77–88. Human Kinetics, Champaign, IL.

Hewett, T.E., Stroupe, A.L., Nance, T.A., Noyes, F.R. (1996) Plyometric training in female athletes. Decreased impact forces and increased hamstring torques. *American Journal of Sports Medicine* **24**, 765–773.

Gilchrist, J., Mandelbaum, B.R., Melancon, H., Ryan, G.W., Silvers, H.J., Griffin, L.Y., Watanabe, D.S., Dick, R.W., Dvorak, J. (2008) A randomized controlled trial to prevent noncontact anterior cruciate ligament injury in female collegiate soccer players. *American Journal of Sports Medicine* **36**(8), 1476–83.

Johnson, R.J. (2001) The ACL injury in female skiers. In L.Y. Griffin (ed.) *Prevention of Noncontact ACL injuries*, pp. 107–111. American Academy of Orthopaedic Surgeons, Rosemont.

Kocher, M.S., Sterett, W.I., Briggs, K.K., Zurakowski, D., Steadman, J.R. (2003) Effect of functional bracing on subsequent knee injury in ACL-deficient professional skiers. *Journal of Knee Surgery* **16**(2), 87–92.

Krosshaug, T., Slauterbeck, J.R., Engebretsen, L., Bahr, R. (2007) Biomechanical analysis of anterior cruciate ligament injury mechanisms: three-dimensional motion reconstruction from video sequences. *Scandinavian Journal of Medicine and Science in Sports* **17**, 508–519.

Lehnhard, H.R., Young, S., Butterfield, S.A. (1996) Monitoring injuries on a college soccer team: the effect of strength training. *Journal of Strength and Conditioning Research* **10**, 115–119.

Mandelbaum, B.R., Silvers, H.J., Watanabe, D.S., Knarr, J.F., Thomas, S.D., Griffin, L.Y., Kirkendall, D.T., Garrett Jr., W. (2005) Effectiveness of a neuromuscular and proprioceptive training program in preventing the incidence of ACL injuries in female athletes: 2-year follow up. *American Journal of Sports Medicine* **33**, 1003–1010.

Myklebust, G., Bahr, R. (2005) Return to play guidelines after anterior cruciate ligament surgery. *British Journal of Sports Medicine* **39**, 127–131.

Myklebust, G., Engebretsen, L., Braekken, I.H., Skjølberg, A., Olsen, O.E., Bahr, R. (2003) A prospective cohort study of anterior cruciate ligament injuries in elite Norwegian team handball. *Scandinavian Journal of Medicine and Science in Sports* **8**, 149–153.

Olsen, O.E., Myklebust, G., Engebretsen, L., Holme, I., Bahr, R. (2005) Exercises to prevent lower limb injuries in youth sports: cluster randomised controlled trial. *British Medical Journal* **330**, 449.

Pfeiffer, R.P., Shea, K.G., Roberts, D., Grandstrand, S., Bond, L. (2006) Lack of effect of a knee ligament injury prevention program on the incidence of noncontact anterior cruciate ligament injury. *Journal of Bone and Joint Surgery Am* **88**, 1769–1774.

Sitler, M., Ryan, J., Hopkinson, W., Wheeler, J., Santomier, J., Kolb, R., Polley, D. (1990) The efficacy of a prophylactic knee brace to reduce knee injuries in football. A prospective, randomized study at West Point. *American Journal of Sports Medicine* 18: 310-315.

Söderman, K., Werner, S., Pietilä, T., Engström, B., Alfredson, H. (2000) Balance board training: prevention of traumatic injuries of the lower extremities in female soccer players? A prospective randomized intervention study. *Knee Surgery Sports Traumatology and Arthroscopy* **8**, 356–363.

Wedderkopp, N., Kaltoft, M., Holm, R., Froberg, K. (2003) Comparison of two intervention programmes in young female players in European handball—with and without ankle disc. *Scandinavian Journal of Medicine and Science in Sports* **13**, 371–375.

Zazulak, B.T., Hewett, T.E., Reeves, N.P., Goldberg, B., Cholewicki, J. (2007) Deficits in neuromuscular control of the trunk predict knee injury risk: a prospective biomechanical-epidemiologic study. *American Journal of Sports Medicine* **35**, 1123–1130.

Further reading

Griffin, L.Y. (ed.) (2001) *Prevention of Noncontact ACL injuries*. American Academy of Orthopaedic Surgeons, Rosemont.

Hewett, T.E., Yearout, K., Manske, R. (2006) Preventing injury to the anterior cruciate ligament. In R. Manske (ed.) *Postsurgical Orthopedic Sports Rehabilitation: Knee and Shoulder*, pp. 319–336. Mosby, St. Louis, MO.

Hewett, T.E. (2007) An introduction to understanding and preventing ACL injury. In Hewett T.E., Schultz, S.J.,

Griffin, L.Y. (Eds) *Understanding and preventing non-contact ACL injury*, p. *xxi-xxviii*. Human Kinetics, Champaign, IL.

Hewett, T.E., Myer, G.D., Ford, K.R. (2007) Theories on how neuromuscular intervention programs may influence ACL injury rates: changing landing techniques and improving balance in intervention studies. In T.E. Hewett, S.J. Schultz, L.Y. Griffin (eds.) *Understanding and Preventing Non-contact ACL Injury,* pp. 75–90. Human Kinetics, Champaign, IL.

Hewett, T.E., Myer, G.D., Ford, K.R., Slauterbeck, J.R. (2007) Dynamic neuromuscular analysis training for preventing anterior cruciate ligament injury in female athletes. *Instructional Course Lectures* **56**, 397–406.

Hewett, T.E., Paterno, M.V., Noyes, F.R. (2000) Neuromuscular contributions to knee kinematics and kinetics: normal versus the pathological state. In S.M. Lephart, F.H. Fu (eds.) *Proprioception and Neuromuscular Control in Joint Stability*, pp. 77–88. Human Kinetics, Champaign, IL.

Hewett, T.E., Zazulak, B.T. (2007) The costs associated with ACL injury. In T.E. Hewett, S.J. Schultz, & L.Y. Griffin (eds.) *Understanding and Preventing Non-contact ACL Injury,* pp. 47–56. Human Kinetics, Champaign, IL.

Hewett, T.E., Zazulak, B.T., Myer, G.D. (2007) Theories on how neuromuscular interventions may influence ACL injury rates: EMG activity, muscle firing patterns, and pre-activation. In T.E. Hewett, S.J. Schultz, L.Y. Griffin (eds.) *Understanding and Preventing Non-contact ACL Injury,* pp. 173–182. Human Kinetics, Champaign, IL.

Chapter 6
Preventing hamstring injuries

Geoffrey M. Verrall[1], Árni Árnason[2] and Kim Bennell[3]

[1]SPORTSMED.SA, Sports Medicine Clinic, Adelaide, Australia
[2]Department of Physiotherapy, University of Iceland, Reykjavik, Iceland
[3]Centre for Health, Exercise and Sports Medicine, School of Physiotherapy, University of Melbourne, Australia

Epidemiology of hamstring injuries in sports

Introduction

The hamstring muscle group consists of three muscles of the posterior thigh, the biceps femoris, semitendinosus, and semimembranosus muscles. Their action is to extend the hip and flex the knee and all three muscles are supplied by the sciatic nerve. In understanding the etymology of the word, ham refers to the hollow on the back of the human knee with string referring to the tendons that are present.

Epidemiology of hamstring injuries in sports

Hamstring muscle strains are common injuries in sports that have movement requirements with sudden acceleration and maximal sprinting. These include sports such as athletic sprinting and all of the football codes. Additionally in sports where the hamstring muscles are stretched beyond the usual movement of the muscles, in particular hip flexion, also have a high frequency of hamstring muscle injury. Sports in this particular group include dancing and waterskiing. Hamstring strains are the first or second ranked injury in terms of injury incidence in the football codes such as soccer, rugby, Australian Rules football, and American football (Table 6.1). The incidence of hamstring muscle strain injuries has changed with studies from the 1980s indicating that ankle sprains were the most common type of injury in soccer, followed by knee sprains or hamstring strains. The more recent soccer studies indicate that the proportion of hamstring strains has increased with most modern studies indicating that hamstring strains are the most common injury in soccer (Hawkins & Fuller, 1999). Where data is available this trend has also been reflected in the epidemiology of injury for all football codes.

Table 6.1 Risk of hamstring strains in different sports. The numbers reported are average estimates based on the studies available.

Sport	Competition incidence[1]	Training incidence[1]	Rank[2]
Sprinting			1 (28.6–38%)
Rugby	5.6	0.3	1–2 (9.7–10.7%)
Australian Rules football	3.7–8.6	NA	1 (13.7–23.8%)
Soccer male	2.4–4.1	0.4–0.7	1–2 (11.0–16.5%)
Soccer female	NA	NA	2 (13.1%)
American football	NA	NA	2 (4.9%)

[1]Incidence is reported for adult, competitive athletes as the number of injuries per 1000 hours of training and competition. NA: Not available.
[2]Rank indicated the relative rank of this injury within the sport in question, as well as the proportion as a percentage of total number of injuries within the sport.

Sports Injury Prevention, 1st edition. Edited by R. Bahr and L. Engebretsen Published 2009 by Blackwell Publishing ISBN: 9781405162449

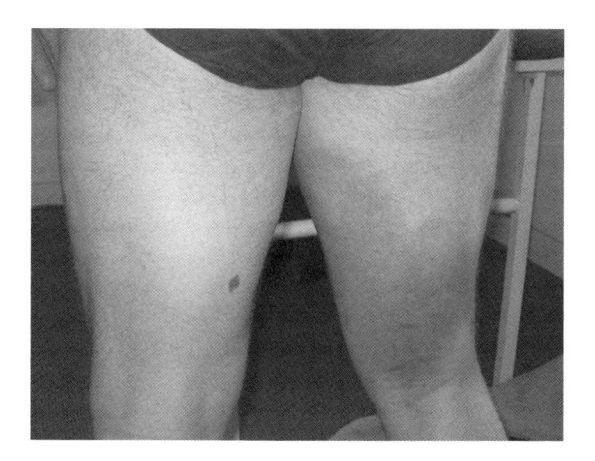

Figure 6.1. Hamstring injury with resultant posterior thigh bruising. This injury, although spectacular in appearance, is uncommon, especially with acceleration/running hamstring injuries

Diagnosis of hamstring injuries

The diagnosis of hamstring muscle strain injury generally involves the sudden onset of posterior thigh pain whilst accelerating/sprinting. Usually the athlete cannot compete further due to the injury and has varying degrees of dysfunction over the subsequent days/weeks depending on the severity of the injury. Pain on resisted hamstring contraction is the most common clinical sign with the frequency of thigh tenderness and the presence of visible bruising being variable (Figure 6.1) (Verrall et al., 2003). Traditionally clinical diagnosis has been used in scientific studies to signify the presence of hamstring muscle strain injury. However recent use of imaging, in particular MRI, has demonstrated that there may be variation in the classical previously accepted clinical picture. Some cases vary by demonstrating a hamstring injury on imaging despite an insidious onset of injury with few clinical signs, whereas others demonstrate no hamstring injury despite classical clinical signs suggesting in these cases a different etiology for the posterior thigh pain (Verrall et al., 2003). From this it can be stated that when reporting research on hamstring injuries, imaging should be used to verify the injury but for general day-to-day management of injured athletes with the common mechanism of injury, clinical judgement should suffice. This may not be the case for elite level athletes as MRI has recently been shown to have some ability in predicting injury prognosis (Slavotinek et al., 2002; Connell et al., 2004). Athletes that have posterior thigh injuries with negative MRI scan results for hamstring muscle injury have a much better prognosis with respect to an earlier return to sport and a marked decrease in injury recurrence rate when compared to athletes with posterior thigh injuries and positive MRI scan results with respect to hamstring muscle injury (Verrall et al., 2003).

Time loss from hamstring injuries

In soccer, Australian Rules football and rugby the average absence from competition due to hamstring muscle strain injury has been shown to be 17–25 days, with athletes generally missing 2–3 weekly matches. However due to the troublesome nature of these injuries the range of days of absence can be considerably higher. These figures are derived from studies on hamstring muscle injury in these sports. Many sports have no available data on the effect on athletes due to hamstring injury. In Australian football there is a high recurrence rate for re-injury with studies demonstrating that this can be as high as 35%. Similar recurrent injury rates can also be seen in soccer with studies demonstrating re-injury rates of between 12% and 35%. Other sports have not completed research in this important area but it is likely that recurrent injuries would be common.

In elite level soccer approximately three injuries can be expected per 1000 playing hours (Árnason et al., 2004). A team playing 50 matches per season results in approximately 800 h of match playing time. Therefore it is expected that on average that each team will have two to three injuries per year during matches, as well as one to two during training (see later). In practice it is demonstrated, and this data derives from Australian Rules football, that there is much variation in the incidence of injury between teams. At this stage it is unclear whether sub-elite or club level results in a lower, or higher, frequency of hamstring injury. Younger teams, underage athletes, have been demonstrated to have fewer hamstring muscle injuries.

The most commonly injured hamstring muscle is the biceps femoris (long head) muscle, followed by the semitendinosus and semimembranosus muscles. This may in part be dependent on the mechanism of the hamstring injury but in many cases more than one hamstring muscle is injured in any single muscle injury. At this time the implications with respect to athlete return to sport and recurrence rate is not known when comparing single or multiple muscle injuries. It is known that the larger the demonstrated muscle injury, the worse prognosis the athlete has (Verrall et al., 2006) but whether for the same size injury to have one muscle injured or more than one muscle injured and affect on athlete prognosis is unclear at this time.

Imaging studies have demonstrated that hamstring muscle injuries, in fact all muscle strain injuries, involve the musculotendinous junction (Garrett, 1996; Slavotinek et al., 2002). Some hamstring muscle injuries only involve the proximal or distal tendons, this is less than 10% of the total number of hamstring strain injuries. With the majority of hamstring muscle strain injuries involving the biceps femoris the injury location is evenly divided to above (proximal muscle injury) and below (distal muscle injury) the short head of biceps insertion into the long head of the biceps femoris (Slavotinek et al., 2002; Connell et al., 2004). Although research is incomplete on this area there does not appear to be a large difference in athlete prognosis when comparing higher injuries to lower injuries. This does not apply to proximal tendon injuries as these athletes do have a significantly worse prognosis with respect to return to sport. The exception to this is where the hamstring muscle is injured in an overstretched type mechanism, such as dancing and waterskiing. These athletes are more likely to have a proximal muscle/tendon injury.

Key risk factors: how to identify athletes at risk

Despite the high incidence of hamstring strains in several popular sports, research on their specific risk factors is limited. Most studies that measure risk factors for hamstring strains have been performed on male subjects in Australian Rules football and soccer. These studies have varied in their size and methodology with differing injury definitions and statistical analyses being used, thereby making it difficult to be conclusive about the findings that these studies have generated. However some findings have been similar in nearly all the studies that have been conducted. In particular the two most consistent findings associated with hamstring strain injury include having a history of a previous hamstring strain injury and being of older age. A summary of internal and external risk factors can be seen in Table 6.2.

Previous hamstring strain injury

Studies on risk factors for hamstring strain injury have consistently demonstrated that previous hamstring strain injury is a principal risk factor for hamstring muscle strain injury. In elite soccer the risk for hamstring injury has been shown to increase by between 3.5 and 11.6 times for previously injured players compared to players without previous hamstring injury (Árnason et al., 2004). In Australian football a previous hamstring injury has been shown to increase hamstring injury risk by 2.1–6.3 times the risk for previously uninjured players (Verrall et al., 2001). Reports from studies of several sports show that re-injury rates are high and this demonstrates the troublesome nature of hamstring muscle strain injuries.

It is considered that the presence of a previous injury predisposes to future injury by changing the muscle properties so that following injury and subsequent athlete rehabilitation and muscle repair the muscle is less able to absorb force making it more prone to re-injury. In effect the scarring of the muscle affects the muscle properties particularly in attenuating force from the muscle to the tendon making the entire muscle at increased risk for re-injury (Taylor et al., 1993). The proposed mechanism of this is considered in more detail later in this chapter. It is also possible that risk factors that originally placed the athlete at risk are still in operation.

Some limitations to this evidence exist in that it is not known for how long a previous hamstring injury will predispose to a future injury and the proposed mechanism of increased injury risk

Table 6.2 Internal and external risk factors for hamstring strains in different sports. The numbers reported are average estimates based on the studies available.

Risk factor	Relative risk/odds ratio[1]	Evidence[2]	Comments
Internal risk factors			
Previous hamstring strain	2.1–11.6	++	Good prospective studies
Previous strains >21.8 cm^3	2.3	+	Measured with MRI
Previous knee injury	5.6	+	
Increased age	1.1–1.4	++	Independent of previous hamstring injury
Race			
Aboriginal descent in Australian football	11.2	+	Single study
Black players in soccer	NA	+	Single study
Decreased hamstring muscle strength	NA	+	Conflicting research results
Hamstring muscle flexibility	NA	0	Poor studies
Gender	NA	0	No research available
External risk factors			
Muscle fatigue	NA	+	Observational studies
Higher level of competition play	NA	+	Observational studies
Insufficient warm-up	NA	0	No evidence
Player position	NA	+	Observational studies

[1] Relative risk/odds ratio indicates the increased risk of injury to an individual with this risk factor relative to an individual who does not have this characteristic. A relative risk of 1.2 times means that the risk of injury is 20% higher for an individual with this characteristic. NA: Not available.

[2] Evidence indicates the level of scientific evidence for this factor being a risk factor for hamstring strains: ++ —convincing evidence from high-quality studies with consistent results; + —evidence from lesser quality studies or mixed results; 0— expert opinion without scientific evidence.

has not been studied in any detail at this point in time.

Older age of athlete

Most studies indicate that increased age is a risk factor for hamstring strains in adult male soccer (relative risk/odds ratio 1.1–1.4) (Árnason et al., 2004) and Australian Rules football (relative risk/odds ratio 1.3) (Verrall et al., 2001). These ratios estimate the increase in risk for the athlete for a 1 year increase in age. Multivariate statistical analyses presented in risk factor studies suggest that this increase in risk with age is independent of whether the athlete had a previous hamstring muscle injury. The incidence of hamstring strains in Australian Rules football has also been shown to be higher in senior players when compared to junior players. It is also interesting to note that in junior level, hamstring strain is the fourth most common injury in terms of injury incidence whereas in the adult level it is the most common injury. Similar results have also been found in soccer.

Studies have shown that with increased age there will be a reduction in the cross-sectional area of skeletal muscles, considered to be primarily as a consequence of a reduction in size and number of Type II muscle fibers. It is muscles with predominance of Type II muscles, such as the gastrocnemius, rectus femoris, and biceps femoris, that are most prone to strain injury. How a reduction in the number of Type II fibers leads to an increased risk for strain injury is not entirely clear. Other studies have also reported denervation of muscle fibers with increased age. These factors could possibly predispose older athletes to hamstring strains. Other possible confounding factors such as previous hamstring strains, decreased flexibility, and increased muscle fatigue could increase the risk of hamstring strains in older athletes compared to younger athletes. Although increased age itself is not modifiable, some of these age-related confounding factors could be modifiable and working with these factors could possibly lower the risk of hamstring strains in older athletes.

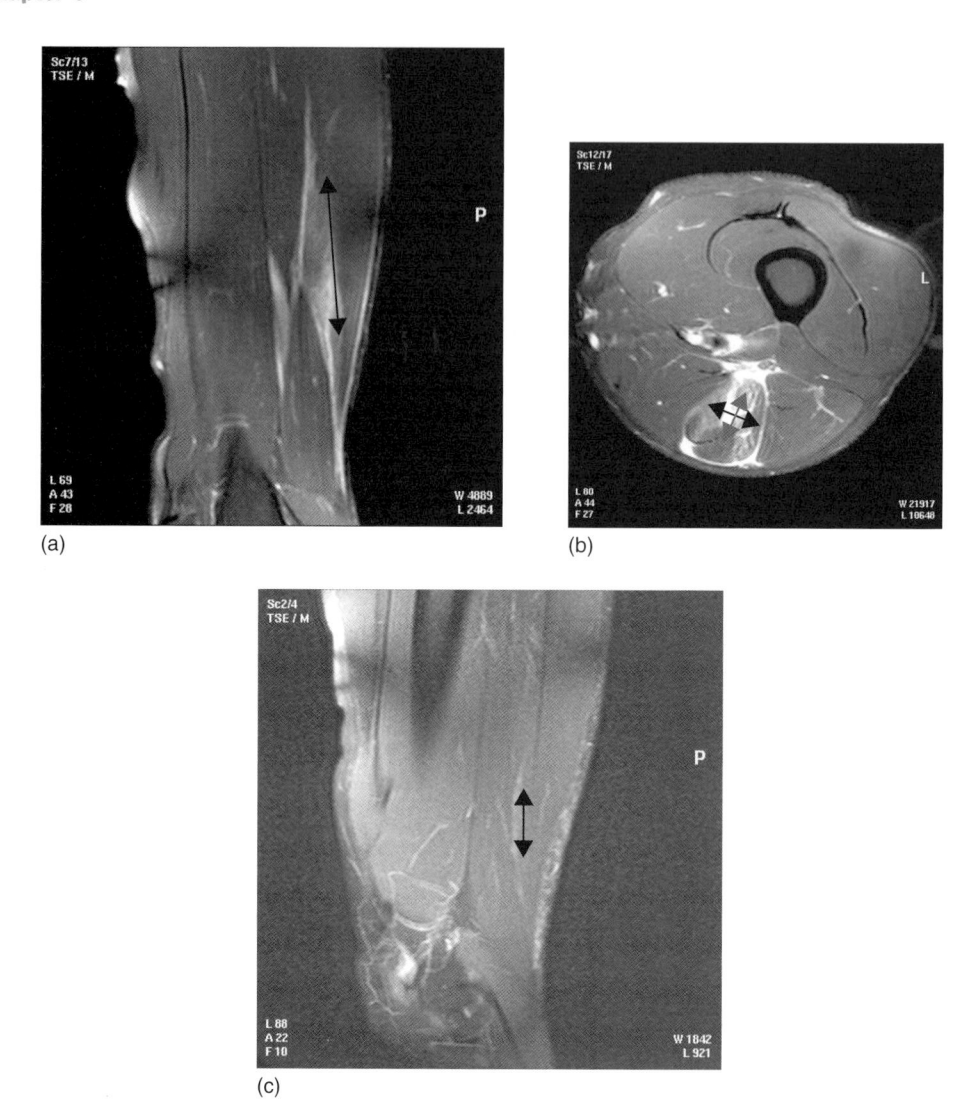

Figure 6.2. MRI investigations of hamstrings injuries; (a) large semitendinosus muscle injury (T2 coronal view, the vertical arrow represents the proximal–distal extent of injury); (b) large semitendinosus muscle injury (T2 axial view, the vertical arrow represents the antero-posterior extent of injury, whereas the horizontal arrow represents the medio-lateral extent); (c) small biceps femoris muscle injury (T2 coronal view, the vertical arrow represents the proximal–distal extent of injury)

Size of hamstring muscle strain injury

Athletes who have incurred hamstring strains of large volume (larger than 20 cm^3 when measured using MRI) have been found to be at an increased risk of re-injury compared to athletes with hamstring strains of less volume (Verrall et al., 2006). Examples of MRI-detected small and large hamstring injuries with their subsequent size measurement can be viewed in Figure 6.2a, b, c. The reason for this high rate of recurrence could be changes in structure or scar tissue formation in or near the muscular tendinous junction after the previous injury, as scar tissue is proposed to be less functional compared to the original tissue (Taylor et al., 1993). Along with the scar tissue formation, atrophy will occur in the muscle as well as changes in viscoelastic properties that can predispose to recurrent injury. Another concern is inadequate rehabilitation as well as too early return to competitive physical activity after the previous hamstring strain. The risk factor, previous injury, is modifiable with optimal rehabilitation after hamstring strains. While the optimal rehabilitation program is not entirely clear, it would seem advisable not to allow athletes to participate too early after hamstring strain in sports that require high demand on speed, jumping, acceleration, deceleration, extreme hamstring flexibility, etc.

Race

Some studies have shown that soccer players of black origin and Australian Rules football players of aboriginal decent sustain significantly more hamstring strains than white players. It has been proposed that these players are generally considered to be the fastest in their particular sport when compared to their white counterparts. This has lead to the conclusion that these athletes have increased risk for hamstring injury due to their muscles having a higher proportion of type II muscle fibers in order to develop faster speed. A faster speed is considered to generate higher hamstring stressors and this maybe the reason for increased injury risk.

Hamstring muscle strength and hamstring/quadriceps strength ratio

Some studies have indicated that decreased hamstring strength, inadequate hamstring/quadriceps strength ratio, and a difference in right/left hamstring strength ratio could be potential risk factors for hamstring strains. This is based on the premise that the hamstring is weak relative to the quadriceps and therefore the leg develops too much leg extension force that needs to be counteracted by the flexion action of the hamstrings leading to subsequent hamstring injury. However it should be noted that other studies have reported results that conflict with these findings. The studies that have been performed all use a dynamometer to measure the concentric and eccentric strength of the hamstring and quadriceps with the resultant production of a Hamstring to Quadriceps (H:Q) strength ratio. The obvious advantage of this is that it is an easily quantifiable ratio and can potentially be modified by specific training of the muscle considered to be deficient in strength. However further research needs to be performed in this area before there will be universal agreement as to the validity of this approach in the possible prevention of hamstring injuries. It is also not possible to be specific about the optimal H:Q ratio and whether this ratio should be calculated using concentric or eccentric force production, as this have not been reliably determined. In recent years there has been more emphasis on the eccentric action of the hamstring muscles and many rehabilitation programs and prevention programs emphasize eccentric strength training and conditioning.

In interpreting the various studies, difficulties arise in comparing methodology on how the strength of the quadriceps/hamstrings were measured, the reproducibility of the method, and, more importantly, what exactly constituted a hamstring injury. These two factors are probably important in explaining conflicting study results (Bennell et al., 1998).

In conclusion, an imbalance in muscle strength between the hamstrings and quadriceps muscles is an area that warrants further research as it possibly a risk factor for hamstring injury. If this was proven to be the case it is also an area where the risk factor may be more easily, relative to other approaches, modifiable.

Flexibility

Many investigators have discussed the possibility that poor hamstring flexibility could be a risk factor for hamstring strains. Different methods are used for testing hamstring muscle flexibility in different studies so comparison between these studies is difficult. In general there is a paucity of evidence and the methodology has been relatively poor thereby not allowing definitive conclusions to be drawn. Although flexibility is not as easy to measure when compared to the hamstring to quadriceps strength ratio, muscle flexibility is also an area that warrants further research. If flexibility, increased or decreased, can be demonstrated to be a risk factor for subsequent hamstring injury, it has the potential to be more easily modified.

Competition versus training

While it is generally accepted that hamstring strains occur more frequently during competition, as opposed to training sessions, this information is only available for a limited number of sports (Table 6.1), as research is incomplete in this area. Hamstring muscle strain injuries occur more commonly in competitive matches compared to training. It has been demonstrated that the likelihood of sustaining a hamstring injury during a competitive match as compared to during training may be increased up to 10 times in high-risk sports such as soccer and Australian football (Garrett, 1996; Verrall et al., 2003). A possible reason for this is that competitive matches usually involve more intense effort over a longer time period when compared to the usual training situation. This may lead to increased fatigue and a larger total amount of load (force) on the hamstring muscle making it more prone to injury.

Muscle fatigue

Studies from soccer show an increased incidence of hamstring strains during the last third of the first and second half of matches (Hawkins & Fuller, 1999). This is generally used to indicate that fatigue may be a risk factor for hamstring injury. Similar results have also been demonstrated in rugby and Australian football with hamstring muscle strain injuries occurring in the latter part of the game or time period.

Fatigued muscles have been demonstrated in laboratory studies to be able to absorb less force than their non-fatigued counterparts (Mair et al., 1996). The absorption (attenuation) of force generated by the moving leg is a very important function of the hamstring muscles during running. It is this reduction in force attenuation that is considered to be the reason why fatigued muscles are at increased risk for injury.

Level of competition play

Studies on players from soccer and Australian Rules football have shown that hamstring strains are more common in higher, more professional leagues. The reasons for this have not been fully elucidated but the increased training and playing demands of the higher levels of competition are considered to in some way increase hamstring strain risk.

Player position on field

Player position on the field of play has been shown to be important in some sports including backs having a higher incidence of injury compared to forward in rugby and wide receivers having a higher incidence in American football. In Australian football and soccer the midfield players are considered to be at higher risk for hamstring muscle strain injury. The reason for this increased risk in these players in these sports is similar to the argument proposed to explain the increased risk seen in some ethnic groups. Players in these positions are usually amongst the fastest for that particular sport.

Insufficient warm-up

It is considered that an insufficient warm-up may increase the risk for subsequent hamstring muscle strain injury. The proposed mechanism for this is that insufficient warm-up leads to muscles being more viscous and less elastic with poorer neuromuscular coordination. There is little or no scientific evidence for this assertion, except animal studies showing that the load to failure is higher after warm-up. However, warm-up should be undertaken to adequately prepare the athlete for competition and not just for an injury prevention role.

Take-home message

Knowledge of potential risk factors for hamstring muscle strains are important for the development of preventive measures. In the majority of cases, the causes of hamstring strains can be considered to be multifactorial with a complex series of events leading to injury. In this regard there are many potential risk factors that may lead given the right set of conditions to a hamstring strain.

Current knowledge suggests players with a previous hamstring injury and older players are almost certainly at an increased risk for subsequent hamstring muscle injury. These athletes in particular should be targeted for prevention programs.

Other substantive risk factors have not as yet been identified but the avoidance of excessive fatigue, identifying athletes with hamstring weakness and considering the playing position and role in the team of athletes demonstrate potential risk factors and these athletes should also be targeted for prevention programs.

Finally it should be considered that different sports, and different athletes within those sports, probably have different risk factors. Therefore it is not surprising that in most studies, measurement of a single potential risk factor almost always fails to predict hamstring muscle strain injury occurrence.

Injury mechanisms for hamstring muscle injuries

Basic principles of hamstring muscle strain injury

The typical injury mechanism for hamstring muscle strains is unknown as there is little scientific literature addressing the topic. As a basic principle it can be stated that hamstring muscle strain injuries result from an increase in biomechanical load that exceeds the tolerance of the hamstring muscle(s). In understanding the mechanism of hamstring muscle strain injuries we need to consider factors that may increase or decrease biomechanical load on the hamstring muscle. In addition factors that change the load tolerance of the muscle(s) also need to be considered.

Intuitively in most cases it is difficult to see how a change in the biomechanical load to the muscle during athletic performance can be affected. The Olympic motto of faster, higher, stronger, and the demands of modern day sport suggest that the demands on the athlete and the muscles that propel the athlete are more likely to increase over time rather than decrease. Therefore in looking at hamstring muscle strain injury mechanisms with a view to prevention, how factors change the load tolerance of the hamstring muscle are probably more important as there is more potential to modify some of these factors. Factors that reduce the load tolerance of the hamstring muscle may render the hamstring muscle more susceptible to injury from what would generally be considered to be normally tolerated biomechanical loads and forces. We also need to examine factors that may increase the load tolerance of the hamstring muscles as this would obviously be useful in the prevention of hamstring muscle strain injuries.

Excessive biomechanical load

In some cases the mechanism, whether increased biomechanical load or decreased load tolerance, can be determined by understanding the nature of the sport and subsequent injury pattern. An example of a hamstring muscle strain injury in a sport where the biomechanical load obviously exceeds the load tolerance of the hamstring muscle(s) is the typical water skiing injury. In this sport the typical injury occurs when the athlete is forcibly pulled over with a forced flexion of the trunk and a fully extended leg, usually during a starting (take-off) maneuver. This results in an excessive load on the hamstring muscles with subsequent injury. In this case the mechanism of injury is indisputable. It is worth noting that these excessive force injuries, when seen in a clinical setting, are often more severe and may involve all three hamstring muscles compared to the typical running sport injury.

Another example where this mechanism (excessive load) may be the predominant mechanism for injury is those sports where the muscle and leg is hyperextended as the athlete attempts a sport-specific movement. Examples can be seen in dance and sports that involve kicking, particularly overhead kicking (Askling et al., 2007).

Reduced load tolerance

The most common situation for a hamstring muscle strain injury occurs when the athlete is sprinting and/or accelerating. This action is common to many sports but especially in track running and in all of the football codes around the world. The considered mechanism for injury in these cases is predominately a reduction in the load tolerance of the hamstring muscle making it more susceptible to the strain injury as opposed to an increase in biomechanical load. This assertion comes from the observation that most injuries occur randomly in the act of running, an event that the athlete performs constantly and where there is no observable increase in biomechanical load. This leads to the conclusion that a decreased load tolerance is the most likely explanation. In other words the load-bearing properties of the muscle are altered in such a manner that the muscle can no longer tolerate a load that it had previously tolerated. This injury event is generally a sudden onset in nature and generally unpredictable. In one stride the athlete and hamstring muscle, are functioning normally and suddenly in the next stride the athlete sustains a hamstring injury.

Factors that may be important in reducing the load tolerance properties of the hamstring muscle are often considered to be risk factors for injury. These have been discussed in the earlier section. However it can be said that in most cases how each of the earlier described risk factors reduces the capacity of the hamstring muscle to resist normally tolerated forces is unclear and the reasons for injury are speculative. Similarly the weighting or importance of each risk factor has not been determined at this time.

It should also be remembered that in the sports involving body contact there exists the possibility that in some cases of hamstring injury, too much load on the hamstring muscle is the predominant mechanism of injury rather than a reduced capacity of muscle to absorb force. This includes sports involving tackling where the athlete tries to force against resistance. In some cases the resistance can result in an excessive force to the hamstring muscle, for example, in an American football or rugby scrimmage line, or when the athletes' leg is fixed (trapped) whilst they are trying to accelerate or sprint.

Predominant hamstring muscle injured

The most common hamstring muscle injured as a consequence of reduced load tolerance of the hamstring muscle is the long head of biceps femoris muscle. This is followed in frequency by the semitendinosus and then the semimembranosus muscles, respectively. The short head of biceps femoris muscle is infrequently injured and at this current time is not considered to be an important muscle in the pathogenesis of hamstring muscle strain injury. We understand the different frequency of muscle injuries from the results of imaging studies undertaken in running athletes (Slavotinek et al., 2002; Connell et al., 2004) where reduced load tolerance is suspected to be a key factor in injury pathogenesis.

At this time little research has been undertaken as to why the biceps femoris (long head) is the most susceptible to muscle stretch injury as a consequence of a reduced ability to resist normal loading forces whilst the athlete is sprinting. Important factors that may be unique to the biceps femoris muscle include the rate (velocity) and the amount of stretch of the muscle that occurs in the muscle and tendon, its anatomical location and the amount of force (load) that needs to be dissipated by this muscle.

In hamstring muscle strain injuries where excessive force is the considered mechanism it is often shown, by imaging studies, that more than one muscle is injured. At this time it is not clear which muscle is the predominant muscle injured.

Musculotendinous junction

The most common anatomical location of hamstring muscle injuries is the musculotendinous junction. The reasons for this are unclear but it may represent a site of comparative weakness. In the case of the biceps femoris muscle, the most commonly injured hamstring muscle, injuries appear to be evenly distributed in proximal and distal sites as defined by whether the injury is above or below the insertion of the short head of the biceps femoris muscle into the long head. Again this has been determined principally by imaging studies performed on running athletes (Slavotinek et al., 2002; Connell et al., 2004).

Stage of gait cycle

For sprinting injuries the muscle is considered susceptible to injury in the swing phase of the gait cycle. At this time the hamstring muscle is acting eccentrically (developing force whilst elongating) to slow the femur and tibia. The typical force length curve of the hamstring muscle is shown in Figure 6.3. The total amount of force that the hamstring muscles generate is described by the

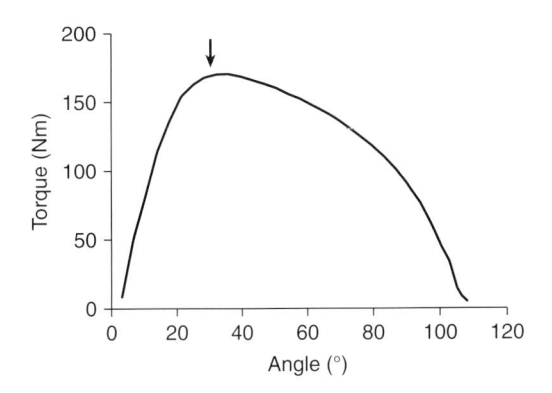

Figure 6.3. Typical torque length curve of the contracting hamstring muscles. The area under the curve represents the total amount of force that the muscle generates. Arrow signifies peak torque.

area under the curve and is considerably more in the eccentric (slowing femur through swing) phase of hamstring action when compared to the concentric (ground contact and pull-through) phase of the gait cycle.

It is also considered that the muscle is most vulnerable in the late phase of the swing cycle but the exact reasons for this as well as the actual biomechanical events leading up to and causing the failure of the muscle are not known at this time. As discussed in the risk factors section, fatigue is considered to be an important factor in the pathogenesis of hamstring muscle injury by reducing the load tolerance that the muscle can withstand (Mair et al., 1996). It is therefore not surprising that many hamstring muscle strain injuries occur late in a game or training when fatigue is at its maximum and in the phase of the gait cycle where the most force needs to be generated by the hamstring muscle, that is, the eccentric swing phase. The consequence of these factors leads to a relative force overload to the hamstring muscle with subsequent injury.

Take-home message

The current state of knowledge suggests the following mechanisms for hamstring muscle strain injury: (1) overwhelming force to the muscle, (2) overstretch of the muscle, and (3) reduced load tolerance of the muscle. The majority of injuries occur during sprinting and/or acceleration and this suggests that reduced load tolerance of the muscle is the most common mechanism of hamstring injury. Reduced load tolerance of the muscle may well be, at least in part, the function of a fatiguing (fatigued) muscle. This fact has implications in the prevention of hamstring injury with the avoidance of muscle fatigue by training the muscle to better tolerate fatigue being the cornerstone of many current hamstring injury prevention programs. Other common risk factors are less able to be influenced. In effect increasing age, having a previous injury, and being a faster player are inherently unchangeable risk factors.

However more research needs to be undertaken on the mechanisms of hamstring muscle strain injuries and it is possible that with better understanding this list may change substantially. Finally, it can be stated that at this time it is not known whether the mechanism of hamstring muscle strain injury is important in the pathogenesis and subsequent recovery of the injury and whether this alters the risk for subsequent re-injury. For example, it is not known whether an overstretch or excessive force injury is better or worse in terms of athlete prognosis than a sprinting/acceleration decreased load tolerance injury.

Identifying risks in the training and competition programs

Little is known about the differing risks between the competitive games and training programs. As stated earlier hamstring injuries are more likely to occur in the competitive match situation compared to training so it is possible that different risks exist for these different situations or more likely the risks are magnified in the competitive match situation. Some other general non-specific observations have been made to identify risks in training and competition, but the reasons for these observations are speculative.

In many sports there is a predominance of hamstring muscle strain injuries in the early part of the competitive season (Orchard & Seward, 2002).

The reasons for this observation are not known. Pre-season training programs have been primarily designed to improve the fitness of the participants. In many cases improving athletes' fitness is done in a manner that is not particularly sport specific with many training regimens not replicating the specific energy demands of the sport. This is especially true for sports, such as the football codes, that have extensive aerobic and anaerobic requirements with multiple sprinting (maximal efforts) being required over an extended time period. An example of this lack of sport specificity is to train a soccer player by running in 5 km time trials in the pre-season. In a competitive game this type of aerobic running is not generally consistent with how the game is played—the running requirements in a typical soccer game involve recurrent interval sprinting with maximal and sub-maximal efforts with each effort generally not lasting more than 6 s in time or 50 m in distance.

It is therefore considered that many early season hamstring muscle strain injuries are the result of the failure of the muscle to adapt to the increased load (force) that is required to be absorbed when there is a transition from predominately aerobic conditioning that is used in the pre-season training program to the actual requirement of the competitive sport—recurrent maximal anaerobic sprinting efforts. Thus when the competitive matches commence (including the late pre-season trial games) more hamstring injuries occur as the muscle has not yet adapted to the increased load requirements that is specific to the running demands of competitive sport. An early season predominance of hamstring injuries has been demonstrated in some sports including Australian rules football (Orchard & Seward, 2002) and soccer (Hawkins & Fuller, 1999). Understanding this transition risk factor can assist in developing an effective prevention program.

It is also clear that aerobic conditioning is an important component in most sports. Recent research suggests that it is even more important in track sprinting than had been previously recognized. Most football codes require predominately interval maximal anaerobic efforts followed by a limited, or in many cases no, recovery period. It is in the limited recovery period where aerobic conditioning is important. Therefore a pre-season conditioning program requires both aerobic conditioning and anaerobic interval sprint conditioning in order to attain maximal sport-specific fitness for the athlete. Current best practice suggests that if a change from a predominately aerobic program to a predominately anaerobic program is considered then this transition should involve a gradual, rather than an abrupt, change from one form of training to another. In this way there may be a reduction in the early season risk of hamstring muscle strain injury. Furthermore once the playing season has commenced it is now considered that the predominant form of fitness undertaken at practice should be in the same manner with respect to anaerobic/aerobic components, as is needed in competitive matches. Recent studies on hamstring injuries in female elite soccer and elite Australian football have demonstrated reduced hamstring injuries in athletes that undertook a pre-season training program that was, in part, undertaken to attempt to decrease hamstring injury occurrence (Mjølsnes et al., 2004; Verrall et al., 2005).

Prevention measures

There have been very few published studies on the prevention of hamstring muscle strain injury. Similarly, very few of the rehabilitation programs have been validated. As such there is limited scientific evidence to assess the results for any prevention programs for hamstring muscle strain injuries. However, analysis of the available evidence demonstrates that some methods for hamstring injury prevention are of probable benefit whereas others demonstrate possible benefit and finally others have been mentioned as being of benefit on the basis of expert opinion.

Improving training specificity and improving fatigue resistance were considered to have probable benefit in preventing hamstring injury. Possible beneficial methods discussed include identifying and modifying at-risk athletes, hamstring muscle strengthening, improving hamstring flexibility, and adequate rehabilitation form hamstring injury. Finally, thermal pants and an adequate warm-up

Table 6.3 Injury prevention matrix for hamstring strains: potential measures to prevent injuries.

	Pre-crash	Crash	Post-crash
Athlete	Improving training specificity Increasing fatigue resistance	Minimizing fatigue	Adequate and comprehensive rehabilitation program Identifying size of hamstring injury so adequate rehabilitation program can be instituted
	Identifying at-risk athletes and implementing targeted prevention programs Hamstring muscle strengthening Improving muscle flexibility Warm-up		
Rules/environment	–	–	–
Material	Thermal pants	–	–

have been considered beneficial to preventing hamstring strain injury and are also discussed. A summary of these methods are presented in the hamstring injury prevention matrix shown in Table 6.3.

Improving training specificity

At the highest level of participation most athletes require an extreme level of fitness especially in sports such as the football codes where the athletes can compete for up to 2 h. In many of the pre-season and in season training programs for these football codes there has been an emphasis on aerobic conditioning as the predominant training. However the energy requirements of most football codes require the athletes to be able to cope with high-intensity anaerobic interval maximal or sub-maximal sprinting efforts. As discussed in the mechanisms section, it is in the process of the intensive anaerobic effort, the sprint, that many hamstring muscle strain injuries occur.

Most sports with similar energy requirements should consider improving the specificity of training so that the athletes are better able to cope with match day, the principal time of hamstring muscle strain injury, running stressors. Thus "training as the game is played" should prevent hamstring injuries by improving hamstring muscle conditioning and developing improved fatigue resistance. There is evidence to support this proposition (Heidt et al., 2000; Verrall et al., 2005).

Improving fatigue resistance

There is evidence that fatigued muscles are able to absorb less energy than non-fatigued muscles. Therefore by improving the specificity of training and muscle conditioning it may be possible to prevent hamstring muscle strain injuries by making the muscle more fatigue resistant and better able to absorb energy loads particularly in the eccentric phase of the gait cycle action where the muscle is most commonly injured.

Identifying at-risk athletes

The principal risk factors for hamstring muscle injury are increasing age of the athlete and the athlete having a previous history of hamstring injury. These risk factors cannot be altered. However identifying these athletes in the team group, informing these athletes of their at-risk status, and then targeting prevention programs to these particular athletes is a strategy that may prove worthwhile in preventing hamstring injuries.

Strengthening

Increased hamstring muscle strength has long been considered to help prevent hamstring injuries, and recent scientific evidence supports this proposition. As the principal role of the hamstring muscles is to eccentrically slow the femur and tibia and is antagonistic to the quadriceps muscle it is felt that

Table 6.4 Eccentric strength training program (Nordic hamstring lowers, see Figure 6.4a, b).

Week	Sessions per week	Sets and repetitions	Comments
1	1	2 sets, 5 repetitions	Adaptation to the exercise. Important to start slowly, this is a demanding exercise. Do not do too many sessions, sets or repetitions in the beginning; it could result in excessive muscle soreness.
2	2	2 sets, 6 repetitions	Try to hold against with the hamstring muscles as long as possible before falling on the arms.
3	3	3 sets, 6–8 repetitions	Increased loading. It is possible to withstand the forward fall longer and perform more sessions, sets and repetitions.
4	3	3 sets, 8–10 repetitions	Near full program.
5 or more	3	3 sets, 12–10–8 repetitions	Full program. When it is possible to withstand the whole range of motion for 12 repetitions, the load can be increased by adding speed to the starting phase of the motion or by having someone to push on the subjects back (in the height of the shoulder blades) at the starting phase.

strengthening the hamstring muscle may assist in improved attenuation of this force thereby decreasing the injury risk. Recently, exercises that may be more specific in increasing eccentric hamstring strength have been studied. An exercise called Nordic hamstring lowers has been introduced as a potential preventive exercise for hamstring strains (Table 6.4). This exercise program has been shown to increase the eccentric hamstring strength (measured at 60°/s) by 11% in a period of 10 weeks of training (Árnason et al., 2008). A 4 year study of 17–30 Norwegian and Icelandic elite soccer teams indicated that teams that used the Nordic hamstring lowers exercise combined with stretching of short duration during warm-up reduced their risk of hamstring strains by 57% compared to teams that did not use the program during the same season (Árnason et al., 2008). The intervention teams also showed a lower incidence of hamstring strains than the same teams during the baseline seasons (58% lower rate).

It has not yet been determined whether strengthening prevents hamstring injury solely by increasing the eccentric strength of the hamstring muscle or whether other factors are as important. These other factors include improving flexibility, improving fatigue resistance, and improving the functional operation of the hamstring muscles. In this manner whenever studies report an increase in strength of the hamstring muscle as being the mechanism of the intervention effect it is difficult to be confident that this is actually the case. Although more research is needed, strengthening remains an important method to consider in preventing hamstring injury.

Flexibility

The role of flexibility in muscle strain injuries has not yet been fully elucidated. The presented studies into this area have been poorly performed with regards to the injury definition used and the reproducibility of the flexibility measures. At this time it is not possible to state the boundaries of normal and abnormal flexibility and thus the amount of flexibility that places an athlete at risk is not clear. Accordingly, it is not clear how to implement prevention programs that may change flexibility.

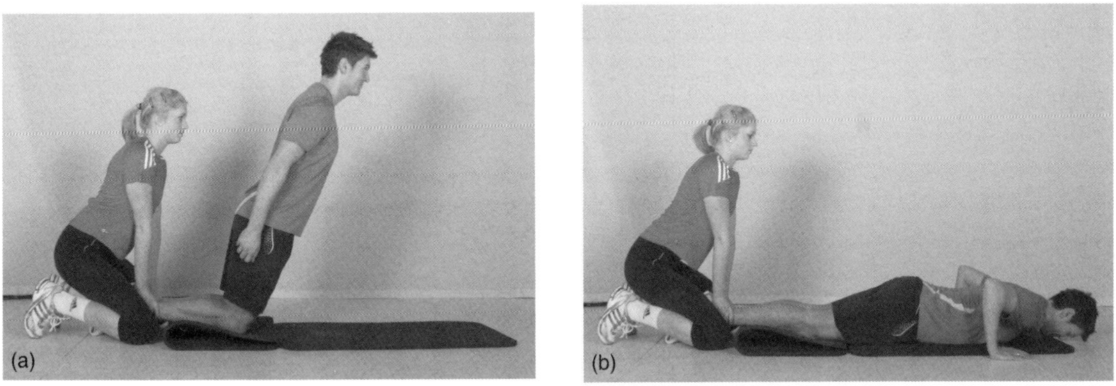

Figure 6.4. Eccentric strength training using Nordic hamstring lowers. Nordic hamstring lowers is a partner exercise. The subject kneels on soft, but firm ground. The partner stabilizes the subject's legs by holding them down at the floor. It is important that she holds tight and does not allow any movement. The subject leans forward, keeping his back straight, slight flexion in hips is allowed. He resists the forward fall with his hamstrings as long as possible and then uses his arms and hands to buffer the landing, going all the way down until the chest touches the ground. Then he uses his arms to push off so she can reach the kneeling position again. Reproduced from Bahr (2004) with permission from the publisher (©Lill-Ann Prøis & Gazette Bok)

Laboratory evidence on animal muscle have demonstrated that muscles have been shown to increase force absorption for any given increase in length (stretch) of the muscle. Thus increasing flexibility may make the muscle more resistant to stretch injury. However, in the study from Norway and Iceland mentioned earlier, no effect was found from flexibility training alone (Árnason et al., 2008).

Rehabilitation of hamstring injuries and the relationship to prevention of injuries

For hamstring muscle strain injuries, in fact for all muscle strain injuries, the rehabilitation program following injury is an important factor in attempting to prevent re-injury. This is due to the observation that the most important risk factor for hamstring muscle injury is previous injury. Hence many hamstring injuries are actually re-injuries, thereby making the components of the original rehabilitation program important in preventing hamstring (re)injury.

Studies of Australian rules football players demonstrate that this risk for re-injury occurs principally for the first 8 weeks following an injury. Unfortunately there are very few studies demonstrating the effects of rehabilitation programs on re-injury risk. Table 6.5 analyzes the components of a typical hamstring injury rehabilitation program and attempts to justify the rationale for each action. An example of a typical rehabilitation program for a sport requiring interval high-intensity sprinting is demonstrated in Table 6.6.

There is little scientific evidence for the intensity, duration, and timing for any exercise that is introduced in the immediate post-injury period. However it is generally accepted that controlled exercise, as opposed to rest, should be introduced early in the rehabilitation period. Histological evidence demonstrates that muscle injury repair involves scar formation at the site of injury. It is considered that the formed scar does not have the same properties as the pre-existing muscle with respect to load attenuation making the injured muscle and surrounding muscle area more prone to further injury (re-injury). By commencing activities early in the post-injury period it is thought that the scar formation at the site of injury will be improved in terms of attaining properties that are more like the pre-existing muscle. This would then result in an increased tolerance of the muscle to load when more strenuous activity is recommenced with a subsequent reduced risk for re-injury. There is some supportive histopathological evidence for this proposition. Further evidence for introducing stretches and activities early in the rehabilitation period comes from studies that examine the length–tension curve of previously injured athletes (Brockett et al., 2004). In effect these demonstrate

Table 6.5 Components of a hamstring muscle strain injury rehabilitation program.

Progression/action	Rationale
At injury	
Remove from field of play	Prevent further injury
Apply ice and compression	Prevent bleeding of injury. Recent evidence from MRI studies of hamstring muscle strain injuries suggests bleeding is not a common outcome of these injuries. If bleeding is demonstrated to be present clinically, usually at day 2 or 3 following injury, by the presence of a bruise, then this generally signifies a higher grade (more severe) hamstring injury. However despite the lack of evidence for ice application for hamstring injuries it is still recommended that it is performed post-injury.
Immediate post-injury period	
Commence stretching and weight-bearing activities	Aids in the healing of the injury with the aim being an earlier and more successful (in terms of a reduction in injury recurrence), return to sport.
Commence non-weight-bearing activities (e.g., cycling, swimming)	Prevent athlete deconditioning in the rehabilitation period.
Introduce anti-inflammatory medication	Overall there is little evidence for this approach and some contention. In support of this it can be considered that the anti-inflammatories can act as an analgesic and therefore allow an earlier commencement of activities in rehabilitation. It should be stated that some authors consider that anti-inflammatories impede healing at the injury site and thus increase the re-injury risk in athletes.
Post-injury period	
Stretching and running progression	A graduated increase in activities is stated to reduce the risk of overloading the injured muscle, and also allow increasing load tolerance, thereby reducing the risk of subsequent re-injury.
Introduction of specific sport skill exercises	To ensure the athlete is ready for return to play.
Commence strengthening	Improve the strength of the muscle making the muscle less prone to re-injury as the muscle is able to absorb more force for any given length or tension. There is however little scientific evidence to support this proposition and therefore many hamstring rehabilitation programs do not have a formal strengthening component. This component of the rehabilitation program is discussed in more detail in the following section.

that the hamstring heals in a shortened position with a reduction in the angle of the knee where the hamstring generates maximal force when compared to athletes who have not had a previous hamstring injury (Figure 6.6). This is considered to be a risk for re-injury and it has been suggested that an early introduction of stretching, including eccentrically based stretches, may be important in preventing this shortening.

Current trends in injury management with the goal of preventing re-injury

Unfortunately, re-injury following rehabilitation is very common. In Australian football the re-injury rate is ~30% (Orchard & Seward, 2002). There is about a one in three risk of an athlete with a hamstring muscle strain injury of sustaining another strain injury on the same side, with a high proportion of these re-occurring in the rehabilitation and/or the immediate return to sport period. In Australian Rules football there is an increased risk for hamstring muscle re-injury for up to 8 weeks after the athlete returns to sport. The re-injury risk drops to less than 4% after the athlete has played eight matches. In many cases this time period can be 3 months from the original hamstring muscle strain injury.

Recent trends in this sport have been to manage these injuries more conservatively. These increasingly conservative measures include:

1. A longer convalescent interval (an increase in time before the athlete returns to competitive matches) after the athlete sustains an injury.

Table 6.6 An example of a rehabilitation program used post-hamstring injury in a sport requiring multiple maximal anaerobic efforts with a short duration of recovery (e.g., soccer, Australian football).

Progression	Program
Upon injury	Ice 20 min every hour; 5 episodes Ice bath optional Elevation Compression bandage
Injury plus 1 day	Examination Full weight bearing Rest from activities
Injury plus 2 days	Stretch to point of pain Pain free walking
Injury plus 3–5 days	Re-examination Stretching Bike, swim, pool running as tolerated Pain free emphasis for all activities on days 0–5 Ultrasound once per day. Gentle massage only when pain free No anti-inflammatory medication (injection/oral/topical) Return to running (see later) when walking pain free Commence weights and eccentric exercises when pain free stretch (see later) is obtained
Running progression	Progression upon completion of two to three sessions in each of the following: 1. Pain free walking—jogging 4×500 m 2. Interval running (Jog, slow speed, run) maximum speed 70%—4×500 m, Avoid rapid acceleration. 3. Commence speed running (No rapid acceleration). 80–90% speed—Commence at 5 times of 40 m for 2 sets. Therefore 10 times total with 15 min break between sets. 4. Speed running—no rapid acceleration—80–90% speed—10 times of 40 m for 2 sets. Therefore 20 times total with 15 min break between sets. 5. Deceleration runs. No rapid acceleration—10 times of 40 m—90% effort for 2 sets—deceleration (complete stop) within 20 m decreasing to 10 m. 6. Acceleration runs—5 times of 40 m for 2 sets 7. Acceleration runs—10 times of 40 m for 2 sets—full acceleration from crouched start
Stretching progression	Progression to next stage when pain free: Passive hamstring stretch—when pain free Active hamstring stretches with physiotherapy supervision (see Figure 6.5a, b) Strength assessment by physiotherapist—if no detectable difference clinically between affected and non-affected side then commencement of eccentric stretching regime—slow Commencement of fast eccentric stretches and closed-chain weights regimen
Return to sports-specific training	Return to sports-specific training when achieved running and stretching progression PLUS normal examination. Normal examination parameters include absence of posterior thigh tenderness, pain free resisted hamstring contractions in prone (straight leg and 20° flexion; internal, neutral and external leg rotation positions) and supine (knee flexion; full extension and 90° knee flexion positions) Return to playing when achieved 1 full week of training Rehabilitation continued after return to sport; continues for 8 weeks post return to sport

2. Less aggressive treatment of the hamstring muscle strain injury in the immediate post-injury period, including less use of anti-inflammatory medication and other controversial strategies such as corticosteroid injections.

3. More emphasis on the introduction of stretching, including eccentric based stretches, in the immediate post-injury period with a decreased use of strengthening programs in the immediate post-injury period.

4. Continuing rehabilitation for some time after the athlete has returned to sport.

5. Attempting to prevent significant muscle fatigue in the immediate return to sport period with increased use of rest periods and if allowable in the sport interchange periods.

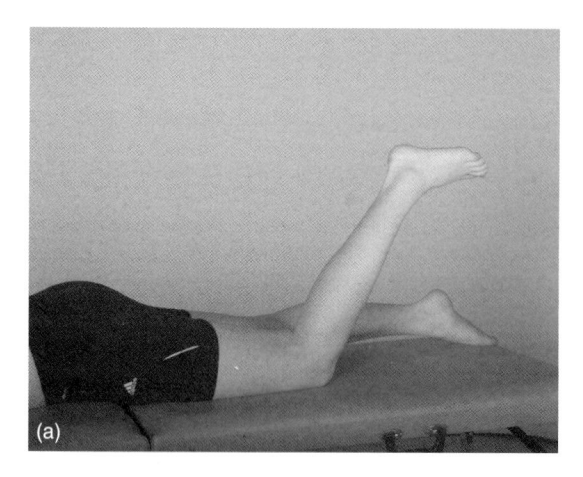

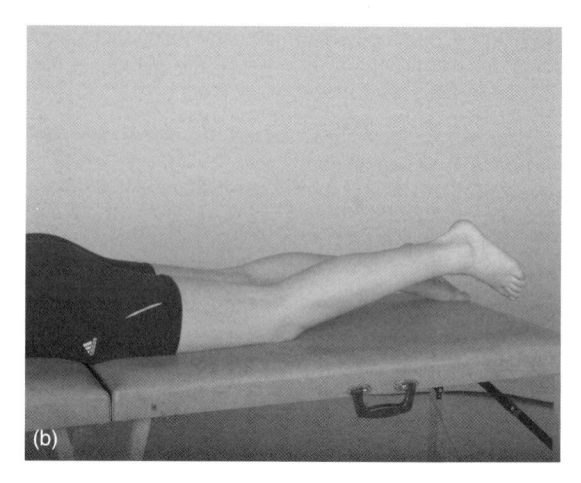

Figure 6.5. Example of eccentric exercise performed during rehabilitation—drop and catch. The athlete is lying on stomach, knee flexed to 90°. The muscles are relaxed allowing the foot to fall to ground ("the drop"). The foot is prevented from touching the ground ("the catch") by contracting the hamstring muscles. Initially gravity is used but later in the rehabilitation pathway ankle weights can be added

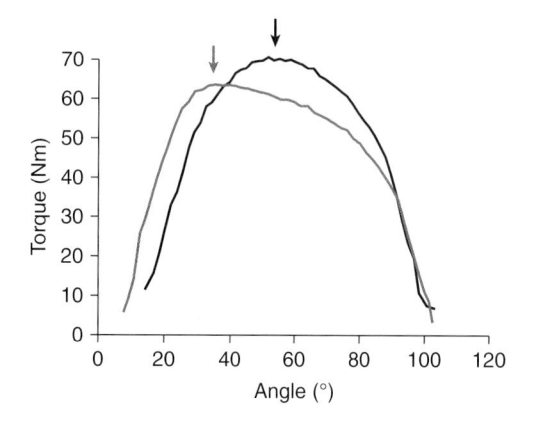

Figure 6.6. Hamstring force production in previously injured and healthy hamstring muscles. The previously injured hamstring muscle is denoted by large black dots. Note that although the total amount of torque generated is approximately the same as for the uninjured side (white dots), the peak force production occurs at decreased knee angle. Effectively the hamstring has healed short. Redrawn with permission from Brockett et al. (2004)

Thermal pants

Expert opinion has suggested that wearing thermal pants to keep the hamstring muscle warm may be useful in hamstring injury prevention, though little evidence exists to prove their efficacy.

Warm-up

Inadequate warm-up has long been considered to be a risk factor for injury though little evidence exists for this assertion. It can be stated that warm-up is probably more useful in preparing the athlete for best performance during competition rather than being useful for injury prevention.

Changing the sport to decrease the number of hamstring injuries

Aside from the inconvenience to the athlete and the team, and in professional sport this inconvenience can be considerable and have a significant impact on the playing level and professional remuneration for the athlete that sustains the injury, in most cases a hamstring muscle strain injury has no long-term negative health consequence for the athlete. These injuries are considered

The evidence for this more conservative approach has not been validated at this time and it remains to be seen whether these strategies can prevent more hamstring muscle strain reinjuries.

Table 6.7 Current trends in implementing hamstring muscle injury prevention program for team sports requiring high-intensity anaerobic interval sprinting and aerobic performance, applicable to sports such as football, soccer, Gaelic football, Australian Rules football, hockey, rugby. The Aussie Rules program.

Progression	Rationale
1. Implementing testing procedures that measure the performance requirements (high-intensity interval sprinting) of the sport	Most team sports particularly at the elite playing level measure athletic performance in the pre-season to gauge the fitness of the athlete. Often the athlete focuses his/her training with an emphasis on performing well at this measure. As "training as the game is played" is the goal of pre-season conditioning, with respect to hamstring injury prevention, then using measures of anaerobic interval performance are preferable to aerobic performance. An example of this is the use of the 20 m repeated shuttle run test (multi-stage fitness testing) rather than the 3 km time trial performance.
2. Implementing specific training drills that more closely reflect match day conditions	Improving muscle conditioning and anaerobic performance and obtaining fatigue resistance.
3. Increasing the number of hamstring muscle stretching regimes whilst muscle is fatigued	Increasing energy absorption of hamstring muscle for any given length of muscle and improving fatigue resistance.
4. Avoiding exercises that may lower the hamstring to quadriceps strength ratio	An example of this is the increasing use of closed kinetic chain exercises for weights training rather than open kinetic chain exercises as these latter exercises are more likely to alter the H:Q ratio. Quadriceps to hamstring strength ratios have been shown to be predictive for hamstring muscle strain injury. Therefore any exercise that may possibly change this ratio should be avoided especially in athletes without previous history of hamstring injury.
5. Avoiding exercises that may change the length–tension curve of the hamstring muscles in a negative fashion	An example of this would be to increase the volume of slow running or cross training using stationery cycling in athletes that require their length–tension curves to be maximal, that is, athletes required to sprint at full intensity. Decreasing the length–tension curve of the hamstring muscles may place the athlete at increased injury risk. This is the postulated mechanism for the high rate of injuries in athletes that have had a previous hamstring injury.

part of the game and hence there is little need for the sports governing bodies to consider rule, or other, changes that may help decrease the hamstring injury rate.

Current trends in implementing hamstring muscle injury prevention (Aussie Rules program)

In a rapidly changing field some of the current trends in training athletes for the purpose of hamstring injury prevention, and their rationale for their introduction, can be seen in Table 6.7. This program has been developed based on some basic principles related to implementing sports-specific testing procedures, specific training drills that more closely reflect the requirements of the sport, increasing hamstring muscle stretching whilst muscle is fatigued, avoiding exercises that may cause a mismatch in hamstring to quadriceps strength, and avoiding exercises that may change the length–tension curve of the hamstring muscles in a negative fashion. There is some evidence that training based on these principles may reduce injury risk significantly (Verrall et al., 2005).

Take-home message

There is a need for more well-conducted research into the area of hamstring injury prevention, but there is however enough evidence to make some recommendations that may be useful in hamstring injury prevention. This includes eccentric strengthening exercises, sports-specific testing and conditioning programs, and appropriate rehabilitation after injury. However, this is a field that is rapidly changing as more evidence about what works (and what does not) emerge. It is important that the physician, trainer, coach, etc. keep up to date with the latest developments and closely monitor the athletes in their care.

References

Árnason, Á., Sigurdsson, S.B., Gudmundson, A., Holme, I., Engebretsen, L., Bahr, R. (2004) Risk factors for injuries in soccer. *American Journal of Sports Medicine* **32**, 5S–16S.

Árnason, Á., Andersen, T.E., Holme, I., Engebretsen, L., Bahr, R. (2008) Prevention of hamstring strains in elite soccer: an intervention study. *Scandinavian Journal of Medicine and Science in Sports* **18**, 40–48.

Askling, C.M., Tengvar, M., Sartook, S., Thorstensson A. (2007) Acute first-time hamstring strains during slow-speed stretching: clinical, magnetic resonance imaging and recovery characteristics. *American Journal of Sports Medicine* **35**, 1716–1724.

Bennell, K., Wajswlner, H., Lew, P., Schall-Riaucour, A., Leslie, S., Plant, D., Cirone, J. (1998) Isokinetic strength testing does not predict hamstring injury in Australian rules footballers. *British Journal of Sports Medicine* **32**, 309–314.

Brockett, C.L., Morgan, D.L., Proske, U. (2004) Predicting hamstring injury in elite athletes. *Medicine and Science in Sports and Exercise* **36**, 379–387.

Connell, D.A., Schneider-Kolsky, M.E., Hoving, J.L., Malara, F., Buchbinder, R., Koulouris, G., Burke, F., Bass, C. (2004) Longitudinal study comparing sonographic and MRI assessment of acute and healing hamstring injuries. *AJR American Journal of Roentgenology* **183**, 975–984.

Garrett Jr., W.E. (1996) Muscle strain injuries. *American Journal of Sports Medicine* **24**, S2–S8.

Hawkins, R.D., Fuller, C.W. (1999) A prospective epidemiological study of injuries in four English professional football clubs. *British Journal of Sports Medicine* **33**, 196–203.

Heidt Jr., R.S., Sweeterman, L.M., Carlonas, R.L., Traub, J.A., Tekulve, F.X. (2000) Avoidance of soccer injuries with pre-season conditioning. *American Journal of Sports Medicine* **28**, 659–662.

Mair, S., Seaber, A., Glisson, R., Garrett Jr., W.E. (1996) The role of fatigue in susceptibility to acute muscle strain injury. *American Journal of Sports Medicine* **24**, 137–143.

Mjølsnes, R., Arnason, A., Østhagen, T, Bahr, R. (2004) A 10 week randomized trial comparing eccentric vs. concentric hamstring strength in well-trained soccer players. *Scandinavian Journal of Medicine and Science in Sports* **14**, 31–37.

Orchard, J., Seward, H. (2002) Epidemiology of injuries in the Australian football league 1997–2000. *British Journal of Sports Medicine* **36**, 39–44.

Slavotinek, J.P., Verrall, G.M., Fon, G.T. (2002) Hamstring injury in athletes: the association between MR measurements of the extent of muscle injury and the amount of time lost from competition. *AJR American Journal of Roentgenology* **179**, 1621–1628.

Taylor, D.C., Dalton, J.D., Seaber, A.V., Garrett Jr., W.E. (1993) Experimental muscle strain injury. Early functional and structural deficits and the increased risk for reinjury. *American Journal of Sports Medicine* **21**, 190–194.

Verrall, G.M., Slavotinek, J.P., Barnes, P.G., Fon, G.T., Spriggins, A.J. (2001) Clinical risk factors for hamstring muscle strain injury: a prospective study with correlation of injury by magnetic resonance imaging. *British Journal of Sports Medicine* **35**, 435–440.

Verrall, G.M., Slavotinek, J.P., Barnes, P.G., Fon, G.T. (2003) Diagnostic and prognostic value of clinical findings in 83 athletes with posterior thigh injury. Comparison of clinical findings with magnetic resonance imaging documentation of hamstring muscle strain. *American Journal of Sports Medicine* **31**, 969–973.

Verrall, G.M., Slavotinek, J.P., Barnes, P.G. (2005) The effect of sports specific training on reducing the incidence of hamstring injuries in professional Australian Rules football players. *British Journal of Sports Medicine* **39**, 363–368.

Verrall, G.M., Slavotinek, J.P., Barnes, P.G., Fon, G.T, Esterman, A (2006) Assessment of physical examination and magnetic resonance imaging findings as predictors for recurrent injury. *Journal of Orthopaedic and Sports Physical Therapy* **36**, 225–233.

Further reading

Bahr, R. (2004) Preventing sports injuries. In R. Bahr & S. Mæhlum (eds) *Clinical Guide to Sports Injuries*, pp. 41–53. Human Kinetics, Champaign.

Bahr, R., Holme, I. (2003) Risk factors for sports injuries—a methodological approach. *British Journal of Sports Medicine* **37**, 384–392.

Geraci, M.C. (1998) Rehabilitation of the hip, pelvis and thigh. In W.B. Kibler, S. Herring & J.M. Press (eds) *Functional Rehabilitation of Sports and Musculoskeletal Injuries*, pp. 216–243. Aspen, Maryland.

Orchard, J., Best, T.M., Verrall, G.M. (2005) Return to play following muscle strains *Clinical Journal of Sports Medicine* **15**, 436–441.

Petersen, J., Hölmich, P. (2005) Evidence based prevention of hamstring injuries in sport. *British Journal of Sports Medicine* **39**, 319–323.

Chapter 7
Preventing groin injuries

Per Hölmich[1] and Lorrie Maffey[2] and Carolyn Emery[3]

[1]Department of Orthopaedic Surgery, Orthopaedic Research Unit, Copenhagen S, Denmark
[2]Faculty of Kinesiology; Community Health Sciences, Faculty of Medicine, University of Calgary, Calgary, Canada
[3]Sport Medicine Centre, Faculty of Kinesiology; Community Health Sciences, Faculty of Medicine, University of Calgary, Calgary, Canada

Epidemiology of groin injuries in sports

Groin injuries in sport are common, yet often difficult to diagnose and treat. Groin injuries may be acute but often become chronic in nature. The most common location (>50%) of groin pain reported in athletes is the adductor muscle tendon region. Acute onset pain in this region is commonly attributable to an adductor longus muscle enthesopathy but may also be related to the iliopsoas and or the abdominal muscles. The differential diagnosis for groin pain in athletes may include incipient hernia (also known as sports hernia or athletic hernia), adductor-related groin pain, abdominal muscle strain, hip joint etiology (i.e., labral tear, osteoarthritis, impingement), iliopsoas-related groin pain, fracture, nerve compression (i.e., obturator or lateral femoral cutaneous nerve entrapment), or osteitis pubis (i.e., inflammation often leading to sclerosis of the pubis symphysis) (Figure 7.1). The unspecific terms "osteitis pubis," "pubalgia," and "pubic bone stress" are sometimes used when a pathoanatomic diagnosis cannot be made. Lesions to the lower abdominal muscles and other structures associated to the inguinal canal can lead to a condition with some similarities of a hernia. The terms "sports hernia"

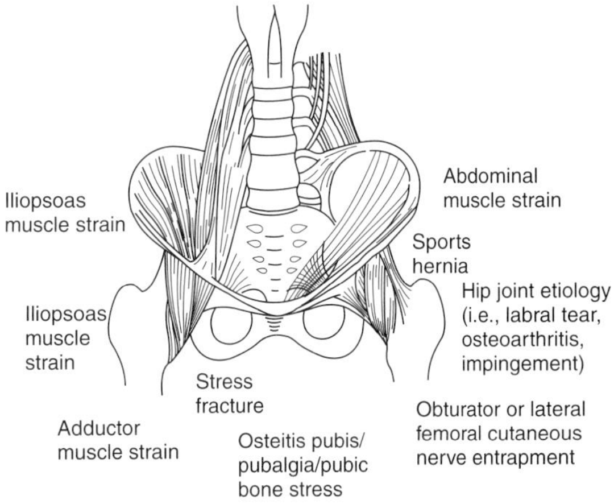

Figure 7.1. The differential diagnosis for groin pain in athletes is widespread and may include any items listed on this diagram

and "incipient hernia" are commonly used. These refer to a condition of groin pain located to the lower part of the abdomen and to the upper and medial part of the groin region, often radiating to the medial thigh and across the pubic symphysis.

Groin injury is among the top one to sixth most common cited injury in the Olympic sports of ice hockey, speed skating, soccer, and athletics. Groin injuries account for 3–11% of all injuries in some Olympic sports including ice hockey, speed skating, soccer, swimming, and athletics. Sport-specific groin strain injury rates vary in the literature from 0.2 to 5 injuries per 1000 participation hours

Sports Injury Prevention, 1st edition. Edited by R. Bahr and L. Engebretsen Published 2009 by Blackwell Publishing
ISBN: 9781405162449

Table 7.1 Risk of groin injury in different sports. The numbers reported are average estimates based on the sport studies with available data.

Sport	Competition incidence[1]	Training incidence[1]	Rank[2]	Comments
Team sports				
Ice hockey	2–5	0.5	2–4 (10%)	Prospective data
Soccer	4	1	2–4 (10–20%)	Prospective data
Individual sports				
Speed skating	NA	NA	5 (10%)	Retrospective data
Swimming	NA	NA	NA	Retrospective data suggests 25/100 elite swimmers/year experience groin pain
Athletics	NA	NA	4–6 (7–9%)	Prospective data

[1] Incidence is reported for adult, competitive athletes as the number of injuries per 1000 h of training and competition.
[2] Rank indicated the relative rank of this injury type within the sport in question, as well as the proportion as a percentage of the total number of injuries within the sport.
NA: Data not available.

or 10–25 injuries per 100 sport participants per year (Table 7.1). Groin strain injuries have been cited to account for 20% of all muscle strain injuries in elite levels of soccer and >40% of muscle strain injuries in ice hockey, specifically. Groin injuries account for >10% of all injuries in elite levels of ice hockey, soccer, and athletics. It should be noted that few studies utilized similar general injury or groin strain injury definitions and even fewer studies actually define groin injury. Future consideration of sport participation exposure when examining injury incidence will facilitate comparisons both between studies in the same sport and across sports.

Typically, severity of injury has been reported in terms of time loss from sport and has been reported for elite levels of ice hockey, soccer, and swimming. In ice hockey, the mean number of sessions missed in the National Hockey League due to a groin injury was reportedly 7–12 sessions (range: 0–180) over two seasons of play. In swimming, the mean number of sessions missed due to cases of groin pain was 11. In soccer, 40% of groin injuries reportedly result in more than 1 week time loss from soccer and 10% result in more than 1 month time loss. Of course, many groin injuries become chronic and many athletes continue to participate despite pain. At this point in time there is little, if any good data on prevalence of groin pain, that is, the percentage of athletes suffering from groin pain at any given time during their sport careers or following sport retirement. As such, time loss may not be the best or only predictor of severity though it is the only indicator of severity in the literature.

Key risk factors: how to identify athletes at risk

Groin injury prevention strategies may be developed and evaluated if there is a good understanding of the athlete population at risk, and the risk factors associated with injury for this population. Groin injury risk factors may be considered intrinsic or extrinsic to the athlete (Table 7.2). These factors can be further identified as modifiable or non-modifiable. Modifiable risk factors are those that can potentially be altered to reduce injury rates through the implementation of injury prevention strategies. There is evidence that modifiable risks such as decreased levels of sport-specific training, endurance, strength, and balance do increase the risk of overall injury in sport. Non-modifiable risk factors are those factors that cannot be altered to reduce injury rates through the implementation of injury prevention strategies but

Table 7.2 Internal and external factors for groin injury in different sports. The numbers reported are average estimates based on the studies available.

Risk factor	Relative risk[1]	Evidence[2]	Comments
Internal risk factors—non-modifiable			
Previous injury	2–7×	++	Ice hockey and soccer
↑ Age	3×	+	Ice hockey evidence clear, conflicting evidence in rugby
Gender	1	+	Ice hockey
↑ Body Mass Index	Greater risk	+	Rugby
Sport specificity—breast stroke	Greater risk	+	In comparison to other stroke specialists
Internal risk factors—modifiable			
↓ Amount of sport-specific training in the pre-season (<18 sessions)	3×	+	Ice hockey
↓ Hip range of motion	1.1×	+	Evidence in soccer, conflicting evidence in ice hockey
↓ Hip adduction strength	1	+	Conflicting evidence
↑ Hip abduction strength	Greater risk	+	Rugby
↓ Hip adduction: abduction strength ratio	Greater risk if ratio <95%	+	Ice hockey
Delayed onset transverse abdominal muscle recruitment	Greater risk	+	Australian Rules football

[1]Relative risk indicates the increased risk of injury to an individual with this risk factor relative to an individual who does not have this characteristic. A relative risk of 1.2× means that the risk of injury is 20% higher for an individual with this characteristic. NA: Not available.
[2]Evidence indicates the level of scientific evidence for this factor being a risk factor for groin injury: ++—convincing evidence from high-quality studies with consistent results; +—evidence from lesser quality studies or mixed results; 0—expert opinion without scientific evidence.

facilitate the identification of the sport population at risk. Examples of non-modifiable risk factors would be age, gender, and previous injury.

Non-modifiable intrinsic risk factors: previous injury

There is evidence that previous groin injury consistently increases the risk of groin injury between 2.5- and 7-fold in both soccer and ice hockey. This is certainly also consistent with the evidence supporting previous injury as the key risk factor for many other injury types, including hamstring strain injury in elite athletes. This finding is likely consistent with persistent symptoms, physiological deficiencies related to the initial injury (i.e., muscle strength, endurance, proprioception) and/or inadequate rehabilitation. If the previous injury has not been sufficiently treated and the athlete returns to sport too early, that is, prior to all the physiological deficiencies being addressed, this could contribute to a reinjury for the athlete. This situation could perhaps occur because of insufficient treatment or because of a wish from the athlete and/or the coach for an early return to sport. Other possible explanations for reinjury might be that a secondary muscular imbalance has occurred following the injury (or possibly prior to the injury that lead to the initial injury), that is, hip muscle strength ratios less than optimal or poor timing of torso muscle recruitment. If this secondary muscle imbalance is not addressed properly it may create a problem for the athlete upon return to sport.

Age and sport experience

Conflicting evidence exists regarding role of age and sport experience as a risk factor for groin injury. Increasing age and/or experience is a risk factor for groin strain injury in the National Hockey League (ice hockey) as demonstrated by a sixfold increase in groin injuries in veterans compared to rookies.

However, another study in Australian Rules Football demonstrated that players under 18 years of age were at greater than two times the risk of groin strain injury than the more veteran players. Increasing age and sport experience as risk factors for groin injury may be rationalized by the idea that the body's collagen tissue changes in its nature with advancing age and therefore it may not be as potentially adaptable to respond to quick force changes or recover from fatigue. Additionally, it has been shown that specific muscle strength decreases with advancing age which may put these muscles more at risk for injury. There is consistency in the literature to support increased age as a risk factor for muscle strains in the hamstring and calf muscles. Decreased age and sport experience as a risk factor for groin injury in Australian Rules football players may be secondary to the study's definition of groin injury that included muscular and unspecified groin injuries such as osteitis pubis, differing from other studies that did not include osteitis pubis. In addition, studies finding an increased risk with increasing age did not include players under age 18 and musculoskeletal immaturity may have played a role in the increased risk in junior Australian football players.

Gender

While there is a paucity of literature examining groin injury specifically in female sport, gender has not been identified as a risk factor for groin strain injury. In varsity level ice hockey, gender was not found to be a risk factor for all injury or groin strain injury specifically. Gender differences have more commonly been reported for ligament sprain injuries.

Body composition

Increased body mass index has been identified as a risk factor for groin injury in rugby players but not in any Olympic sports.

Sport specificity

In swimmers, specifically, stroke specificity is a risk for groin strain injury with a greater risk of groin injury in breaststroke specialists, followed by individual medley and finally those specializing in a combination of non-breaststroke/individual medley. This is not surprising given the unique eccentric adductor muscle activity and abduction ROM required in breast stroke kick compared to that in other strokes.

Modifiable intrinsic risk factors: range of motion

Conflicting evidence exists for the role of decreased hip abduction ROM as a risk factor for groin strain injury. In one study, a protective effect (10% risk reduction) related to greater hip abduction and extension (i.e., players identified as being in the top 1/3 of players based on flexibility) in soccer players has been identified. However, there has been no evidence of hip abduction ROM as a risk factor for groin strain injury in other sports. A possible explanation between decreased ROM of the hip (as well as or in addition to decreased ROM of the lumbar spine and or pelvis) and groin injury may be that decreased ROM of the hip joints might lead to a change in the biomechanics related to sprinting, skating, tackling, kicking, and jumping. This could in turn lead to an increase of the load on the related muscles and tendons. An example could be decreased internal rotation of the hip joint leading to a need for changing the axis of rotation when kicking a ball or tackling. This would increase the load on the oblique muscles of the lower abdomen and thereby putting more stress on the conjoint tendon (i.e., where the tendons of the transverse abdominal muscle and the internal oblique muscle join and insert into the pubic tubercle). This could result in an inflammatory response and/or degeneration of the tendon leading to pain by itself or to a strain, a tear, or an avulsion.

An explanation for the conflicting evidence regarding the connection between decreased hip ROM and groin injury is that there is evidence that most muscle injuries occur during eccentric contractions within the normal range of joint motion and not the end of range and that stretching is not significantly associated with a reduction in total injuries. This ongoing debate over

ROM or flexibility may have to do more with the inconsistent methods of testing and definitions in the literature. Additionally, there is a growing body of evidence that is pointing toward stretching being functional to the activity demands of the sport as well as the individual body concerns of the athlete. The contradiction in the evidence regarding the role of stretching in sport performance and injury prevention may be explained by differences between sport activities. In sports involving "explosive" type skills, stretching may result in an increased capacity for the tendon to absorb energy and thereby be a prophylactic measure for injury prevention. The demands on different players (i.e., position of play) within the same sport may also differ, resulting in potentially divergent effects from the same flexibility program. The evidence-based debate regarding muscle flexibility and its role in injury prevention continues. A recent study of community level Australian football players suggested that decreased quadriceps flexibility was an independent predictor of hamstring injury in this group of athletes. This finding further fuels the discussion that it may not be adductor muscle length that is the important factor in groin injury prevention but rather the muscle length of its synergistic and opposing muscles such as the abductor and hip flexor muscles. Additionally, when traumatic osteitis pubis is considered as a potential source of groin pain, a reduction hip range of motion (ROM) is demonstrated in athletes with chronic current and recovered groin injury. As insertional tendinopathy and osteitis pubis are often clinically difficult to diagnostically separate (and may even be the same injury where the changes in the pubic symphysis are a reflection of the increased stress across the joint because of the disturbed pelvic stability combined with the strain imposed by the sport itself), it may be that some studies on groin strain injury are including athletes with a past injury of osteitis pubis as study participants. Past injury has already been demonstrated to be a risk factor for groin strain injury and this could be confused with the role of hip flexibility as a risk factor for groin strain injury. Future work in the area of flexibility may shed new light on its importance with regard to injury prevention.

Training background

Decreased levels of pre-season sport-specific training was clearly a risk factor for groin strain injury in the National Hockey League, with players training less than 18 sport-specific sessions in the pre-season demonstrating a threefold increase risk (Emery & Meeuwisse, 2001). An increase in pre-season sport-specific training and a subsequent decrease in groin injury may be supported by eccentric training of the thigh muscles as well as abdominal supporting muscular training. Pre-season sport-specific training may allow for further contraction and function-specific recruitment of these muscles which might allow for their more effective utilization and less onset of fatigue as the season progresses. Fatigue has been noted in the literature to be a contributing factor for muscle injury.

Muscle strength and function

With respect to hip muscle strength, while there was no evidence that peak isometric adductor strength was a risk factor for groin injury in ice hockey, the adductor to abductor isometric strength ratio might be a risk factor for groin strain injury in ice hockey. In one study, the pre-season adductor strength was 18% less than the abductor strength in those players sustaining a subsequent groin injury, compared to those uninjured during the season (Tyler et al., 2002). In rugby players there has been some support for non-dominant limb peak abductor torque and peak torque later in abduction ROM with isokinetic testing being predictive for groin strain injury (Cusi et al., 2001). It is hypothesized that the mechanism of injury associated with groin injuries in ice hockey players is the eccentric force of the adductors attempting to decelerate the leg during a stride. A systematic review examining muscle strength as a risk factor for acute muscle strain, also found decreased muscle strength and/or muscle ratios to be predictive of strain injury, consistent with the findings related to groin strain injury. It may be that the adductor strength (i.e., concentric and eccentric) throughout its length as well as the adductor to abductor strength ratio are important factors for injury prevention.

There is also evidence that the onset of transversus abdominal muscle recruitment activity (EMG) is delayed during an active straight leg raise while no differences occurred in the other abdominal muscles in Australian Rules Football players with long-standing groin pain versus controls suggesting a possible associated risk. A strength imbalance between the propulsive muscles and the stabilizing muscles of the hip and pelvis has been proposed as a mechanism for adductor strains in athletes. A large percentage of groin pain may actually be due to inability to properly load transfer from the legs and or torso to the pelvis. Restoring load transferability by restoration of the stabilizing role of the pelvis by abdominal contraction may be important in athletic injury management and possibly injury prevention. There is some support for "core stability" interventions targeting abdominals and gluteals in reducing the risk of hamstring and groin injury in rugby players but further research is required to support these findings. Such findings lead to inquiry regarding the role of the muscles of the torso (i.e., transverse abdominus, obliques, diaphragm, multifidus, pelvic floor) in stabilizing the pelvis such that the abductors and adductors can work explosively and not get strained. Perhaps it is the balance of all the torso muscles that is a critical factor in groin injury. It may be that the adductor strength (i.e., concentric and eccentric) throughout its length, with a balanced and strong torso, may be important for injury prevention.

Risk factors beyond the groin region alone, including torso musculature, require further examination. The role of load transfer and torso stabilizing muscles, eccentric isokinetic strength including strength ratios of the adductors to abductor muscles, and muscle length of the adductors and opposing muscle groups (i.e., abductor and hip flexor muscles) require further consideration.

Take-home message: how to identify athletes at risk

There is evidence that the risk factors for groin injury that can potentially be altered to reduce injury rates through the implementation of injury prevention strategies are decreased hip abduction ROM, decreased levels of pre-season sport-specific training and abdominal muscle recruitment. Inconsistent evidence exists regarding muscle strength as a risk factor for groin injury. Arguably, however, there is some evidence that hip adductor:abductor strength ratio may be of importance. Additionally there is evidence that there are non-modifiable risk factors that cannot be altered to reduce injury rates through the implementation of injury prevention strategies such as age or sport experience, gender, sport-specific movement (i.e., breast stroke in swimming), and previous injury.

An annual musculoskeletal preparticipation examination is often done by physiotherapists working with athletic teams to anticipate and preclude physiological and biomechanical problems for athletes prior to the commencement of a sport season activities. As such, the ultimate goal of such a preparticipation examination is injury prevention. Such a comprehensive examination should identify both the sport-specific biomechanical and physiological requirements for training and competition, as well as when there are possible biomechanical and physiological deficits that might be a precursor to injury. Preparticipation examinations consistently include athlete questionnaires including questions that might identify an increased risk for groin injury such as previous injury, levels of pre-season sport-specific training, age or sport experience, gender, and sport-specific movements (i.e., swimming stroke) (Table 7.3). In addition, standard neuro-musculoskeletal examinations and some form of functional testing are components of this preparticipation examination.

The standard neuro-musculoskeletal examination which tests for strength in the form of isometric, concentric, and/or eccentric testing contribute to the identification of such strength ratios (i.e., hip adductor:abductor muscle strength ratio which is a potential risk factor for groin injury). The standard neuro-musculoskeletal examination should also include a neurological examination, active and passive ROM testing (decreased hip ROM is another potential risk factor for groin injury), articular testing in the form of joint glides, muscle recruitment testing especially around the torso and pelvis (deficits here may lead to an increased risk for groin injury), static and dynamic postural and balance investigations, and appropriate

Table 7.3 Preparticipation examination: identifying risks for groin injury.

Identified risk for groin injury	Preparticipation examination: Subjective questionnaire	Preparticipation examination objective examination (specific test)
Previous injury	X	
Age or sport experience	X	
Gender	X	
Sport-specific movement	X	
Decreased levels of pre-season sport-specific training	X	
Decreased hip abduction range of motion		Joint ROM: • active • passive
Abdominal muscle recruitment		Modified double straight-leg lowering test Flexor endurance test Real time ultrasound testing EMG testing Observational scoring
Hip muscle strength		Muscle strength tests: • isometric (manual muscle testing) • concentric (isokinetic testing) • eccentric (isokinetic testing)

functional tests. Functional performance tests for the sport in question are recommended for inclusion in a preparticipation examination. It is suggested that not only the clinical test outcome be scored (i.e., side lunge repetitions) but also the form and efficiency of the underlying functional movement involved in the test should be rated. For example, it is not only important to take note of the weight that an athlete can load with during a one-legged bench side step up test but how the athlete's body was aligned during the test. As few validated scoring systems exist the examiner is advised to develop scoring methodologies and to submit this scoring method to future research scrutiny. Upon recognition of potentially modifiable risk factors by the physiotherapist, sport-specific injury prevention strategies designed to reduce such risks can be implemented (Table 7.4 and Boxes 7.1–7.3).

Injury mechanisms

Acute versus chronic injury

The injury mechanism associated with groin injuries is in many cases difficult to identify with certainty. Groin injury often has the characteristics of an overuse injury and the exact moment of injury (the inciting event) can be hard to establish.

The typical history presented by the athlete with a groin injury comes in two versions: (1) 40% have experienced an acute painful incident during training or competition or (2) 60% present with a gradually developing pain in the groin region often typical of an overuse injury. The acute strain usually involves one or more muscles. In most cases, the lesion is in the musculotendenious junction, but in some cases the tendon itself or the entheses where the tendon inserts into the bone is the site of the injury. These injuries happen during forceful action and the athletes are usually not in doubt that something happened: It hurts, the function of the limb is affected and sometimes a discoloration of the skin is immediate. In most cases, the athlete will have to stop the activity and leave the field. In some cases the athlete describes a snapping feeling in the groin and sometimes even accompanied by a sound. If not attended to appropriately, these injuries might develop into a more long-standing and sometimes chronic injury. The other typical history is when the athlete gradually realize,

98 Chapter 7

Table 7.4 Injury prevention matrix for groin injuries: potential measures to prevent injuries.

	Pre-injury	Injury	Post-injury
Athlete	Preparticipation examination (Table 7.3) Neuromuscular balance: 1. Hip range of motion 2. Hip muscle strength 3. "Core"/trunk recruitment Full rehabilitation from previous injuries Pre-season sport specific training Ice or field friction	Training status Falling/tackling/checking techniques Safe technique and biomechanics	Treatment Rehabilitation Restoration of neuromuscular function
Surroundings	Playing rules	Playing surfaces (ice, field) in good shape, that is, no holes in field or ice	Emergency medical coverage Diagnosing expertise Rehabilitation team (physiotherapy, athletic therapy)
Equipment	Shoe friction and torsional resistance with the playing surface Appropriate boot and blade on skate to support the ankle	Groin pressure wraps or tension shorts	First-aid equipment Ice

---

Box 7.1 Stretching program for the hip muscles

#1. Stretch for hip flexors

Ensure that the pelvic floor, deep transversus abdominus and deep multifidus muscles are recruited while the athlete is quietly abdominal breathing. This will help to keep the back in the required neutral position (not lordotic or kyphotic). While kneeling on the right knee and with the left hip and knee at a 90° angle and the foot flat on the floor (not allowing the medial arch of the foot to collapse), translate the pelvis forward thereby allowing the right hip to extend and stretching the right hip flexors. Maintain this hold for 5–10 slow and gentle breaths. Do not force the movement or move into or through pain with this movement. Repeat 2–4 times each leg.
Common errors: the low back sags into a lordosis, the left knee and leg rotates inward, the left foot medial arch collapses, loss of the recruitment of the pelvic floor and deep transversus abdominus resulting in over activity of the more superficial abdominal muscles as well as breath holding.

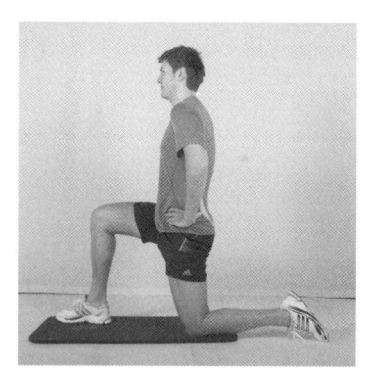

#2. Stretch for hip adductors

Ensure that the pelvic floor, deep transversus abdominus, and deep multifidus muscles are recruited while the athlete is quietly abdominal breathing. This will help to keep the back in the required neutral position (not lordotic or kyphotic or side bent into side flexion). With equal weight on each foot, stand with the feet apart in abduction (slightly wider than the shoulder width if your range of motion allows for this). Flex the right knee and shift more weight onto the right leg while you keep the left hip and knee in neutral flexion and extension thereby allowing the left hip to further abduct and stretching the left hip adductors. Maintain this hold for 5–10 slow and gentle breaths. Do not force the movement or move into or through pain with this movement. Repeat 2–4 times each side.
Common errors: the low back sags into a lordosis and or side flexion, the right or left knee and leg rotates inward, the right

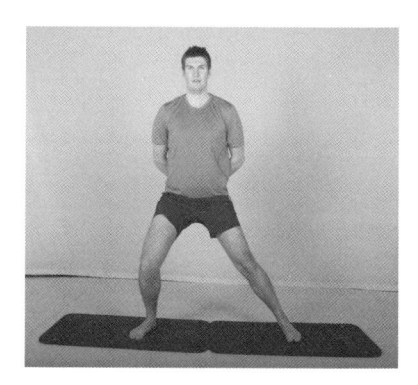

(Continued)

Box 7.1 (Continued)

or left foot medial arch collapses, left knee and hip flexes, loss of the recruitment of the pelvic floor and deep transversus abdominus resulting in over activity of the more superficial abdominal muscles as well as breath holding.

#3. *Stretch for hip adductors/extensors*
Ensure that the pelvic floor, deep transversus abdominus and deep multifidus muscles are recruited while the athlete is quietly abdominal breathing. This will help to keep the back in the required neutral position (not lordotic or kyphotic or side bent into side flexion). With the right hip in abduction and flexion and the right knee in flexion (like the crossed leg sitting position for the right leg) let the left hip go into full extension with the knee extended as well. Shift your weight toward the right leg and each hand thereby allowing the left hip to further extend and stretching the left hip flexors and adductors. Maintain this hold for 5–10 slow and gentle breaths. Do not force the movement or move into or through pain with this movement. Repeat two to four times each side.

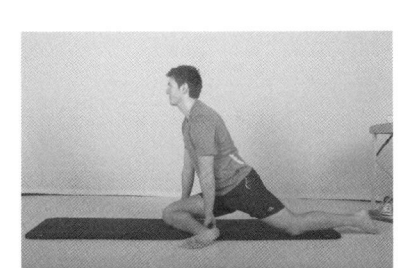

Common errors: the low back sags into a lordosis and or side flexion, the left knee and leg rotates inward, loss of the recruitment of the pelvic floor and deep transversus abdominus resulting in over activity of the more superficial abdominal muscles as well as breath holding.

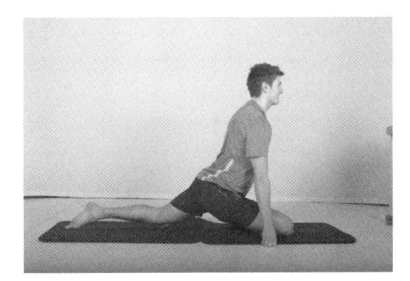

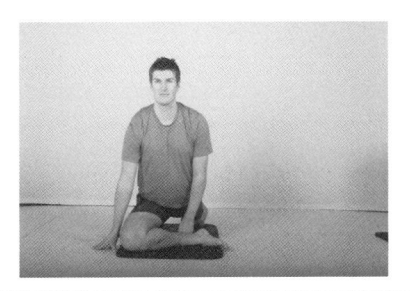

Box 7.2 Exercises for restoring the recruitment of the torso muscles as well as the strengthening abductor and adductor muscles

Isometric contraction of adductors (a) without and (b) with torso movement

(a) Ensure that the pelvic floor, deep transversus abdominus and deep multifidus muscles are recruited while the athlete is quietly abdominal breathing. This will help to keep the back in the required neutral position (not lordotic or kyphotic or side bent into side flexion). With the both knees extended, squeeze a soccer ball between your ankles and then flex both hips to approximately 30°. Maintain this hold for 5–10 slow and gentle breaths. Do not force the movement or move into or through pain with this movement. Repeat 5–20 times.

Common errors: the low back lordosis, the legs rotate inward (medially), the hands counter push into the floor, the head counter pushes into the floor, loss of the recruitment of the pelvic floor and deep transversus abdominus resulting in over activity of the more superficial abdominal muscles as well as breath holding.

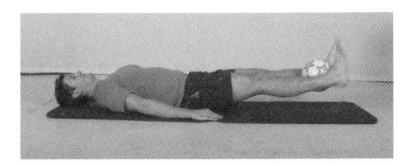

(b) Ensure that the pelvic floor, deep transversus abdominus and deep multifidus muscles are recruited while the athlete is quietly abdominal breathing. This will help to keep the back in the required neutral position (not lordotic or kyphotic or side bent into side flexion). With the both knees flexed, squeeze a soccer ball between your knees.
Cross your hands in front of your chest and contract your oblique and rectus abdominus thereby raising your torso from the floor approximately 4 inches. Ensure that your head and neck stay in line with your thorax. Then flex both hips up toward your chest. Maintain this hold for 5–10 slow and gentle breaths. Do not force the movement or move into or through pain with this movement. Repeat 5–20 times.

Common errors: the low back lordosis initially then kyphosis as the low back counter pushes into the floor, the legs rotate inward (medially), the head and neck shear forward from the alignment of the thorax (lower neck flexion and upper neck extension), gritting of the teeth, loss of the recruitment of the pelvic floor, and deep transversus abdominus resulting in over activity of the more superficial abdominal muscles as well as breath holding.

(Continued)

Box 7.2 (Continued)

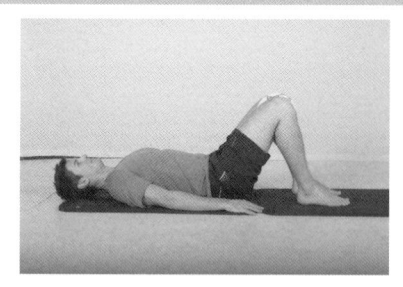

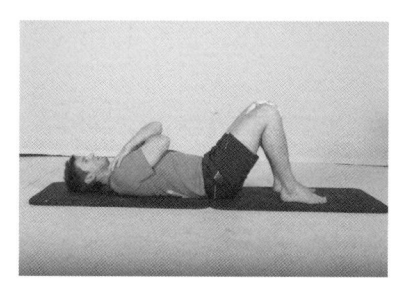

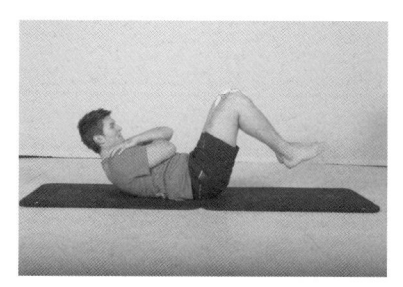

abducts, the arms counter balance by flexing or abducting, loss of the medial arch of the left foot, dorsi or plantar flexion and eversion of the right foot, loss of the recruitment of the pelvic floor and deep transversus abdominus resulting in over activity of the more superficial abdominal muscles as well as breath holding.

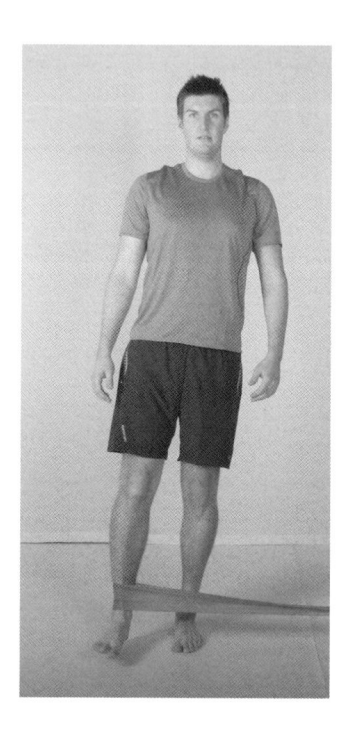

Standing with a stable pelvis, that is, good torso control using tubing or cables and perform concentric abduction or eccentric adduction

Ensure that the pelvic floor, deep transversus abdominus and deep multifidus muscles are recruited while the athlete is quietly abdominal breathing. This will help to keep the back and the rest of the spine in the required neutral position (not lordotic or kyphotic or side bent into side flexion). With the both hips in a neutral posture, both knees extended and the tubing around the right ankle, abduct the right leg to 15° while maintaining the spine posture and the left leg posture as well as maintaining an elevated medial arch of the left foot. Maintain this hold for 5–10 slow and gentle breaths. Slowly return back to the start position (both hips in a neutral posture). Do not force the movement or move into or through pain with this movement. Repeat 5–20 times each side.

Common errors: the low back lordosis, thoracic kyphosis, chin poked forward head and neck posture, the left leg rotate inward (medially), the right leg rotates outward (laterally) and flexes as it

Standing with a stable pelvis, that is, good torso control using tubing or cables and perform concentric adduction or eccentric abduction

Ensure that the pelvic floor, deep transversus abdominus and deep multifidus muscles are recruited while the athlete is quietly abdominal breathing. This will help to keep the back and the rest of the spine in the required neutral position (not lordotic or kyphotic or side bent into side flexion). With the right hip in a neutral posture and the left hip in 15° abduction, both knees extended and the tubing around the left ankle, adduct the left leg to neutral abduction/adduction posture while maintaining the spine posture and the right leg posture as well as maintaining an elevated medial arch of the right foot. Maintain this hold for 5–10 slow and gentle breaths. Slowly return back to the start position. Do not force the movement or move into or through pain with this movement. Repeat 5–20 times each side.

Common errors: the low back lordosis, thoracic kyphosis, chin poked forward head and neck posture, the left leg rotate inward (medially) and flexes as it adducts, the right leg rotates outward

(Continued)

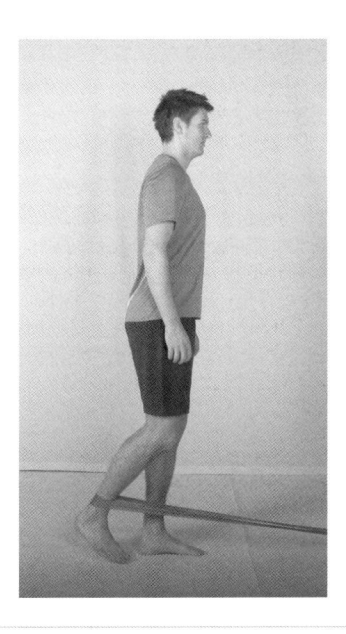

Box 7.2 (Continued)

(laterally), the arms counter balance by flexing or abducting, loss of the medial arch of the right foot, dorsi or plantar flexion and inversion of the left foot, loss of the recruitment of the pelvic floor and deep transversus abdominus resulting in over activity of the more superficial abdominal muscles as well as breath holding.

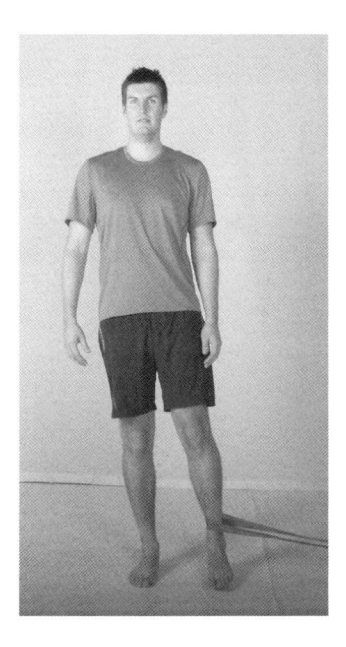

Standing with a stable pelvis, that is, good torso control using tubing or cables and perform concentric flexion
Ensure that the pelvic floor, deep transversus abdominus and deep multifidus muscles are recruited while the athlete is quietly abdominal breathing. This will help to keep the back and the rest of the spine in the required neutral position (not lordotic or kyphotic or side bent into side flexion). With the hips in a neutral posture, both knees flexed approximately 15° and the tubing around the left ankle, flex the left hip to approximately 15° while maintaining the spine posture and the right leg posture as well as maintaining an elevated medial arch of the right foot. Maintain this hold for 5–10 slow and gentle breaths. Slowly return back to the start position. Do not force the movement or move into or through pain with this movement. Repeat 5–20 times each side.
Common errors: the low back lordosis, thoracic kyphosis, chin poked forward head and neck posture, the left leg rotate inward (medially) and adducts as it flexes, angle of knee flexion changes in one or both knees, the right leg rotates outward (laterally), the arms counter balance by flexing or abducting, loss of the medial arch of the right foot, dorsi or plantar flexion and inversion of the left foot, loss of the recruitment of the pelvic floor and deep

transversus abdominus resulting in over activity of the more superficial abdominal muscles as well as breath holding.

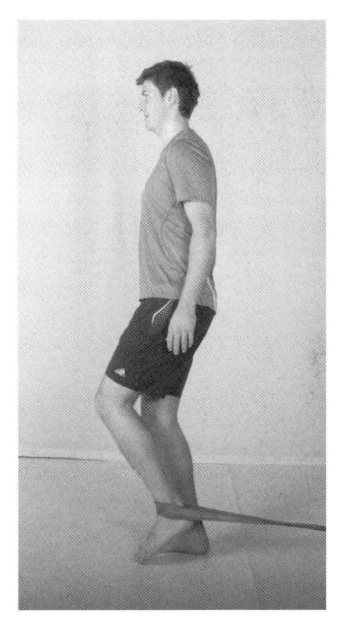

Standing with a stable pelvis, that is, good torso control using tubing or cables and perform concentric extension
Ensure that the pelvic floor, deep transversus abdominus and deep multifidus muscles are recruited while the athlete is quietly

(Continued)

Box 7.2 (Continued)

abdominal breathing. This will help to keep the back and the rest of the spine in the required neutral position (not lordotic or kyphotic or side bent into side flexion). With the hips in a neutral posture, both knees flexed approximately 15° and the tubing around the right ankle, extend the right hip to approximately 5° while maintaining the spine posture and the left leg posture as well as maintaining an elevated medial arch of the left foot. Maintain this hold for 5–10 slow and gentle breaths. Slowly return back to the start position. Do not force the movement or move into or through pain with this movement. Repeat 5–20 times each side.

Common errors: the low back lordosis, thoracic kyphosis, chin poked forward head and neck posture, the right leg rotate inward (medially) and adducts or abducts as it extends, angle of knee flexion changes in one or both knees, the right leg rotates outward (laterally), the arms counter balance by flexing or abducting, loss of the medial arch of the left foot, dorsi or plantar flexion and inversion of the right foot, loss of the recruitment of the pelvic floor and deep transversus abdominus resulting in over activity of the more superficial abdominal muscles as well as breath holding.

Box 7.3 Progression of exercises for restoring the recruitment of the torso muscles as well as the strength of the abductor muscles and the adductor muscles: (a) Speed of exercise: (i) Slow (ii) Medium (iii) Fast; (b) ROM: (i) Inner range of motion (ROM) (ii) Mid to Outer ROM; (c) Load/resistance: (i) Low load (ii) Moderate (iii) High load; (d) Base of support: (i) Stable (ii) Unstable (See #1 and #2); (e) Functional specific positions (See #3, #4, #5)

#1. Standing with a unstable pelvis with good torso control using tubing and performing concentric abduction or eccentric adduction

Ensure that the pelvic floor, deep transversus abdominus and deep multifidus muscles are recruited while the athlete is quietly abdominal breathing. This will help to keep the back and the rest of the spine in the required neutral position (not lordotic or kyphotic or side bent into side flexion). With the both hips in a neutral posture, both knees extended and the tubing around the right ankle, abduct the right leg to 15° while maintaining the spine posture and the left leg posture as well as maintaining an elevated medial arch of the left foot. Maintain this hold for 5–10 slow and gentle breaths. Slowly return back to the start position (both hips in a neutral posture). Do not force the movement or move into or through pain with this movement. Repeat 5–20 times each side.

Common errors: the low back lordosis, thoracic kyphosis, chin poked forward head and neck posture, the left leg rotate inward (medially), the right leg rotates outward (laterally) and flexes as it abducts, the arms counter balance by flexing or abducting, loss of the medial arch of the left foot, dorsi or plantar flexion and eversion of the right foot, plantar flexion and eversion of the left foot, loss of the recruitment of the pelvic floor and deep transversus abdominus resulting in over activity of the more superficial abdominal muscles as well as breath holding.

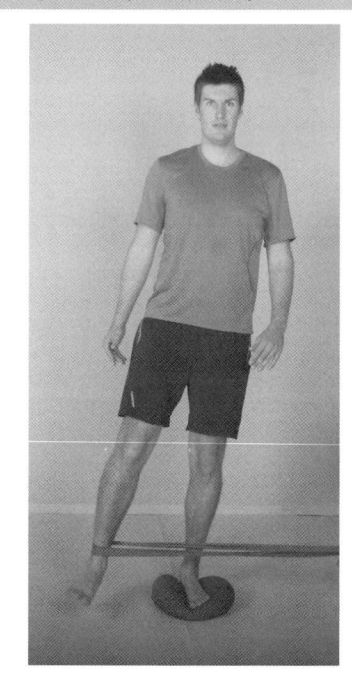

(Continued)

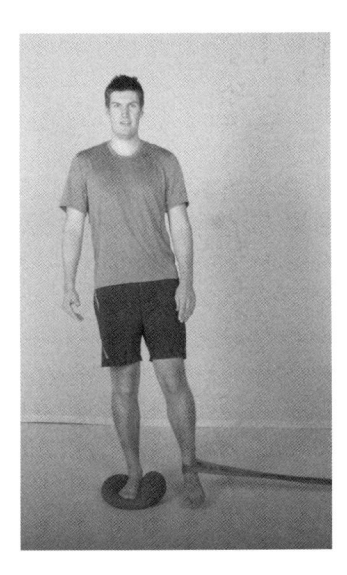

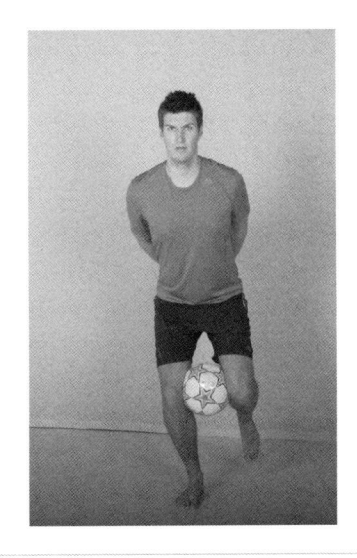

Box 7.3 (Continued)

#2. Standing with a unstable pelvis with good torso control using tubing and performing concentric adduction or eccentric abduction

Ensure that the pelvic floor, deep transversus abdominus and deep multifidus muscles are recruited while the athlete is quietly abdominal breathing. This will help to keep the back and the rest of the spine in the required neutral position (not lordotic or kyphotic or side bent into side flexion). With the right hip in a neutral posture and the left hip in 15° abduction, both knees extended and the tubing around the left ankle, adduct the left leg to neutral abduction/adduction posture while maintaining the spine posture and the right leg posture as well as maintaining an elevated medial arch of the right foot. Maintain this hold for 5–10 slow and gentle breaths. Slowly return back to the start position. Do not force the movement or move into or through pain with this movement. Repeat 5–20 times each side.

Common errors: the low back lordosis, thoracic kyphosis, chin poked forward head and neck posture, the left leg rotate inward (medially) and flexes as it adducts, the right leg rotates outward (laterally), the arms counter balance by flexing or abducting, loss of the medial arch of the right foot, plantar flexion and eversion of the right foot, dorsi or plantar flexion and inversion of the left foot, loss of the recruitment of the pelvic floor and deep transversus abdominus resulting in over activity of the more superficial abdominal muscles as well as breath holding.

#3. Functional position: Isometric adduction with or without superimposed squats on the leg

Ensure that the pelvic floor, deep transversus abdominus and deep multifidus muscles are recruited while the athlete is quietly abdominal breathing. This will help to keep the back and the rest of the spine in the required neutral position (not lordotic or kyphotic or side bent into side flexion). Arms behind your back resting lightly on the back. With the hips and knees flexed approximately 20° squeeze a soccer ball between your knees as well as maintaining an elevated medial arch of the foot. Maintain this hold for 5–10 slow and gentle breaths. Slowly return back to the start position. Note this can be made more difficult by maintaining this position as you do a deeper squat on your leg. Do not force the movement or move into or through pain with this movement. Repeat 5–20 times each side.

Common errors: the low back lordosis and side flexion with or without rotation, thoracic kyphosis, chin poked forward head and neck posture, the left leg rotate inward (medially) and adducts, right leg abducts and laterally rotates, the arms lose their position (often extend off the back), loss of the medial arch of the left foot, dorsi or plantar flexion and inversion of the right foot, loss of the recruitment of the pelvic floor and deep transversus abdominus resulting in over activity of the more superficial abdominal muscles as well as breath holding.

(Continued)

Box 7.3 (Continued)

#4. Functional position: simulated running position note the athlete is to move between positions in photo (a) and (b) repetitively and at various speeds and with various limb ROM
Ensure that the pelvic floor, deep transversus abdominus and deep multifidus muscles are recruited while the athlete is quietly abdominal breathing. This will help to keep the back and the rest of the spine in the required neutral position (not lordotic or kyphotic or side bent into side flexion). With the hips flexed approximately 20° and the right knee flexed approximately 20° and the left knee flexed approximately 80°, extend and straighten your right knee while maintaining an elevated medial arch of the right foot. Note this can be made more difficult by deeper squatting on your right leg as well as alternately swinging your arms as if you were running or skating. Do not force the movement or move into or through pain with this movement. Repeat for 30 s to 2 min each side.

Common errors: the low back lordosis and side flexion with or without rotation, thoracic kyphosis, chin poked forward head and neck posture, the right leg rotate inward (medially) and adducts, left leg abducts and laterally rotates, the arms lose their position and coordination with the leg movement, loss of the medial arch of the right foot, dorsi or plantar flexion and inversion of the left foot, loss of the recruitment of the pelvic floor and deep transversus abdominus resulting in over activity of the more superficial abdominal muscles as well as breath holding.

#5. Functional position: skating side to side jumps—note the athlete is to move between positions in photo (a) and (b) repetitively and at various speeds and with various limb ROM
Ensure that the pelvic floor, deep transversus abdominus and deep multifidus muscles are recruited while the athlete is quietly abdominal breathing. This will help to keep the back and the rest of the spine in the required neutral position (not lordotic or kyphotic or side bent into side flexion). Arms behind your back gentle resting on the low back. With the left hip in a neutral posture and the left knee in approximately 20° flexion as well as the right hip abducted approximately 30° and the right knee extended, adduct the right leg to neutral and flex the right knee approximately 20° while maintaining the spine posture and while the left leg abducts approximately 30° and the left knee extends. Repeat for the other leg. All the while maintaining an elevated medial arch for each foot. Repeat for 30 s to 2 min. Do not force the movement or move into or through pain with this movement.

Common errors: the low back lordosis, thoracic kyphosis, chin-poked forward head and neck posture, loss of the leg posturing especially inward (medially) rotation of the leg that is in neutral abduction–adduction, the arms counter balance by flexing or abducting, loss of the medial arch of the feet, loss of the recruitment of the pelvic floor and deep transversus abdominus resulting in over activity of the more superficial abdominal muscles as well as breath holding.

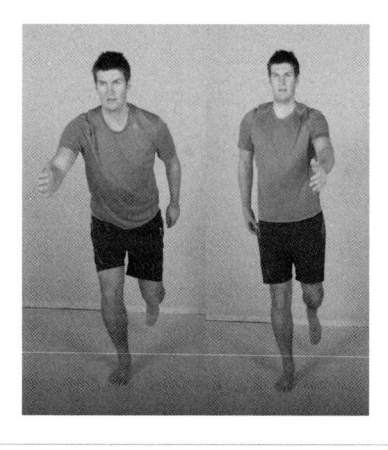

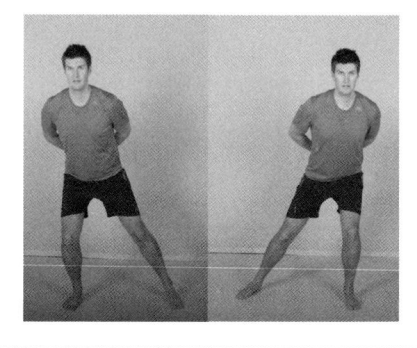

that the groin is getting increasingly sore after exercise and becomes an increasing problem even during the sports activity. The symptoms are those of a typical overuse pattern. In the beginning, there is only pain after activity with stiffness of the muscle group and a decreased ROM of the hip joint, developing to pain in the groin at the commencement of sport activity. The pain will often disappear as the athlete warms up, but will recur during the sport as fatigue occurs. If the athlete does not get appropriate treatment and instead continues to participate in the sport, the pain-free periods will become shorter and finally all sport activity will cause pain, and even activities of daily living might be a problem. Frequently, there is no recollection of a single incident causing the pain, but often an increase or change in activity level, technique or likewise has happened. This

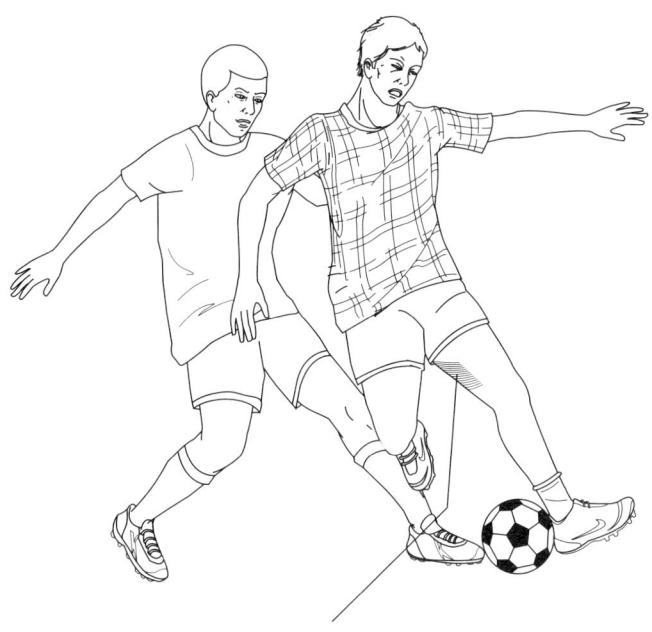

Proximal adductor muscle group at risk here as left leg is in adduction, external rotation and extension.

Figure 7.2. The groin muscles can be forcefully loaded from external and internal forces such as a soccer/football/rugby player in a sliding tackle

same pattern can be seen in athletes returning to sport after an initial acute groin injury without receiving appropriate and/or sufficient treatment and rehabilitation.

Considering mechanism by structure injured

The three most commonly mentioned structures involved in groin injury in the literature are the adductor muscles (usually adductor longus), the iliopsoas muscle, and the abdominal muscles. Decreased ROM of the hip joints, dysfunction of the sacroiliac joints, sacrotuberal ligaments, and low back are often seen concomitant to the muscle-related groin injuries. Their role in the both risk factors and a mechanism of groin injury is not clear (see Section "Key risk factors: how to identify athletes at risk").

When the adductor muscles are acutely strained it is often during an eccentric contraction (e.g., in a forced abduction, most likely when the limb is in some amount of abduction which is the position where this muscle is the weakest and as such more prone to sustain an injury) (Figure 7.2). This could be a sudden resistance of an opponent's foot in an attempt to reach a ball or a sliding tackle in soccer or the eccentric force of the adductor muscles attempting to decelerate the leg during a stride in ice hockey. In many cases some degree of hip joint rotation is involved. It can also happen in a forceful concentric adduction contraction for instance in soccer during a kick after a ball in the air or as the result of a direct blunt trauma from contact with an opponent.

The iliopsoas muscle, being a very important and strong hip flexor, can be acutely strained if a forceful hip flexion is interrupted suddenly. This could happen when the player is tackled in the moment of a forceful hip flexion during running, skating, jumping, or kicking (Figure 7.3) or when by mistake kicking into the ground instead of the ball. It can also be injured during an eccentric contraction as when the thigh is suddenly forced into

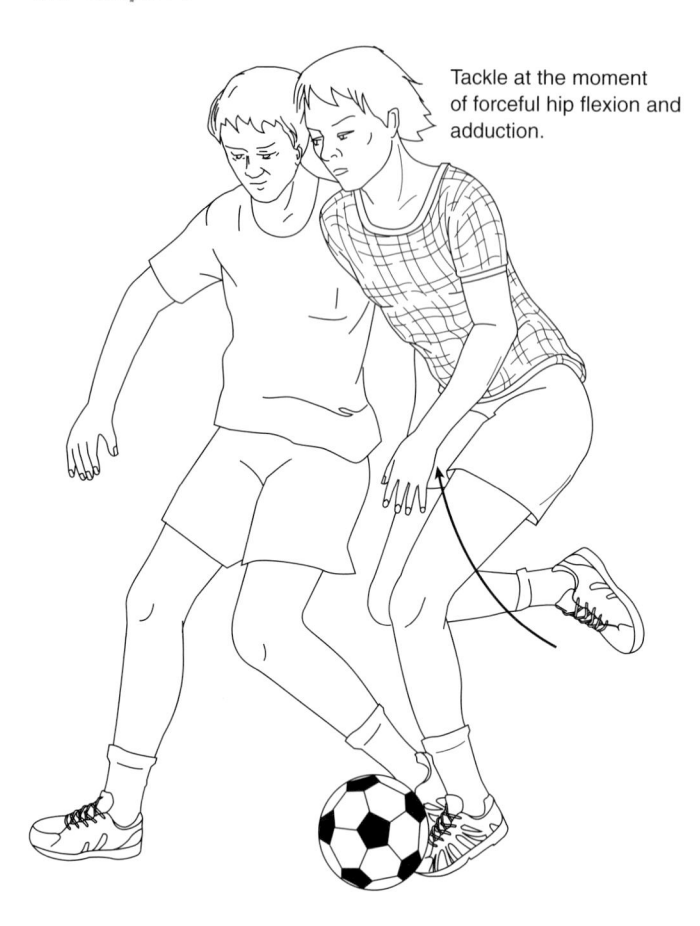

Figure 7.3. An athlete being tackled in the moment of a forceful hip flexion during running and kicking can potentially put the groin muscles at risk of injury

extension and the iliopsoas will try to decelerate the movement by an instantaneous eccentric muscle action.

An acute strain of the lower abdominal muscles usually involves either the conjoint tendon (falx inguinalis) where the tendons of the transverse abdominal muscle and the internal oblique muscle join and insert into the pubic tubercle or the rectus abdominis muscle usually in the entheses at the pubic bone or in the distal myotendendinous junction. The typical mechanism is a traumatic episode where the athlete over-stretches the front of the groin and lower abdomen as in a forceful sliding tackle in soccer or an uncontrolled fall backward where the hip is extended and the abdominal muscles are working hard to stop the fall by contracting with great speed and force, often with an eccentric contraction (Figure 7.4). The more rotation involved in the fall either in the hip joint or in the torso, the more likely it is the conjoint tendon that will sustain the lesion. In this situation the hip flexors (iliopsoas, rectus femoris, and tensor facia latae) are also at risk of sustaining an injury.

Lesions to the lower abdominal muscles and other structures associated to the inguinal canal can lead to a condition with some similarities of a hernia (i.e., often called "sports hernia" or "incipient hernia"). A predisposition for hernia development might be present, but the primary mechanism of injury is probably an acute trauma as described earlier, or a period of overuse as a result of a misbalance of the muscles acting on the pelvis and an intense strenuous activity often involving exercises with many fast reactions including sprinting, jumping, kicking, and sudden changes of direction. The nature of the lesion is not always clear. It may be a strain or tear, inflammation or degeneration at certain points of excessive stress, an avulsion, hemorrhage or edema. It is probably the result of the structural lesion to

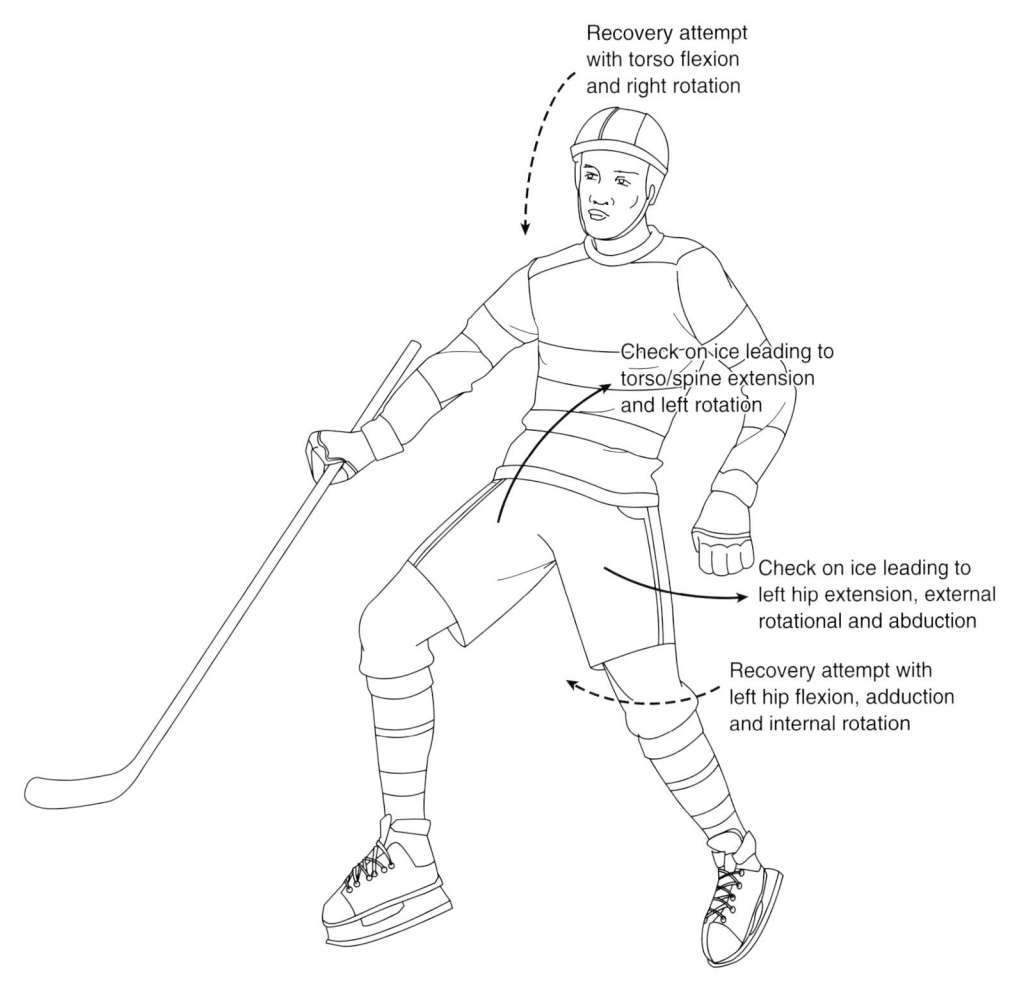

Figure 7.4. Secondary to a tackle or check on the ice, an athlete can put the groin muscles at risk resulting in overstretching the front of the groin and lower abdomen. Injury can occur with the initial insult or with the athlete's attempts to recover

the muscles and/or tendons (i.e., rectus abdominis muscle or insertion, the external oblique, internal oblique and/or transversalis muscle or aponeurosis and the conjoint tendon) involving a weakness of the posterior inguinal wall without a clinically obvious hernia.

The pelvis is the centre of load transfer from the upper extremities and the torso to the lower extremities and vice versa. As such it is dependent of both skeletal and articular stability as well as good neuromuscular stabilization. A number of muscle groups interact on the pelvis and hip and as mentioned earlier the adductors, iliopsoas, and abdominal muscles are primarily at risk of being injured. The adductor muscle group have been shown to be very important as stabilizers of the hip joint, and the interaction of the abdominal muscles (in particular the transverse abdominis muscle), the multifidi muscles deep in the low back and the pelvic floor muscles have been shown to be important for the stability of the low spine and pelvis. The precise functions of the iliopsoas are not fully understood, but the muscle seems to work both as an important hip flexor

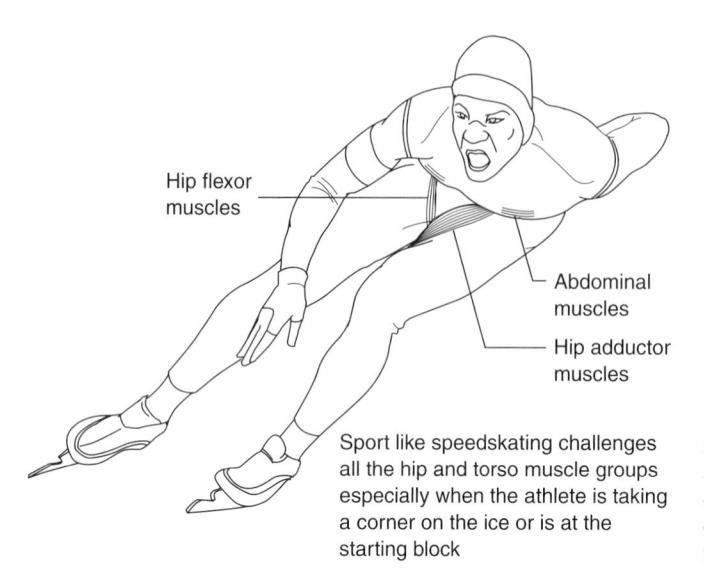

Figure 7.5. Many field and ice sports challenge all the hip and torso muscle groups. In the sport of speed skating, these muscles are challenged especially when an athlete is taking a corner or taking off from the starting block

(Figure labels: Hip flexor muscles; Abdominal muscles; Hip adductor muscles. Caption within figure: Sport like speedskating challenges all the hip and torso muscle groups especially when the athlete is taking a corner on the ice or is at the starting block)

and as a pelvic stabilizer as well as a stabilizer for the lumbar spine. These lumbar and pelvis stabilizing muscles are all constantly involved in most sports-activities contributing with a considerable amount of both eccentric and concentric work and fast changes between these work forms. This makes them highly important but are also at risk of sustaining an injury (Figure 7.5).

The injury mechanism for developing groin injuries with an insidious onset has not been proven, but it seems reasonable that fatigue, overuse or acute overload of any of the muscles previously discussed may lead to disturbance of the interaction between these muscles leaving some of the structures with loads exceeding their ability. This may in turn lead to injuries with structural damage to tissue and a need for repair. The athlete will often try to compensate for this situation and although they might succeed for a while, gradually the pain and loss of function will take over, and the athlete is not able to continue sport participation. The ability to react fast is impaired, and sudden changes of direction, sprinting and strenuous sudden abdominal contractions as when coughing and sneezing become painful. In some athletes this impaired pelvic stability put an increased stress on the symphysis joint leading to a stress reaction that combined with the bony changes seen with the enthesopathy of the adductor longus insertion leads to an increased signal when examined with bone scan and with MRI and to irregularities on X-ray. This is sometimes called "osteitis pubis like changes" as it looks like the changes seen with infection of the joint. The changes are not diagnostic of groin injury since they primarily are related to the amount of soccer or other sports undertaken.

Ice hockey player groin injuries may be caused by the eccentric force of the adductors attempting to decelerate the leg during a stride. However, a large percentage of groin pain in these athletes may actually be due to inability to properly load transfer from the legs and or torso to the pelvis. Studies examining healthy adults suggest that the central nervous system deals with stabilization of the spine and pelvis by contraction of the abdominal and multifidus muscles in anticipation of reactive forces produced by lower limb movement. The transversus abdominis and the oblique abdominal muscles appear to contribute to a function not related to the direction of lower limb movement forces. A strength imbalance between the propulsive muscles and the stabilizing muscles of the hip and pelvis has been proposed as a mechanism for adductor strains in athletes (see Section "Key risk factors: how to identify athletes at risk"). The role

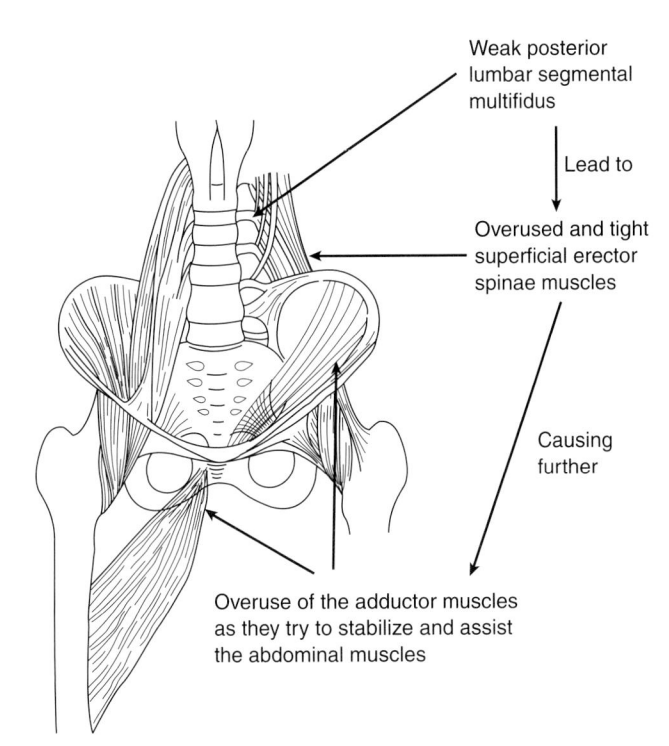

Figure 7.6. As possible cause of strength through length issues of the adductor muscle group leading to further potential for groin strain injury

of the muscles of the torso (i.e., transverse abdominus, obliques, diaphragm, multifidus, pelvic floor) in stabilizing the pelvis such that the abductors and adductors can work explosively and not get strained remains unclear. Perhaps it is the balance of all the torso, pelvis, and hip muscles that is a critical factor in groin injury. For example, weak posterior lumbar segmental multifidus muscles may lead to overused and resultant tight superficial erector spinae muscles causing further potential overuse of the adductor muscles as they try to stabilize and assist the anterior torso muscles, that is, abdominals (Figure 7.6). This situation might lead to strength through length issues of the adductor muscle group leading to further potential for groin strain injury.

Identifying risks in the training and competition program

Groin injury prevention strategies may be developed and evaluated if there is a good understanding of the athlete population at risk, and the risk factors associated with injury for this population (Table 7.4). Age and sports experience are factors that are in nature non-modifiable, but it is tempting to assume, that if increasing age is a risk to sustain groin injury, focus should be to look for methods to take off load and programs that could strengthen the specific structures, that most frequently are injured in the "mature" athletes. If on the other hand decreased age and/or sports experience are risk factors, care must be taken to implement preventive programs for this group, probably including both specific strengthening as well as exercises for pelvic stability and educating the young athletes (and their coaches) in using common sense in the progression of sport specific training and in handling exercise related pain.

Sport specificity has been shown to be a risk factor in swimmers, who are at a risk of getting adductor-related groin problems, if they are breaststroke specialists. A similar connection between groin injury and the specific activity of certain positions or disciplines has not been shown in other sports, most likely because the number of studies investigating this until now is very limited. To prevent sport specificity related groin injuries development of modified techniques that decrease the load on the specific structures could probably decrease the risk of groin injury. Another way would be to strengthen the structures at risk.

Too few sessions of pre-season sport specific training have been shown to be a risk factor in ice hockey. This is probably a reflection of an increased risk of sustaining an injury when participating in sports at a higher level and a higher intensity that you are generally fit for. An increase in pre-season sport-specific training and a subsequent decrease in groin injury may be supported by eccentric training of the thigh muscles as well as abdominal supporting muscular training. Pre-season sport-specific training may allow for further contraction and function-specific recruitment of these muscles, which might allow for their more effective utilization and less onset of fatigue as the season progresses. Fatigue has been noted in the literature to be a contributing factor for muscle injury. As the research data available does not adequately differentiate training and competition groin strain injury one can only insert a "clinical opinion" here. Clinically, there appears to be three main time frames that groin strains appear to be more likely. These times are during the pre-season training when heavy training loads are being done, during the first competitions of the year for explosive speed sports, that is, sprinters and during the last half of the competition year for endurance type sports. Adequate pre-season and continued through season assessment and training of hip ROM as well as hip muscle strength/muscle balance and torso muscle recruitment timing may further minimize the risk of groin injuries.

Preventive measures

A number of more or less well-established risk factors have been mentioned earlier in this chapter (previous groin injury, age, sport experience, sport specificity, pre-season sport specific training, hip ROM, hip muscle strength, and abdominal muscle recruitment), unfortunately there are very few studies that have examined the effect of possible preventive measures (Table 7.4). This section will summarize "best practices" for groin injury prevention in sport, considering the limited but best evidence available identifying risk factors and prevention strategies for groin injury to date. Globally, development of a sport-specific prevention strategy to reduce the risk of groin injury in sport will include components of adequate rehabilitation for previous injury, early identification of sport-specific ROM and strength deficits, and achieving sport-specific ROM and strength as well as muscle timing of recruitment requirements.

Adequate rehabilitation of previous injuries

Previous groin injury is one of the best established risk factors and it is generally considered a non-modifiable factor. However, despite the fact that a previous injury has occurred and this in itself is non-modifiable, there are other related factors that are highly relevant and potentially modifiable. These factors may include how this injured athlete was treated, if there was specific treatment for the injury, if the treatment was functional for the demands of the athlete, and if the athlete returned to the sport including competition with complete rehabilitation of this injury (i.e., full pain free and functional ROM regained, full strength on resisted testing, concentric and eccentric muscle specific function retrained). It is important to use specific treatment methods that treat both the dysfunction related to the specific structural damage that caused the groin pain (i.e., adductor tendon entheses as well as to restore associated pelvic muscular instability by retraining the muscles of the torso as well as the muscles of the hip and pelvis). It is not enough to treat a damaged tendon insertion with steroid injections and time off from the sport and then return when the pain is gone. Likewise, only treating with "core stability" exercises to stimulate the abdominal and low back muscles and then return to sport is not a sufficient treatment and rehabilitation of a damaged tendon insertion to prevent recurrence of the groin injury.

To prevent recurrence of previous groin injuries, treatment aiming at healing the structural damage should be combined with an exercise program to re-establish the pelvic stability and a rehabilitation program gradually including the demands and skills needed to participate in the particular sport before allowing the athlete to return to full participation. Otherwise there is a risk that the factors that originally led to the structural damage will again "take over" and combined with fatigue because of lack of sport-specific rehabilitation may eventually lead to groin re-injury and as often encountered a risk of other injuries as well.

Increasing hip ROM

The ROM of the hip joint is suggested as a risk factor for groin injuries. There are many reasons for pathologic changes of the hip joint ROM, some of which are easily modifiable whereas others are more difficult. Acquired tightness of the rotators, flexors, extensors, abductors or adductors of the hip joint are all potentially able to be loosened with stretching exercises, soft tissue release techniques (manual therapy, massage, dry needling, proprioceptive neuromuscular facilitation techniques), as well as balanced muscle training addressing both the affected muscles and the antagonist muscles. One study found an increased hip abduction ROM after an exercise program including both concentric and eccentric adductor exercises but no stretching exercises for the adductor muscles. Generally there is no evidence that stretching can prevent groin injuries. However there are indications that a normal ROM of the muscles and joints probably is important. In Box 7.1 some stretching exercises for the muscles around the hip joint are described.

Capsular tightness of the hip joint can be found due to post-injury fibrosis reaction, as the result of adaptation to decreased ROM for other reasons during long periods of time or as an inherent general capsular tightness. The collagen tissue in the capsule is probably possible to stimulate to adaptation to a larger ROM with exercises and manual therapy.

Decreased ROM of the hip joint related to bony abnormalities is another and much more difficult problem to treat. Dysplasia of the hip joint can be found in a number of variations and many of these include abnormalities in the ROM of the hip joints, in most cases reducing ROM. In the last decade more attention has been given to the impingement problems of the hip joint. This problem includes groin pain and in most cases some degree of decreased ROM of the hip joint. The two most prominent impingement diagnoses are known as Cam impingement and Pincer impingement. In both cases bony abnormalities lead to potentially further structural damage to the hip joint. They can both be found in athletes without groin or hip pain but with decreased ROM of the hip joints and potentially they are probably a risk factor for developing groin pain. If the impingement problem is symptomatic with hip joint and groin pain, damage to the acetabular cartilage as well as to the labrum of the hip joint is often found. These osseous hip problems need in most cases to be treated surgically if symptomatic, followed by a closely monitored rehabilitation program to re-establish muscle strength and coordination related to the pelvis. In some more rare types of hip dysplasia surgery can be indicated to prevent the development of osteoarthosis in the hip joint. It is not clear, whether any prevention is indicated in cases of pain-free impingement, but theoretically there is a risk, that these patients develop groin injury and intra-articular damage of the hip joint. How these athletes should be advised regarding further sports activities is not clear and is currently a subject for discussion and ongoing scientific studies.

Strength training

The strength of the abductor and the adductor muscles have been debated as possible risk factors earlier in this chapter. One study suggests that the ratio between adductors and abductors are important and that pre-season strength training of the adductor muscles in ice hockey players with adductor/abductor strength ratio <80% could decrease the number of adductor related groin injuries (Tyler et al., 2002). The study however had some methodological concerns and since other studies have been conflicting regarding the strength of the adductor and abductor muscles, the study does not provide conclusive evidence for this method of prevention. If, however, we also consider the protective effect of pre-season sport-specific training in ice hockey, this also has implications for supporting eccentric adductor strength activity to reduce the risk of groin injury.

The combination of strengthening of the adductors and the abductors with abdominal and low back muscle recruitment is probably the area where some of the most likely possibilities are available. A randomized treatment study including specific training of the adductor muscles (static, concentric, and eccentric), as well as exercises for the muscles related to the pelvis including the core stability principles, showed a highly significant effect in the treatment of adductor-related groin injuries (Hölmich et al., 1999). In another randomized controlled trial including 1022 male soccer players, the possible preventive value of such an exercise program has been examined. The exercises (Box 7.2) consisted of the following: (1) static isometric adduction exercises squeezing a soccer ball between the feet and between the knees in the supine position, (2) dynamic adductor and abductor strengthening exercises (concentric and eccentric) done with a partner, (3) coordination of the hip joint related muscles and the muscles of the torso using a dynamic exercise combining sit-up, hip flexion and adduction, (4) dynamic proprioceptive exercise stimulating both concentric and eccentric strength utilizing the principles of core stability (i.e., including the muscles of the torso as well as the muscles of the lower extremities), and (5) stretching exercises for the iliopsoas muscle given the nature of secondary involvement of this muscle in the presence of groin pain. The trial found that the risk of sustaining a groin injury was decreased 31%, but the difference was not statistically significant. Despite the inconclusiveness of this study, the 31% reduction in the risk of getting a groin injury would be a considerable advantage, which probably would make it worth while for the soccer players to do the program.

Take-home message

The best means to identify an athlete at risk for a groin injury may be for the athlete to undergo a preparticipation physiotherapy examination. This could help to identify established risk factors (previous groin injury, age, sport experience, sport specificity, pre-season sport specific training, hip ROM, hip muscle strength, and abdominal muscle recruitment). Development of a sport-specific prevention strategy to reduce the risk of groin injury in sport should include components of adequate rehabilitation for previous injury, early identification of sport-specific ROM and strength deficits, and achieving sport-specific ROM and strength as well as muscle timing of recruitment requirements especially in the torso and hip region. Additionally, pre-season sport-specific training may allow for further contraction and function-specific recruitment of these muscles which might allow for their more effective utilization and less onset of fatigue as the season progresses. Adequate pre-season and continued through season assessment and training of hip ROM as well as hip muscle strength/muscle balance and torso muscle recruitment timing many further minimize groin injuries.

References

Cusi, M.F., Juska-Butel, C.J., Garlick, D., Argyrous, G. (2001) Lumbopelvic stability and injury profile in rugby union players. *New Zealand Journal of Sports Medicine* **29**, 14–18.

Emery, C., Meeuwisse, W. (2001) Risk factors for groin injuries in hockey. *Medicine and Science in Sports and Exercise* **33**, 1423–1433.

Hölmich, P., Uhrskou, P., Ulnits, L., Kanstrup, I.L., Nielsen, M.B., Krogsgaard, K. (1999) Active physical training is an effective treatment of adductor related groin pain in athletes—results of a randomised clinical trial comparing two interventions. *The Lancet* **353**, 439–443.

Tyler, T., Nicholas, S., Campbell, R., Donellan, S., McHugh, M. (2002) The effectiveness of a preseason exercise program to prevent adductor muscle strains in professional ice hockey players. *American Journal of Sports Medicine* **30**, 680–683.

Further reading

Brukner, P., Khan, K., Bradshaw, C., Hölmich, P. (2006) Acute hip and groin pain. In P. Brukner & K. Khan (eds.) *Clinical Sports Medicine*, pp. 394–404. McGraw-Hill, Sydney.

Brukner, P., Khan, K., Bradshaw, C., Hölmich, P. (2006) Longstanding groin pain. In P. Brukner & K. Khan (eds.) *Clinical Sports Medicine*, pp. 405–426. McGraw-Hill, Sydney.

Hölmich, P., Renström, P., Saartok, T. (2003) Hip, groin and pelvis. In M. Kjær, M. Krogsgaard, P. Magnusson, L. Engebretsen, H. Roos, T. Takala, & S.L-Y. Woo (eds.) *Textbook of Sports Medicine—Basic science and clinical aspects of sports injury and physical activity*, pp. 616–637. Blackwell Science Ltd, London.

Maffey, L., Emery, C. (2007) What are the risk factors for groin strain injury in sport? A systematic review of the literature. *Sports Medicine* **37**, 881–894.

Chapter 8
Preventing low back pain

Adad Baranto[1], Tor Inge Andersen[2] and Leif Swärd[3]

[1]Department of Orthopaedics, Sahlgrenska University, Göteborg, Sweden
[2]National Center of Spinal Disorders, National Center of Pain and Complex Disorders, Trondheim University Hospital, St Olav, Norway
[3]Department of Orthopaedics, Sahlgrenska University, Göteborg, Sweden

Epidemiology

Increased training levels

In the 1970s some studies showed positive effects of regular training among adolescents in physical fitness, technique, and coordination. This has led to a common opinion that high doses of training for long periods of time at a young age are required in order to become an elite athlete. Historically, this has resulted in a trend to start training, competition and specialization in one sport at a very young age. This means that many sports require training with high intensity and with high load, often from a very young age. In many sports, it has been found that athletic training with the aim of perfection requires monotonous and repetitive strenuous exercises, leading to an increased risk of musculoskeletal morbidity and/or disturbed growth. A result of this is that overuse injuries are an increasing problem in sports and have also been more noticed among young athletes.

It has also been shown that the growing spine is highly vulnerable to trauma, especially during the adolescent growth spurt (Baranto et al., 2006). In many sports, such as gymnastics, wrestling, and weight lifting, the growing spine is exposed to high loads and in some situations to extreme loads. It is therefore not surprising that a "red flag" has been raised for the early selection of one sport and the early start of specialized training.

Low back pain in young athletes

Back pain symptoms in children and adolescents are different from those in adults and in many cases also have other causes than in adults (Sassmannshausen & Smith, 2002). The symptoms in children are less distinct and they rarely have neurological deficits as in adults. Physicians diagnosing back pain in young athletes must have a specific understanding of these differences in order to avoid incorrect diagnosis and harmful delays in proper treatment. Therefore, diagnosis should be accurate and prompt in pediatric and adolescent athletes, as most have a specific etiology. Back injuries account for 5–8% of all athletic injuries and low back pain has experienced by 10–90% in young elite athletes (Table 8.1) (Swärd et al., 1991; Baranto et al., 2006). In one study it was found that 46% of adolescent athletes reported low back pain compared to 18% of non-athletes (Kujala et al., 1996), and another study found a significantly higher frequency of low back pain in young elite gymnasts (79%) than in controls (37%) (Swärd et al., 1991). In a study on divers the lifetime prevalence of back pain was 89% (Baranto et al., 2006), which is significantly higher than in previous reports (49%) on competitive divers. They also did study the probability that back pain would appear within 1 year (if there was no back pain history earlier)

Sports Injury Prevention, 1st edition. Edited by R. Bahr and L. Engebretsen Published 2009 by Blackwell Publishing ISBN: 9781405162449

Table 8.1 Prevalence of radiological abnormalities on X-rays and MRI, and of symptoms of back pain among athletes (young and adults) in different sports. The results are estimates based on data from different studies.

	Radiological abnormalities (%)	Thoracolumbar back pain (%)
Weightlifting	62–100	23–67
Wrestling	32–86	54–69
Orienteering	71	50
Ice hockey	100	86
Diving	71	89
Gymnastics	42	46–85
Soccer	36	36–58
Tennis	47	32–50
Skiing	–	63
Rowing	–	55

and found that almost on in two divers who did not have any history of back pain would suffer from back pain within 1 year (Figure 8.1).

It has been reported that athletes with abnormalities in the thoracolumbar spine have more back pain than other athletes and non-athletes (Kujala et al., 1996; Sassmannshausen & Smith, 2002; Baranto et al., 2006). Low back pain among athletes may result from acute macro-trauma, repetitive micro-trauma, or stress (Jackson, 1979; Swärd et al., 1991).

Low back pain in adult athletes

The lumbar spine of athletes usually performs demanding and extreme tasks without problems.

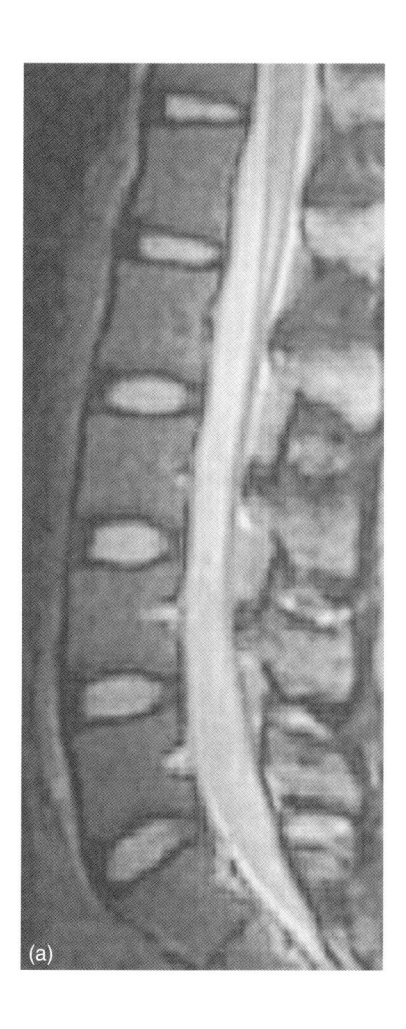

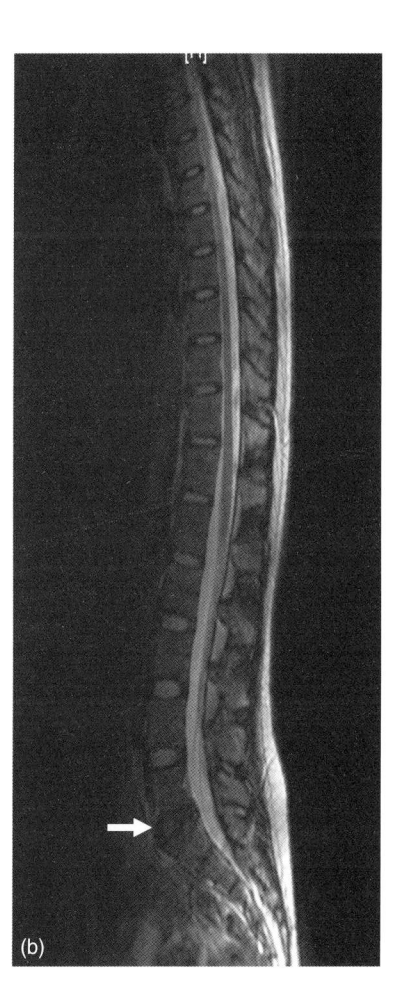

Figure 8.1. (a) Baseline T2 weighted MRI examination in a 20-year-old female diver. (b) T2 weighted MRI at follow-up 5 years later shows moderate disc signal reduction of the L5–S1 disc (arrow)

But the poorly conditioned athlete places himself at great risk for back injury.

Studies have shown prevalence of low back pain in athletes from 1% to 85% and that low back pain is influenced by sport type, gender, training intensity, frequency, and technique (Bartolozzi et al., 1991; Kujala et al., 1996). The literature shows conflicting results on which athletes are at higher risk for low back pain or not, although low back pain is clearly more frequent in some sports than in others. The lifetime prevalence of low back pain in wrestlers has been reported to 59%; significantly higher than that of an age-matched control group (31%). A significantly higher frequency of low back pain has also been reported in elite gymnasts (79%) than in controls (37%) (Swärd et al., 1991). In a prospective study of 134 former top athletes with mean age 33.2 years, it was found that wrestlers had the highest frequency of severe low back pain (54%) as compared to tennis players (32%), soccer players (36%), female and male gymnasts (29%), and non-athletes (32%) (Lundin et al., 2001). However, athletes as a group did not have a higher frequency of back pain than non-athletes, despite significantly more radiological abnormalities among the athletes. In fact, low back pain was less common in former elite athletes (29%) than in non-athletes (44%). Low back pain has also been reported to be more frequent among cross-country skiers (63%) and rowers (55%) than orienteerers (49%) and a control group of non-athletes (47%) (Bahr et al., 2004).

Disc degeneration and spondylolysis are the most common structural abnormalities associated with low back pain in athletes (Bono, 2004). Muscle strains and interspinous ligament sprains have been reported in only one study to be the most common injuries causing low back pain in athletes at any age. However, there are no other studies showing evidence for muscle strains being the most common cause for low back pain in athletes.

One of the most common reasons for missed playing time by professional athletes is pain and dysfunction of the lumbar spine. Other studies have also reported that back pain in many cases was significant enough to interfere with training and competition (Jackson, 1979).

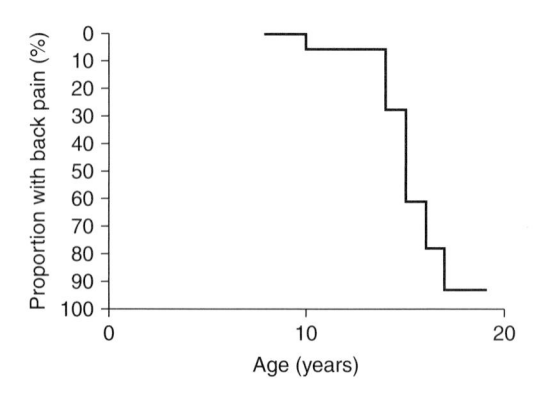

Figure 8.2. The probability of back pain in elite divers. The probability that back pain will appear within 1 year (if there was no back pain history earlier) is about 45%, that is, almost every other diver who has not had any back pain history will suffer from back pain within 1 year

Radiological abnormalities in the spine of athletes

Several studies of the thoracolumbar spine among athletes in sports with great demands on the spine, have reported high frequencies of radiological abnormalities, on plain X-rays and magnetic resonance tomography (MRI) (Figure 8.2), compared to other athletes and non-athletes (Table 8.1) (Alexander, 1977; Goldstein et al., 1991; Swärd et al., 1991; Kujala et al., 1996; Lundin et al., 2001; Baranto et al., 2006). Typical findings are disc degeneration and abnormalities affecting the vertebral endplates and the vertebral ring apophyses. Injury rather than the duration of athletic loading seems important in the etiology of an early degenerative process in the thoracolumbar spine among athletes (Swärd et al., 1991; Kujala et al., 1996).

Abnormalities in the spine among top-level athletes are relatively uncommon before the adolescent growth spurt but thereafter found in increasing frequency (Goldstein et al., 1991; Kujala et al., 1996; Baranto et al., 2006). This is an indication that the growing spine is highly vulnerable to trauma. There is limited knowledge on the effects of high physical loading and development of injuries in the spine during growth and as to whether these injuries contribute to low back pain, progression of disc degeneration or other injuries into adulthood. Despite the long-known fact that intervertebral disc degeneration is more frequent among adolescent athletes than in non-athletes, little has been done to advise the individual athletes or the sports-governing societies to prevent such injuries.

An MRI study of the lumbar spine of professional fast bowlers in cricket showed that they have a relatively higher prevalence of multi-level disc degeneration, a unique pattern of non-dominant side muscular hypertrophy and non-dominate side stress lesions of the lumbar posterior elements. It was found that disc degeneration was not a precursor to lumbar stress changes, but individuals with bilateral stress fractures had severe disc degeneration in all fast bowlers who had a chronic bilateral L5 stress fracture. It was also showed that acute bony stress can be reliably identified using an MRI. An MRI can also detect other structures associated with low lumbar injury, such as intervertebral discs, facet joints, lumbar muscles, and ligaments to be injured (Ranson et al., 2005).

Spondylolysis

Spondylolysis is a radiological diagnosis and means a defect within the bone of the posterior part of neural arch, that is, pars interarticularis. The frequency of spondylolysis in the general population is found to be 4–6% (Figure 8.3). However, the incidence in athletes is much higher, especially in athletes with low back pain where, in one of these studies, spondylolysis was found in 47% of the cases (Sassmannshausen & Smith, 2002). Risk factors are positive family history and co-existing spinal anomalies. Repetitive hyperextension has been shown to be a major risk factor, particularly in gymnastics, figure skating, dancing, and among football linesmen. Spondylolysis was found in a higher frequency than expected among young (range 17–25 years) elite athletes representing female gymnastics (19.2%), male gymnastics (11.5%), tennis (10.0%), wrestling (6.7%), soccer (6.5%), and non-athletes (3.3%). Other authors have reported a high prevalence of spondylolysis in other sports, that is, gymnasts, American football players, divers, wrestlers, weight lifters, rowers, tennis players, soccer players.

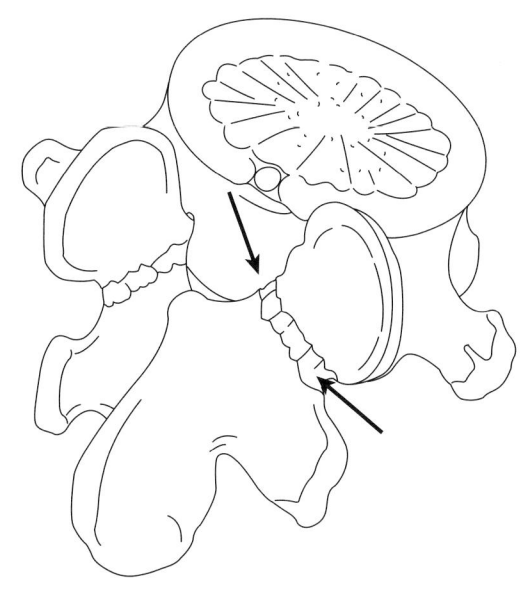

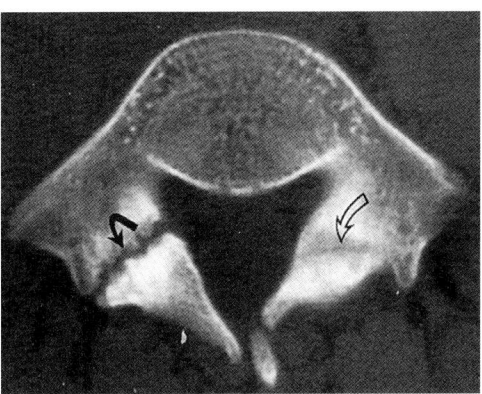

Figure 8.3. Schematic and CT scan showing spondylolysis. Spondylolisthesis is also showed on the drawing to the left as the anterior movement of the upper vertebra in relation to the lower

Anatomy and function of the spine

Development of the spine

The vertebral column consists of a series of linked segments, which serve as the main supporting structure of the body. It also allows sufficient physiological motion between the body parts and also protects the spinal cord from damaging forces. The spine is composed of vertebrae, intervertebral discs, facet joints, ligaments, and muscles.

Development of the spine starts in early life. The vertebra consists of the vertebral body and the neural arch containing transverse, articular, and spinous processes. The growth of vertebral bodies proceeds from the osseous surface of the cartilaginous epiphyseal plates that cover the end plates. These growth plates are, unlike the growth plates of the long bones, not covered by a bony epiphyseal plate. At the periphery of the epiphyseal endplates, in the growing vertebrae, there are recesses where the vertebral ring apophyses are formed. They are the insertion site for the annulus fibrosus of the discs. The area between the ring apophyses and the vertebral body are the weakest part of the spine during growth. The ring apophysis starts to ossify at about 13 years of age and begins to fuse with the vertebral body at about 17 years of age. At completed growth, each vertebra has an elevated rim and a central depression of the endplates.

The etiology and development of intervertebral disc degeneration and abnormalities affecting the vertebral endplates and ring apophyses are not fully known. The etiology of disc degeneration is believed to be multifactorial. As evidenced by the high frequency of abnormalities in the spine of adolescent athletes, mechanical trauma at a young age appears to be a factor of importance especially in sports with great demands on the back (Jackson, 1979; Swärd et al., 1990; Goldstein et al., 1991; Lundin et al., 2001; Baranto et al., 2006).

Little is known about the biomechanics and strength of the degenerated disk. In an experimental study, a degenerative disc was created by drilling a hole through the cranial endplate of a lumbar vertebra into the disc. The results in this study were that twice the axial load was required to create failure of the degenerated discs as compared to non-degenerated discs.

Muscles of the lumbar spine

For descriptive purposes, the spine muscles may be divided into three groups: superficial, intermediate, and deep. The superficial (trapezius, latissimus dorsi, levator scapulae, and rhomboid muscles) and intermediate (serratus posterior superior and inferior muscles) groups are extrinsic back muscles that are concerned with movements of the limbs. The deep group (semispinalis, multifidus, rotators, interspinales, and intertransversarii muscles) constitute the intrinsic back muscles that are concerned with control of the vertebral column. The muscles quadratus lumborum, iliopsoas and the abdominal muscles are also important lumbar spine muscles.

Core stability/neuromuscular control

The term stability is a mechanical concept that most be relate to, but which can be difficult to explain when applied to the body in motion. The term is borrowed from traditional mechanics and describes the ability of a body to remain in the same position while forces are being exerted on it. However, when performing in sports, body configuration is rarely static; in fact, it constantly and rapidly changes. Thus, the athlete must be sufficiently stable and at the same time mobile in order to adapt to the demands placed on them during various movement patterns. The stability and mobility of a joint is primarily dependent on three factors: passive structures (bones, ligaments, joint capsules), active structures (muscles), and the ability to successfully coordinate information and activate the muscles (the central and peripheral nervous system) (Figure 8.4). Thus,

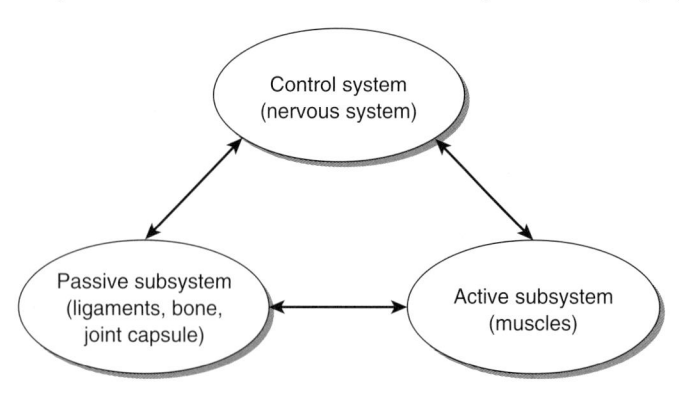

Figure 8.4. Panjabi's model of stability

efficient coordination of the joint systems is required for the athlete to be able to adapt to the demands of sports. This ability is also often referred to as neuromuscular (motor) control. In training terminology this is often referred to as stability, and when referring to the low back pelvis and hip region, "core stability."

Based on recent research, it has become common to categorize the muscles according to their function and location in the body. More simply put, the deep paraspinal muscles, with high endurance and fine motor skills, stabilize the joint systems (here the lower back, pelvis, and hip), whereas the superficial muscles, with less endurance, produce propulsion. The larger the forces produced, the greater the importance of the ability to stabilize, both for the effective utilization of muscle activity (effective technique), and for preventing injuries. Thus, the paraspinal muscles can have a direct influence on segmental stability and control of the lumbar spine due to their attachments to the spinal column. Coordinated contraction of the lumbar paraspinal muscles with the abdominal wall muscles is thought to have a stabilizing effect on the lumbar spinal segments, and therefore providing a safe platform for trunk movement. Dysfunction of these muscles has been suggested to be a significant risk factor in the etiology and chronicity of low back pain.

Key risk factors: how to identify athletes at risk

Improper technique

Improper sport technique and weak abdominal and leg muscles have been shown to increase the risk for spinal injuries. In a study of volleyball players as an example, Bartolozzi et al. (1991) found that only 21% of athletes using proper technique and did not overtrain had degenerative findings in the spine, compared to 62% of athletes using improper technique and overtraining.

Posture

Lower back pain has a strong relationship to posture and it is well known that poor posture is often a result of muscular imbalance. This imbalance can cause low back pain during training cycles and sports competition. Ideal posture, analyzed from the side, has been described as the perfect distribution of weight around the center of gravity in which the agonist and antagonist muscles should be in perfect balance regarding flexibility and strength. Perfect muscular balance in relation to posture will provide for optimum efficiency during movement of sports and daily activities. This perfect balance is however difficult to achieve.

Hyperlordosis or excessive curvature of the lower spine

Another cause of low back pain in adolescent athletes is hyperlordosis or a lordotic lumbar back, which is most commonly due to a forward tilting of the pelvis (Sassmannshausen & Smith, 2002). Forward tilting of the pelvis causes high loads on the intervertebral discs and the facet joints, resulting in high stress in the pars interarticularis of the neural arc of the lower lumbar spine.

It was found in a study on young athletes that the sacro-horizontal angle was larger in athletes with spondylolysis as compared to those without. They, therefore, suggested that an increased sacro-horizontal angle may predispose the individual to spondylolysis and spondylolisthesis, especially in combination with the high mechanical loads sustained in certain sports.

The posture of a forward tilting pelvis causes an increase in the effective curve of the spine. The pathomechanism behind hyperlordosis in children is that the thoracolumbar fascia becomes tight during the adolescent growth spurt due to more rapid growth of the axial skeleton than the fascia. The thoracolumbar fascia consists of three layers of fascia that envelop the muscles of the lumbar spine, effectively separating them into three compartments. Pathologic tightness occurs when the skeletal growth exceeds the capacity of the soft tissues to remain limber. This tightness may cause traction apophysitis at the iliac crest and spinous processes or impingement of adjacent spinous processes. The risk factors are rapid growth and sports that require strong hamstrings, which could exacerbate tightness. The symptoms caused by hyperlordosis are activity-related low back pain.

Age

During growth the nucleus pulposus has a high water content, thereby giving the disc a higher mobility, which accepts movements that put high stresses on the facet joints and posterior elements of the vertebra including pars interarticularis. As the degeneration of the disc starts early in life the elasticity decreases, after the growth spurt the disc will therefore quickly become stiffer.

The degenerative changes found in adolescence in divers may be related to acute spine injuries occurring during the pubertal growth spurt early in the athletic career (Baranto et al., 2006). The results from the several studies suggest that degenerative changes are common among young elite athletes and that trauma to the thoracolumbar spine during the growth spurt is particularly harmful (Goldstein et al., 1991; Kujala et al., 1996; Baranto et al., 2006). The degenerative changes are probably caused by repeated acute injuries, which earlier in the literature has been reported to be of etiological importance for the early degenerative process in lumbar spine among athletes, rather than several years of heavy loading on the spine (Hellström et al., 1990; Goldstein et al., 1991; Swärd et al., 1991; Kujala et al., 1996; Lundin et al., 2001). In divers, the abnormalities were found from the age of 12 years and deterioration was found in only one of the divers under 16 years, but in 73% of those over 16 years (Baranto et al., 2006). This supports the statement that degenerative abnormalities occur at early age, probably due to acute injuries, and deterioration of the abnormalities is due to the duration of heavy loading on the spine.

Although there are clearly sports which put the child and adolescent spine at high risk of injuries, such as gymnastics and competitive diving, it would be expected that the risk of low back problems increases with age as degenerative changes become more prevalent. When examining groups of adult competitive athletes in sports characterized by repetitive low back flexion (cross-country skiing) or extension (rowing) loads, age is an independent risk factor for injury. In fact, the risk of reporting low back pain within a 12-month period increases by 19% for every 5-year increase in age.

Sex

As girls are more flexible and have more joint laxity, they may also have greater risk spine injuries, such as disc degeneration, spondylolysis, and facet joint syndrome. The same study on rowers and cross-country skiers showed that sex was an independent risk factor for low back pain. Women were 35% more likely to report low back pain episodes during the previous 12 months than men.

Previous injury

It has been found that spondylolysis increases the risk for disc degeneration. It has also been shown that back pain results in decreased muscle volume and strength. Therefore a thorough rehabilitation is mandatory after every episode of back pain or back injury.

Typical injury mechanisms: examples from high-risk sports

Acute trauma or repetitive stress

Acute macro-trauma, repetitive micro-trauma/stress, or a combination of these two mechanisms can result in spine injuries in adolescent athletes, resulting in low back pain (Jackson, 1979; Swärd et al., 1991). Repetitive bending (e.g., in gymnastics and diving) and twisting (e.g., in tennis and baseball) of the back increases the risk for spinal injuries in athletes.

In an acute trauma situation, the injury patterns are different in growing individuals when compared to the injury patterns of adults. This was highlighted in a study on cervical spine injuries in traffic accident victims. They found in spines of adolescent victims that they had an avulsion injury of the vertebral endplate (the growth plate), whereas the adult spines had a vertebral body fracture or a rupture of the disc. This indicates that the weakest part of the growing spine is the vertebral growth zone.

Regarding repetitive stress we have performed an experimental study on functional spinal units from young porcine spines where they were vibrated with 20,000 cycles and then axially compressed to failure. The cycling load was chosen to be equivalent to a soccer game or a long distance race. In this study there were no statistically significant differences between specimens exposed to vibrations and non-vibrated specimens with respect to ultimate axial compression strength. The endplate and the growth zone were the weakest parts in both cases.

Loading patterns associated with injury

A combination of different kinds of load is responsible for injuries in the spine of athletes. A single load may cause a specific injury, but in the majority of injuries there are combinations of loads. Heavy loads on the growing spine are the key risk factor for causing injuries in young athletes. The following describes the different loading patterns on the athletic spine.

Compression loads

Compression loads may cause injury of the intervertebral disc (degeneration, low signal intensity on MRI), the ring apophysis, and the endplate (growth abnormalities such as Schmorl's nodes and Scheuermann's disease).

During various athletic activities, high loads are produced on the spine and every different sport places unique demands on the spine (Bono, 2004). For example, in a professional golf player, a swing produces 7500 N of compressive force across the L3–L4 disc. In another study, the average compression loads measured were >17,000 N in the L4–L5 disc in competitive weightlifters (Table 8.2). Cappozzo et al. found in a similar study that when a person performed half-squat exercises with weights ~1.6 times the body weight, the compression forces across the L3–L4 disc were about 10 times the body weight. In these studies, the authors found that increasing lumbar flexion was the most influential factor affecting compressive loads (Bono, 2004).

In several studies we have analyzed the strength of the vertebral functional complex and also described the injury pattern at overload. In radiographic and MRI studies it has been found abnormalities that can be explained by these experiments, for example, the over representation of vertebral growth disturbances found in athletes in the thoracolumbar junction. The most probable explanation for this is that the loads are highest in the anterior part of the vertebral bodies resulting in an injury to the area of the ring apophyses and that the energy in a rotation overload, due to the brute change in facet joint orientation in the lower thoracic spine from allowing to restricting rotation, is transformed from the stable facet joints to the mobile weaker anterior part of the vertebrae. This causes an injury affecting the ring apophysis and thereby a disturbance growth, resulting in wedged vertebrae and a Scheuermann kyfosis, which is also called traumatic form of Scheuermann's disease.

Alexander (1977) suggested in the 1970s that abnormalities such as endplate changes, Schmorl's nodes, apophyseal ring fractures and abnormal configuration of the vertebral body are traumatic forms of Scheuermann's disease and a common finding in athletes. The traumatic form of Scheuermann's disease involves in many cases only one vertebra and has its peak incidence at the thoracolumbar junction (Alexander, 1977). These findings are frequent in sports with repetitive flexion, extension, and rotation of the spine, such as gymnastics and wrestling. The symptoms are low back pain in high frequency accentuated in flexion (Sassmannshausen & Smith, 2002).

Flexion and extension compression

Flexion and extension compression loads also cause injury of the intervertebral disc, the ring apophysis, the endplate (growth abnormalities such as Schmorl's nodes and Scheuermann's disease) and of the facet joints. There is experimental

Table 8.2 Spinal loads have been measured or estimated in different sports.

Sport	Maximum compressive force (N)
Golfers	6,000
Rowers	6,000
American football (linemen)	15,000
Weightlifters	15,000

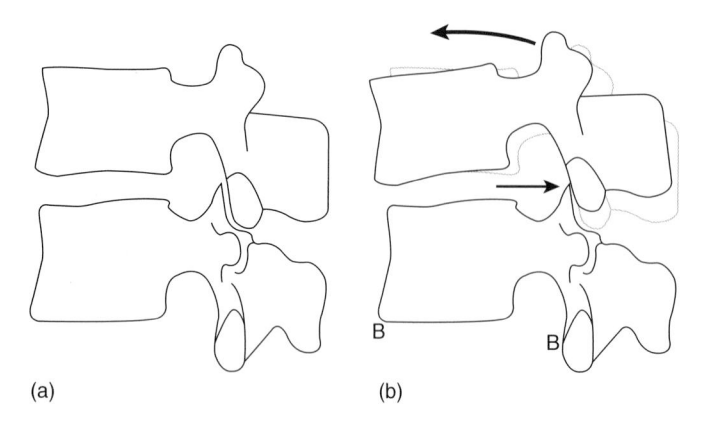

Figure 8.5. The role of the facet joints during flexion (a) Neutral position, (b) sagittal rotation causes the inferior articular process of the facet joint to lift upward, leaving a gap between it and the superior articular process. Anterior sagittal translation is allowed due to this gap. Finally, upon translation, the inferior articular process again impacts the superior articular process, limiting additional flexion

evidence that the spine is more sensitive for injuries during bending movements and especially during extension compression.

The extension movements in the intervertebral joints behave conversely to movements in flexion. The vertebral bodies rotate posteriorly and also undergo a small posterior translation in the sagittal plane. In addition to the tension in the disc, extension movement is resisted by bony impact between the spinous and articular processes, the laminae and also by the capsule of the facet joint. The posterior ligaments are not critical for limiting extension. However, the well-developed anterior longitudinal ligament and the anterior portion of the annulus fibrosus and the facet joints are important inhibitors of hyperextension and posterior translation.

In an experimental study performed on functional spinal units from adolescent male pigs, which were exposed to flexion–compression or extension–compression loading to failure, fractures/separations were seen in the growth zone anteriorly and more frequently, posteriorly in spines exposed to flexion–compression. In extension–compression such injuries occurred only anteriorly. In another experimental study we found that the experimentally degenerative discs in the flexion–compression group required four times more compression load before failure than normal adolescent spine units, while the degenerated extension–compression group required only 60% more load than normal. These results support the clinical impression that compression in extension or flexion is more likely to cause spinal injuries than axial compression alone, and that the spine is more vulnerable in extension–compression than in flexion–compression. These studies showed that, when compressed in flexion or extension, the weakest part was the growth zone, and, to a lesser extent, the endplate, and the injury was more extensive in extension loading than during flexion loading.

The facet joints play a great role in maintaining the stability of the lumbar spine in flexion. To understand these mechanisms it is important to recognize that flexion involves both anterior sagittal rotation and anterior sagittal translation (Figure 8.5). During flexion, the highest pressure is recorded at the antero-medial part of the lumbar facet joint. Each facet joint capsule, acting as a ligament, can resist about 600 N and the tension developed in it during flexion is enough to bend the inferior articular processes downward and forward about 5°. During flexion, the weight of the trunk exerts compressive and shear forces on the intervertebral disc, which are proportional to the angle of inclination of the inter-body joint.

Rotation compression

Rotation compression loads also cause injury of the intervertebral disc, the ring apophysis, the endplate and of the facet joints.

Rotation of the lumbar spine involves torsion of the intervertebral discs and the impact of the facet joints. All the fibers of the annulus fibrosus that are inclined toward the direction of rotation during axial rotation will be strained and the others will be relaxed. It has been calculated that the maximum range of rotation of an intervertebral disc is about 3° and rotation beyond this range will result in micro-injuries in the collagen fibers. The facet joints and,

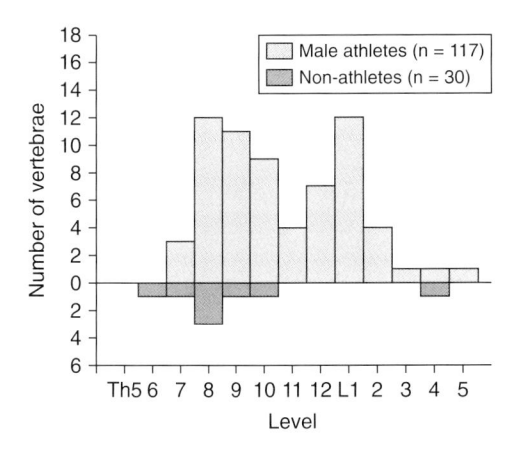

Figure 8.6. Athletes have degenerative abnormalities on X-ray and MRI in the thoracic spine and also in the junction between the thoracic and lumbar spine in contrast to non-athletes.

to a certain degree, the posterior ligaments protect the intervertebral disc from excessive rotation.

Rotation injuries cause injuries mainly in the thoracolumbar junction due to the facet joint configuration. The facet joints from Th12 to S1 are formed to restrict rotation. Therefore repetitive rotation in flexion or extension in sports, such as tennis, creates overuse injuries in this part of the spine, traumatic form of Scheuermann's disease or Mb. Swärd (Swärd et al., 1991; Baranto et al., 2006). Swärd was one of the first who found these degenerative abnormalities in athletes (Figure 8.6). The traumatic form of Scheuermann's disease involves only one vertebra and has its peak incidence at L1 (Alexander, 1977). These findings are frequent in sports with repetitive flexion and extension, such as gymnastics, tennis, and wrestling (Lundin et al., 2001). The symptoms are low back pain accentuated in flexion (Sassmannshausen & Smith, 2002).

Injury mechanism in diving and acrobatic sports

Competitive diving puts high demands on the spinal column. The exposure of axial load on the spine of competitive divers is well described. Flexion and extension bending occur in most diving maneuvers and axial loading, shearing and torsional stresses act through multiple spinal segments, creating a potential for injuries (Badman & Rechtine, 2004).

The injury mechanism is related to the takeoff, flight and the entry phases, and each phase can cause different spine injuries (Badman & Rechtine, 2004). The average entry speed into the water is between 8.4 m/s (1 m springboard) and 14.0 m/s (10 m springboard). At impact a speed reduction of more than 50% within a fraction of a second has been demonstrated, resulting in tremendous axial load on the spine creating significant potential for injuries. This means that tremendous axial forces are generated upon impact, creating significant potential for spinal injury. Inadequate body roll can ultimately result in lateral flexion and rotation through the lumbar spine, during this phase.

Several clinical studies have shown that injuries to the growing spine are common and it can be assumed that these injuries commonly occur during the adolescent growth spurt. Experimental studies indicate that certain loads in extension and flexion compression with or without disc degeneration result in predictable injury patterns involving the disc and adjacent growth zones. These results may serve as a basis for further clinical studies of injury mechanisms in sports with heavy loads on the spine. However, this will require sophisticated standardized analysis of movements and loads on the spine during the execution of the sports activities in training and competition, perhaps similar to the automated kinematic and kinetic computer-analyzed gait analyses systems that have gained acceptance. Such motion analyses must be matched with the injury patterns of the particular sport, in order to define the critical movements with regard to risk for injury of the spine. Also the influence of age, gender, training intensity and individual technique on the development of back pain, and spinal injuries needs to be studied further.

Injury mechanisms for spine injuries in other sports

There are different maneuvers and some times a combination of maneuvers causing spinal injuries in different sports. In tennis, rotation, flexion and extension loads cause spinal injuries. In gymnastics, it is the extreme flexion- and extension–compression loading and axial–compression loading that are responsible for injuries. In weightlifting axial–compression loads cause spinal injuries.

Heavy loads in the spine are obvious in other sports, such as wrestling and gymnastics, where forceful bending movements are exerted at high speed. Other sports involve mainly one-sided stress and loads, such as in tennis, American football, rowing, and soccer.

This is supported by the findings in the spine of athletes in sports involving "flight." During these activities, the athlete is airborne and lands on a hard surface, such as the floor in gymnastics, or the water, such as in diving maneuvers. Other activities associated with spinal injuries include blocking in football, takedowns in wrestling, swinging a bat in baseball, tackling in ice hockey and use of heavy weights and attempts at complex free-weight lifts in weight training.

In baseball, the players are prone to trunk rotation injuries as well as the less common trunk flexion injuries. Loads generated through swinging a bat and accelerating a baseball produces disc and posterior element injuries. Injuries seen in infielders in baseball are mainly of the flexion bending and lifting type.

In American football, tackling, blocking, running, and throwing the ball all involve contact between opponents that can cause a multitude of spine injuries. For example, when a player is reaching for a pass as his opponent drives a shoulder into the flank he may be subjected to a quick forced hyperextension, when the spine is most vulnerable to trauma. The facet joints are at risk with hyperextension of the lumbar spine. As well as protecting the spine against flexion injuries the increased paraspinal musculature causes an unbalanced hyperextension force, which puts the pars interarticularis at great risk.

The etiology of lumbar stress injury in fast bowlers in cricket has been shown to be multifactorial. Asymmetrical development of the paraspinal musculature, particularly quadratus lumborum, was associated to lumbar stress injuries in elite fast cricket bowlers.

The lumbar spine was found to be the most commonly injured site in swimmers, divers, and water polo players and synchronized swimmers. Freestyle and backstroke increase lumbar segmental axial rotation and therefore increase torque forces most, which puts the annulus fibrosus at risk for injury. Top swimmers are at an increased risk for injuries because of exaggerated movements that increase flexion and extension. The lumbar facet pain increases with strokes that accentuate lumbar spine extension, such as breaststroke and butterfly. Finally, in supine swimming extension of the cervical spine induces lumbar extension, resulting in increased stress on the pars interarticularis and the facet joints.

Identifying risks in the training and competition program

The amount of training and competition is of great importance for overuse injuries of the spine in athletes. Goldstein et al. (1991) reported a strong correlation between development of degenerative changes and back pain in gymnasts, and the frequency of back pain was suggested to correlate to the level of activity. In contradiction to these findings, Lundin et al. (2001) found, in a study of elite athletes representing wrestling, gymnastics, soccer, and tennis, that the athletes did not report more back pain than non-athletes (all athletes 60%, non-athletes 61%, female gymnasts 67%), despite significantly more radiological changes. The difference between these two studies may be due to the fact that in the study by Goldstein et al. (1991) the athletes were younger (mean age in female gymnasts 16.6 years) and still active in their sport, while in the study by Lundin et al. (2001) the individuals were older (mean age in female gymnasts 30.6 years, all athletes 33.1 years) and they were mostly former, rather than active, elite athletes.

Goldstein et al. (1991) found that 57% of the gymnasts who trained 15 h or more per week had degenerative changes on MRI, as compared to 13% in those who trained less, and they concluded that the amount of training is of importance for the development of spinal injuries.

Prevention methods

Low back injuries in adolescent athletes are a serious problem. However, if diagnosed and treated properly, the athlete usually can return also to vigorous activities. Many of the sport injuries are the result of inadequate training, pore technique, but also structural anatomical weaknesses in the body. Unfortunately, there is a lack of scientifically documented prevention methods for preventing spinal injuries in athletes. The following are best-practice recommendations based on our current understanding of risk factors and injury mechanisms discussed earlier.

Only when critical motion patterns and loads in specific sports can be identified, prevention may be possible. In order to avoid harmful motion patterns, rules and regulations, as well as scoring systems in esthetic sports, may have to be modified. Since sport rules and regulations usually have historical origin and governing bodies tend to be very protective regarding new or modified age-related rules in sports, considerable efforts and convincing evidence will be needed in order to implement modifications of rules and regulations when needed. Presently, little scientific evidence of this kind is available. Until such information is available, prevention must be based on indirect evidence, such as the overrepresentation of certain injuries in a sport. Thus, more general restrictions can be applied, for example, appropriate (biological) age limits for advanced muscular strength training with weights, limitations of repetitions of strenuous activities at a young age, and avoidance of inappropriate exercises that carry increased risk of injury. All this requires improved education of trainers, coaches, and sport-governing bodies, as well as education of the young athletes themselves, little of which exists today. Medical personnel, including physicians and physical therapists, need to take a more active role in preventing sports injuries, by educational and other activities at all levels, including young athletes.

As described in the earlier section the spine is in great risk for injuries due to extreme loads on the spine in axial compression, hyperflexion and hyperextension bending, rotation, and finally a combination of the loads. It is also well documented that the spine is most vulnerable to trauma during the growth spurt. Furthermore, the amount of training and competition is of great importance for overuse injuries of the spine in athletes. To prevent spinal injuries the most important factor is to avoid high loads on the spine of athletes before the spine is fully grown, which means at least until after the age of 18 years. It is also important to avoid extreme bending movements of the spine in sports when it is possible, even if this is probably not realistic in many sports. The amount of training is of fundamental importance to reduce and avoid overuse injuries on the spine in athletes. Competition schedules should also be adjusted to the biologic age of the athletes. Young athletes should concentrate on coordination, techniques, and balance before the growth spurt.

Adults can help adolescent athletes prevent spinal injury. For example, coaches can institute shorter practices. Properly trained coaches, athletic trainers, parents, or other adults can supervise training sessions and mostly be aware of the weakness of the growing spine and the relation to the growth spurt. They also can teach proper technique for weight training and various exercises. The athlete with back pain must have a rehabilitation concentrating on technique, flexibility, and muscle control to withstand the high demands of their sport.

Prevention principles

On the basis of our current understanding of risk factors and injury mechanisms, the following four principles are recommended to prevent back problems:

1. Avoid exercise straining the back with weights until the spinal column has stopped growing.
2. Avoid heavy strain in extreme positions whenever possible.
3. Develop sufficient strength, stability, and coordination in the back/pelvis and hip to meet the demands of the various characteristics of the different sports.
4. Emphasize training that improves techniques, balance, and coordination.

Unfavorable techniques may be due to insufficient strength, stability, coordination, etc. One example of this may be a handball player who is weak in the lower part of the abdominal muscles, resulting in hyperextension of the lower back when executing a pass/shot on goal. The player will be particularly at risk if the hip flexors are short, causing reduced mobility in the extension of the thoracic spinal column. A large part of the strain is thus put on the lower back. In order to prevent problems in athletes like this, it is important to strengthen the lower abdominal muscles and increase mobility in the hip and thoracic spine.

Another example is cross-country skiing, where many athletes also have lower back problems (Bahr et al., 2004). One reason for this may be unfavorable technique in the double-pole push, where the athlete moves too far forward, causing extreme flexion in the lower back. This places a strain on the back, especially if the athlete does not have sufficient strength and stability in the back/pelvis and hips. A shorter forward motion, where the back is kept in more of a mid-position is likely to both prevent injuries and be a more efficient technique.

The selection of exercises to prevent low back problems should reflect the demands of the sport, designed to enable the athlete to meet the biomechanical demands placed on the lower back. Although different sports have different demands, the principles of preventive training are similar and the exercises can be grouped into three categories.
1. Awareness exercises
2. Stability training/neuromuscular control
3. Dynamic strength training of the muscles in the abdomen and back.

Awareness exercises (Box 8.1)

Awareness exercises are intended to improve control of the pelvic area in order to find a favorable position for the lower back. The objective is to make the athlete aware of the position and angle of the pelvis, to avoid putting the spinal column in a position where it is at increased risk for injuries. The term pelvic position denotes the position of the pelvis in relation to the other body sections. The position of the pelvis may be changed without changing the curvature of the back. If the pelvis is tilted forward, lumbar lordosis will increase. The pelvic angle and the curvature of the spine are thus interrelated. This may be influenced by mobility and strength in the muscles of the back, abdomen, and hip joint. Control of the pelvic region is critically important, since it represents the center of the transfer of force between the upper body and the legs.

Stability training/neuromuscular control (Box 8.2)

Neuromuscular control training (often referred to as "core stability" training) aims to make the athlete able to maintain a favorable position for the lower back, pelvic area, and hip area during various loading conditions. By maintaining a favorable position, the impact on the tissues and structures of the lower back is reduced.

The exercises are also well suited for revealing reduced neuromuscular control and reduced strength in the muscles ("weak links"). The term "weak link" denotes a weak point in a muscle synergy. The objective of core stability exercises is to optimize control and force transfer in the lower back, pelvis, and hips with the least amount of force lost and the least amount of strain on the back.

There are several different ways of training stability/neuromuscular control. Studies have shown that two effective ways of improving/restoring neuromuscular control is to:
1. Train in a closed kinetic chain.
2. Train on an unstable surface.

Training in a closed kinetic chain means that the part of the body being trained is the one bearing weight. One example is the squat exercise. One example of the contrary, a training exercise in an open kinetic chain, is working the quadriceps in a knee extension machine. The squat is the more functional of these exercises. Any training in an open kinetic chain, such as knee extension, is effective for isolating a certain muscle group, but less effective to develop neuromuscular control. Changes in joint position and muscle tension are recorded and transmitted to the central nervous system. This information is vital for the muscles to be able to successfully activate and maintain control of joint position.

Exercising on an unstable surface further challenges the neuromuscular control. Studies indicate that exercises done on unstable surfaces activate

Box 8.1 Introduction to awareness exercises, examples of exercises

Pelvis tilt lying on back
Starting position: Lying on back with bent hip and knees.
Execution: Tighten abdominal muscles so that the lower back touches the floor. Then tighten the muscles in the back to curve the lower back and lift it off the floor.
Note: Athlete produces a flexing motion in the pelvis.

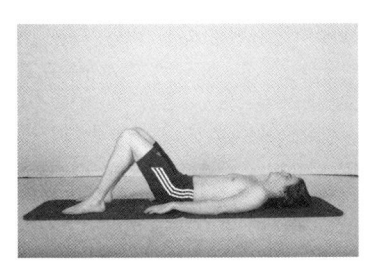

Pelvis flex in standing position
Starting position: Standing up.
Execution: Tighten abdominal muscles to that the lower back curves outward. Then tighten the muscles in the back to curve the lower back inward.
Note: Athlete produces a flexing motion in the pelvis.

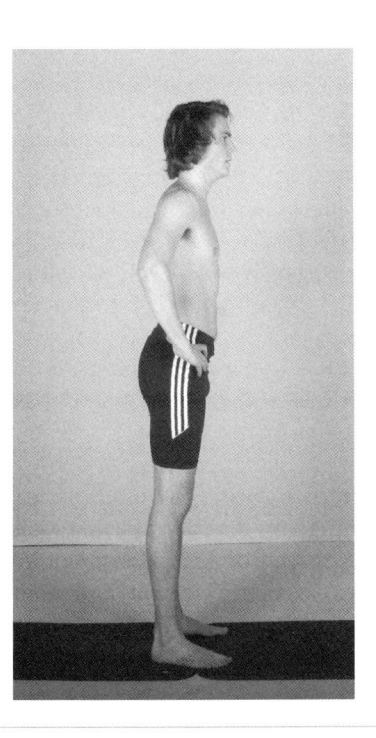

Flexing lower back sideways
Starting position: Lying on the back with legs straight.
Execution: First pull the iliac crest on one side upward, and then the other side.
Note: Athlete flexes lower back sideways

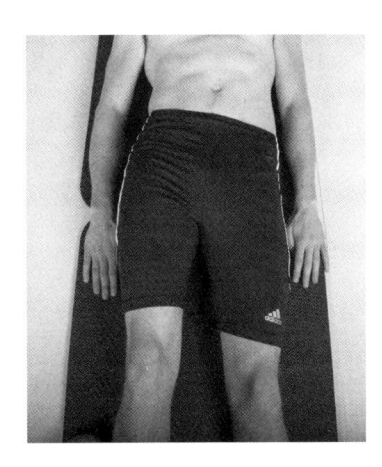

Flexing lower back sideways
Starting position: Standing.
Execution: First pull the iliac crest on one side upward, and then the other side.
Note: Athlete flexes lower back sideways.

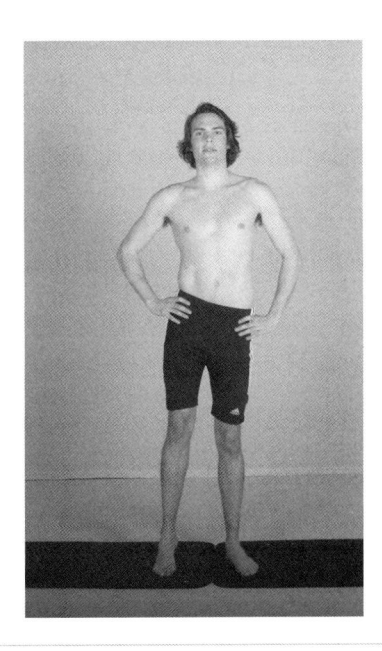

Box 8.2 Stability exercise program

Stability with knee and underarm support
Starting position: Standing on all fours, supporting the body on knees and underarms.
Execution: Maintain position.
Note: Discontinue exercise when "tremors" or deviation from mid-position occur.

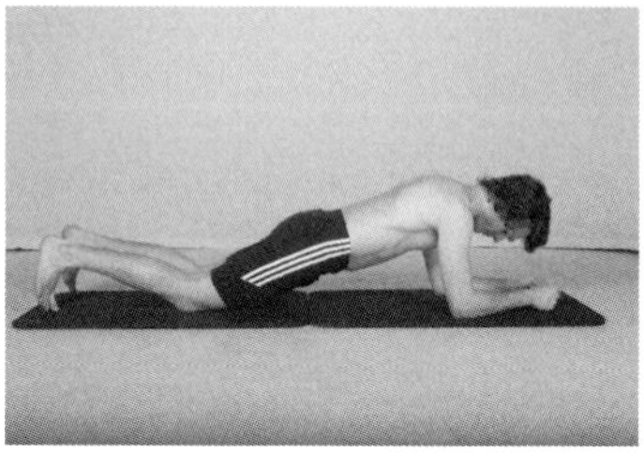

The plank—Stability with knee and underarm support
Starting position: Standing on all fours, supporting the body on toes and underarms.
Execution: Maintain position.
Note: Discontinue exercise when "tremors" or deviation from mid-position occur.

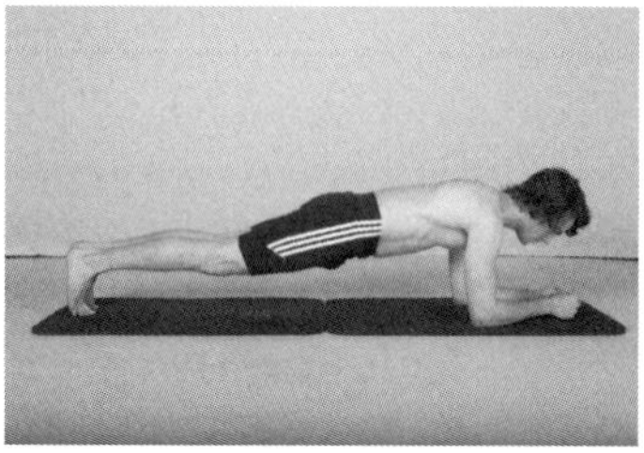

"Wheelbarrow," without additional motion
Starting position: Athlete assumes same starting position as for push-ups. Assistant grabs athlete's ankles and lifts. Throughout the execution of the exercise the athlete maintains the same position of the hands.
Execution: Assistant tries to push the athlete gently forward and then pulls the athlete gently toward himself. The athlete maintains the same curvature of the back and the same position of the hands.
Note: Discontinue exercise when "tremors" or deviation from mid-position occur.

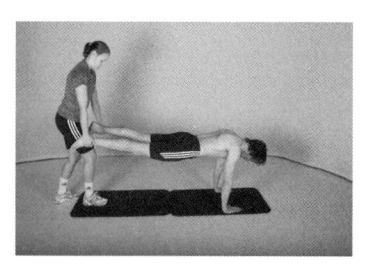

Support on one arm, sideways
Starting position: Lie on side with legs straight and support the body on a straight arm. Attach other arm to hip. Place one foot slightly in front of the other.
Execution: Keep the body straight and the back in the mid-position.
Note: Discontinue exercise when "tremors" or deviation from mid-position occur.
Progression: Feet are placed one on top of the other. Same exercise as above.

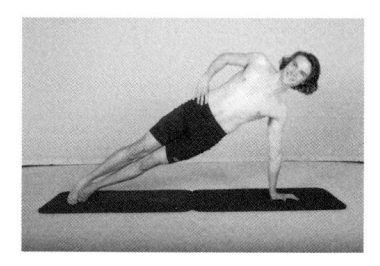

Unstable—Foot and underarm support
Starting position: Standing on all fours supporting the body on feet and underarms. Feet and underarms on balance mats.
Execution: Maintain position.
Note: Discontinue exercise when "tremors" or deviation from mid-position occur.

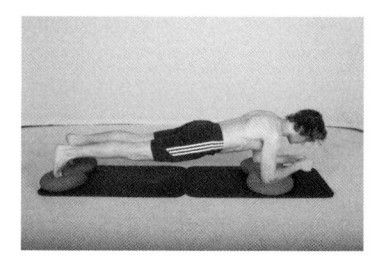

Stability with rotational element—Foot and underarm support
Starting position: Standing on all fours supporting the body on feet and underarms.
Execution: Move one leg out to the side and back.
Note: Discontinue exercise when "tremors" or deviation from mid-position occur.

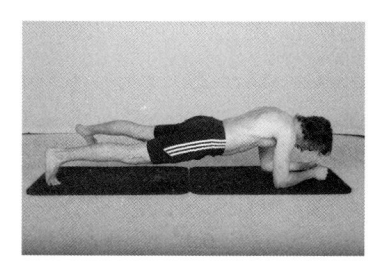

(Continued)

Box 8.2 (Continued)

Body lift with shoulder support
Starting position: Lying on back with arms to the side. Assistant is one step away in front of the athlete. Assistant holds on to athlete's ankles and lifts to hip height.
Execution: Lift buttocks to back mid-position. Only shoulders, neck, head, and arms are in contact with the floor. Assistant lets go off one leg. Move leg to the side. Maintain same low back position.
Note: Discontinue exercise when "tremors" or deviation from mid-position occur.

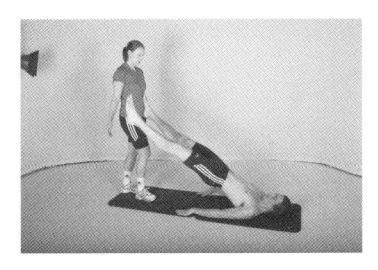

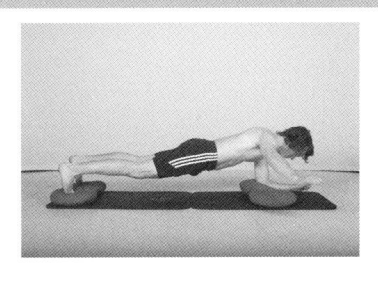

The plank—unstable platform with rotation
Starting position: Standing on all fours supporting body on feet and underarms. Arms supported on balance cushions.
Execution: Move one leg to the side and back. Maintain position.
Note: Discontinue exercise when "tremors" or deviation from mid-position occur.

The plank—unstable platform
Starting position: Standing on all fours supporting the body on feet and underarms. Hands and feet supported on balance cushions.
Execution: Move one arm to the side and back. Maintain position.
Note: Discontinue exercise when "tremors" or deviation from mid-position occur.

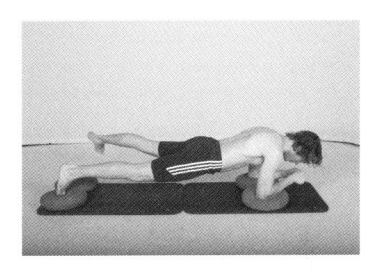

more muscle fibers than if the same exercise is done on a stable surface.

If an athlete is experiencing difficulty with stability exercises, the problems may be due to several causes: (1) Insufficient muscle strength for effective stabilization. If the athlete is not strong enough, it is necessary to, in addition, engage in targeted dynamic strength training of muscle groups that are too weak. Suggested exercises are described under "Dynamic strength training." (2) Insufficient neuromuscular control. If this is the problem, it may be due to a lack of awareness of which muscles are necessary to activate for effective stabilization. If finding the neutral mid-position is difficult, it may be necessary to focus on awareness exercises first. Athletes often experience rapid progress in stability training. It is important to increase the degree of difficulty, so that the athlete continues to be challenged This can be done by introducing unstable surfaces, increasing the load with longer balance arms, and by introducing rotational elements.

When training stability, the athlete should maintain the exact natural mid-position of the lumbar region and pelvis. The athlete is ready to progress to the next level when he is able to maintain this position for 20–30 s without "tremors" or deviations.

This may seem paradoxical, but it is important that the athlete tries to execute the exercises as relaxed as possible. Good stability must not be confused with a static and restricted execution of the exercises.

Dynamic strength training of the muscles in the abdomen and back (Box 8.3)

Dynamic strength training has two main objectives:
1. Increasing the strength in the muscles in the abdomen and back.

Box 8.3 Dynamic strength exercises. In most exercises the athlete should aim to execute the movements as explosively as possible in the concentric phase. To increase muscle strength we recommend ~10 repetitions in each series, for 3–5 series. To improve muscle endurance the athlete may opt to work less explosively with more repetitions in each series. The execution of the exercises should be pain free.

Buttock lift
Starting position: Lying on back with hip and knees bent at 90° angles. Hands behind head.
Execution: Lift knees toward ceiling, lifting buttocks from the floor. Avoid pulling thighs toward chest, this makes the exercise easier.

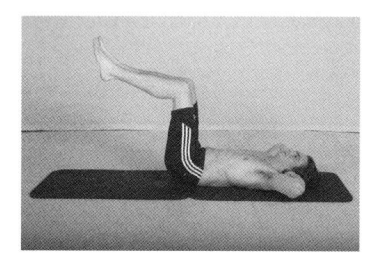

Sit-ups, oblique abdominal muscles, unstable
Starting position: Lying partly on the side, with left buttock on floor. Slightly bent hip and knees. Arms rotated toward the right side.
Execution: Pull arms toward the right side, and lift torso as with sit-ups. Change sides and repeat exercise.

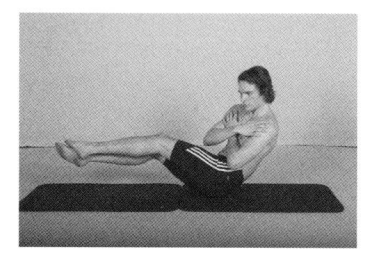

Oblique abdominal muscles, from below
Starting position: Lying on back. 90° bend in hip and slightly bent knees. Legs together. Arms to the side.
Execution: Move legs diagonally to floor and back. Maintain midposition in lower back! Repeat exercise on other side.

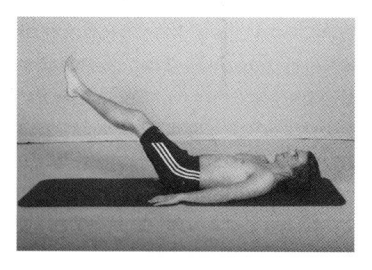

Sit-ups with fixed foot position and rotation
Starting position: Lying on back with bent hip and knees. Arms across chest. Feet on floor. Assistant holds athlete's ankles.
Execution: Lift torso toward thighs, combined with elbow to knee.

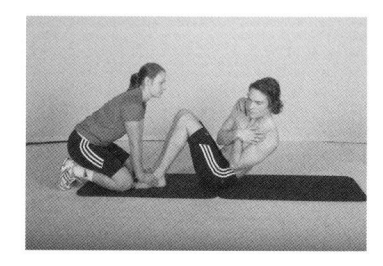

Throwing sit-ups
Starting position: Lying on back with straight hip and knees. Assistant standing ~1.5 m from athlete's feet. Assistant holding medicine ball.
Execution: Assistant throws medicine ball toward athlete's chest. Athlete initiates sit-up motion toward ball, and catches it right before it reaches the chest. Continues the motion up to a sitting position and throws the ball to the assistant before he reaches the sitting position. Exercise is repeated from starting position.

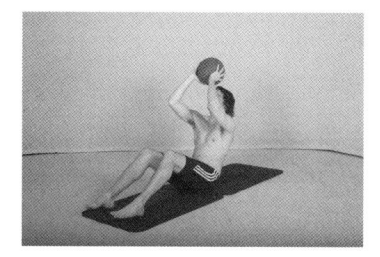

Sideways throwing
Starting position: Sitting ~1 m from assistant. Side facing assistant. Bent hip and knees. Thighs and calves not touching floor. Holding a medicine ball.
Execution: Throw medicine ball sideways to assistant. Exercise is to be executed explosively.

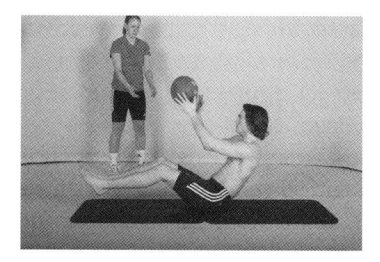

(Continued)

> **Box 8.3 (Continued)**
>
> **Diagonals**
> Starting position: Standing on all fours.
> Execution: Bring left hand together with right knee. Then extend arm and leg diagonally to a horizontal position. Repeat exercise for opposite diagonal.
>
> **Sideways pelvis lift**
> Starting position: Lie on the side supporting the body on one arm. Attach the other arm to hip. Place one foot slightly in front of the other.
> Execution: Move pelvis toward floor and then back to starting position.
> Progression: Place feet one on top of the other. Same procedure as above.
>
> **Maximal throwing**
> Starting position: Standing, facing a wall. Holding medicine ball.
> Execution: Bending knees with an explosive motion, concluding with throwing the medicine ball against the wall.
> Note: Lean forward with lower back in mid-position.

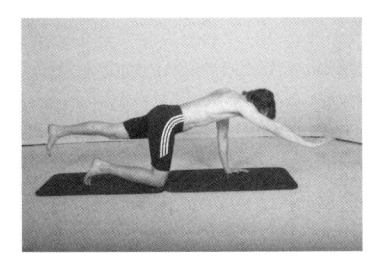

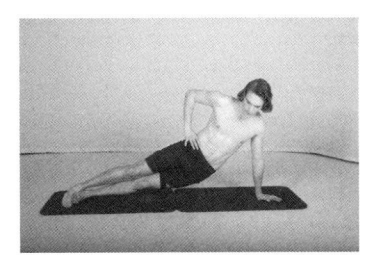

2. Normalizing any "weak links" uncovered during the execution of the stability exercises. Exercises focusing on the lower parts of the abdomen and back are particularly important. In order to be able to tolerate the loads athletes are exposed to, good muscle strength, and muscle endurance in these regions are important. Increased muscle strength results from two mechanisms:

1. Muscle fiber hypertrophy, that is, increasing the cross-sectional area of the muscles.

2. Nervous adaptation, that is, activating more muscle fibers, faster activation and more simultaneous activation.

When a new strength exercise program is started, the initial strength increase over the first few weeks is almost exclusively due to nervous adaptation. Hypertrophy occurs later, and in order to maximize hypertrophy, sub-maximal loads (60–90% of maximal load) with 8–12 repetitions in several series (often 4–6) until exhaustion is recommended. Movements are performed relatively slowly, particularly in the eccentric phase.

Increased muscle strength based on nervous adaptation occurs when several muscle fibers are activated simultaneously, particularly the fast-twitch fibers, which are harder to activate than slow-twitch fibers. In order to activate the highest possible number of motor units, it is critical that the athlete attempts to execute the motion as fast as possible. The same principles apply to the muscles in the abdomen and back. However, for this region one must consider both anatomical and mechanical factors in order to avoid excess strain and injuries resulting from the exercises themselves.

Many athletes have problems achieving the intended strength increase in the lower part of the abdominal muscles. This may be due to the fact that many atheletes worry about injuring their back during exercises intended to strengthen the muscles in their abdomen and back. Therefore, they are cautious during abdominal exercises, taking particular care not to activate the hip flexors. What appears to be the most common abdominal exercise is the "sit-up" without securing the legs, lifting the shoulder blades off the ground. This exercise does not sufficiently challenge the muscles of the abdomen, back, and hip area, and this particular area requires a strong muscle corset. The exercise program suggested in Box 8.3 emphasizes working both the upper and the lower part of the abdominal muscles.

Secondary prevention

In terms of secondary prevention, a certain amount of new knowledge has emerged, which should be implemented. Studies have revealed a connection between changes in neuromuscular control mechanisms and back problems. Changes in the recruitment patterns for both abdominal and back muscles are apparent in most back pain patients, irrespective of the cause of the problems. Muscular dysfunction in low back pain has been described for both the deep and the superficial muscle systems. Locally, it is expressed as a dysfunction in the recruitment and control of deep segmental stabilizing muscles (Hides et al., 1996; Hodges & Richardson, 1996; O'Sullivan et al., 1997; Jull & Richardson, 2000). Dysfunction in the local muscle system in low back pain patients has been shown to include segmental atrophy of deep layers of the lumbar multifidus muscles on the painful side (Hides et al., 1994). This appears soon after acute low back pain, and will not automatically normalize when pain subsides. Studies have also found delayed recruitment and changed function of the transverse abdominis muscles in persons with lower back pain.

Some studies show good effects on lower back pain from targeted exercises of the muscular support system in the lumbar vertebral column, including the transverse abdominis, lumbar multifidii, and pelvic floor muscles. The aim is to isolate the function of these muscles, creating a stabilizing "corset" of "deep stabilizing muscles." This has proven to be beneficial both in the short and in the long run in terms of improved function and decreased pain, and such training is probably critical to avoid reinjuries in athletes with a history of low back pain, although this hypothesis has not been tested in formal trials.

Take-home message

It is important to be aware of the weakness of the growing spine and the relation to the growth spurt. To prevent spinal injuries the most important factor is to avoid high loads on the spine of athletes before the spine is fully grown, which means at least until after the age of 18. It is also important to avoid extreme bending movements of the spine in sports whenever possible. Competition programs should also take the age of the athletes into account.

The amount of training is of fundamental importance to reduce and avoid overuse injuries on the spine in athletes. The young athletes ought to concentrate on coordination, techniques, and balance before the growth spurt. Including specific exercises to improve awareness, core stability training, and dynamic strength of the low back, abdomen, pelvic, and hip region is highly recommended. In particular, athletes with a history of back pain should be targeted with rehabilitation training concentrating on technique, flexibility, and muscle control to withstand the high demands of their sport.

References

Alexander, J. (1977) Scheuermann's disease. A traumatic spondylodystrophy? *Skeletal Radiology* **1**, 209–221.

Badman, B.L., Rechtine, G.R. (2004) Spinal injury considerations in the competitive diver: a case report and review of the literature. *The Spine Journal* **4**, 584–590.

Bahr, R., Andersen, S.O., Løken, S., Fossan, B., Hansen, T., Holme, I. (2004) Low back pain among endurance athletes with and without specific back loading—a cross-sectional survey of cross-country skiers, rowers, orienteerers, and nonathletic controls. *Spine* **29**, 449–454.

Baranto, A., Hellström, M., Nyman, R., Lundin, O., Swärd, L. (2006) Back pain and degenerative abnormalities in the spine of young elite divers: a 5-year follow-up magnetic resonance imaging study. *Knee Surgery Sports Traumatology and Arthroscopy* **14**, 907–914.

Bartolozzi, C., Caramella, D., Zampa, V., Dal Pozzo, G., Tinacci, E., Balducci, F. (1991) The incidence of disk changes in volleyball players. The magnetic resonance findings. *La Radiologica Medica* **82**, 757–760.

Bono, C.M. (2004) Low-back pain in athletes. *Journal of Bone and Joint Surgery (American)* **86**, 382–396.

Goldstein, J.D., Berger, P.E., Windler, G.E., Jackson, D.W. (1991) Spine injuries in gymnasts and swimmers. An epidemiologic investigation. *American Journal of Sports Medicine* **19**, 463–468.

Hellström, M., Jacobsson, B., Swärd, L., Peterson, L. (1990) Radiologic abnormalities of the thoraco-lumbar spine in athletes. *Acta Radiologica* **31**, 127–132.

Hides, J.A., Stokes, M.J., Saide, M., Jull, G.A., Cooper, D.H. (1994) Evidence of lumbar multifidus muscle wasting ipsilateral to symptoms in patients with acute/subacute low back pain. *Spine* **19**, 165–172.

Hides, J.A., Richardson, C.A., Jull, G.A. (1996) Multifidus recovery is not automatic following resolution of acute first episode low back pain. *Spine* **21**, 2763–2769.

Hodges, P.W., Richardson, C.A. (1996) Inefficient muscular stabilization of lumbar spine associated with low back pain. A motor control evaluation of transversus abdominis. *Spine* **21**, 2640–2650.

Jackson, D.W. (1979) Low back pain in young athletes: evaluation of stress reaction and discogenic problems. *American Journal of Sports Medicine* **7**, 364–366.

Jull, G.A., Richardson, C.A. (2000) Motor control problems in patients with spine pain: a new direction for therapeutic exercise. *Journal of Manipulative and Physiological Therapeutics* **23**, 115–117.

Kujala, U.M., Taimela, S., Erkintalo, M., Salminen, J.J., Kaprio, J. (1996) Low-back pain in adolescent athletes. *Medicine and Science in Sports and Exercise* **28**, 165–170.

Lundin, O., Hellström, M., Nilsson, I., Swärd, L. (2001) Back pain and radiological changes in the thoraco-lumbar spine of athletes. A long-term follow-up. *Scandinavian Journal of Medicine and Science in Sports* **11**, 103–109.

O'Sullivan, P.B., Phyty, G.D., Twomey, L.T., Allison, G.T. (1997) Evaluation of specific stabilising exercise in treatment of chronic low back pain with radiological diagnosis of spondylolysis and spondylolisthesis. *Spine* **15**, 2959–2967.

Ranson, C.A., Kerslake, R.W., Burnett, A.F., Batt, M.E., Abdi, S. (2005) Magnetic resonance imaging of the lumbar spine in asymptomatic professional fast bowlers in cricket. *Journal of Bone and Joint Surgery (British)* **87**, 1111–1116.

Sassmannshausen, G., Smith, B.G. (2002) Back pain in the young athlete. *Clinical Sports Medicine* **21**, 121–132.

Swärd, L., Hellström, M., Jacobsson, B., Peterson, L. (1990) Back pain and radiologic changes in the thoraco-lumbar spine of athletes. *Spine* **15**, 124–129.

Swärd, L., Hellström, M., Jacobsson, B., Nyman, R., Peterson, L. (1991) Disc degeneration and associated abnormalities of the spine in elite gymnasts. A magnetic resonance imaging study. *Spine* **16**, 437–443.

Further reading

Adams, M., Bogduk, N., Burton, K., Dolan, P. (2002) *The Biomechanics of Back Pain*. Churchill Livingstone, Edinburgh.

Bogduk, N.L.T. (1997) *Clinical Anatomy of the Lumbar Spine and Sacrum*, 3rd edn. Churchill Livingstone, New York.

Richardson, C., Hodges, P., Hides, J. (2004) *Therapeutic Exercise for Lumbopelvic Stabilization: A Motor Control Approach for the Treatment and Prevention of Low Back Pain*. Churchill Livingstone, Edinburgh.

Chapter 9
Preventing shoulder injuries

Michael R. Krogsgaard[1], Marc R. Safran[2], Peter Rheinlænder and Emilie Cheung[3]

[1] Department of Orthopedic Surgery, Copenhagen University Hospital Bispebjerg, Denmark
[2] Department of Orthopaedic Surgery, Stanford University, Stanford, CA, USA
[3] Department of Orthopaedic Surgery, Clinic for Physiotheraphy, Frederiksberg, Denmark.

Epidemiology of shoulder injuries in sports

Shoulder injuries are common in sports and can be traumatic, microtraumatic, or overuse in origin. Detailed information on the prevention of shoulder injurie is lacking, however. According to a study in the United States, of the general population, shoulder injuries accounted for 8.1% of all sports injuries. Of these, 9.4% precluded participation on at least one occasion, 5.7% precluded participation for at least 1 month, and 10.7% resulted in the participant giving up the sport permanently. Therefore, the potential to prevent shoulder injuries should be optimized, and some chronic overuse-related injuries, as well as acute injuries, may be avoided.

Table 9.1 provides an overview of available epidemiological data on shoulder injuries in sports. Baseball and softball account for the highest percentage of shoulder injuries, relative to other locations in the body, and these tend to be overuse injuries. In the United States, it has been estimated that 18% of all injuries in baseball to people over 6 years of age who play are to the shoulder, second only to elbow injuries. It is estimated that 5.8 shoulder injuries occur per 100 participants a year. In softball 17.4% of all injuries involve the shoulder, making it the most common injury location, with an incidence of 6.4 injuries per 100 participants over a 1-year period. In tennis, the general annual incidence of shoulder pain and injury has been estimated at 2.5 injuries per 100 people playing per year, with 3.3% of all tennis injuries involving the shoulder (#7 of all musculoskeletal injuries in tennis). The prevalence of shoulder pain in competitive junior tennis players was found to be 24% in boys and 35% in girls over a 3-year study. Further, it has been found that 50% of expert players had a history of shoulder pain and 74% of professional male tennis players and 60% of professional female tennis players had shoulder or elbow pain that affected their tennis at some point in the past.

Swimming is another sport where shoulder pain is so prevalent that the term "swimmer's shoulder" has become commonly accepted, though the exact pathology may be argued. It has been shown that the longer one swims, the higher the prevalence of shoulder pain and swimming intensity and distance are most associated with shoulder pain. Studies have shown that the prevalence of shoulder pain increases with age. In a study of age group national level competitive swimmers, it was found that 11% of male and 9.4% of female competitive swimmers, aged 13–14 years had current shoulder pain that interfered with their training, while 21% of male and 25.5% of female competitive swimmers aged 15–16 years had pain at the time of questioning that interfered with their swimming, and 17.7% of male and 35% of female swimmers with an average age of 19 years had shoulder pain limiting their swimming practice and competition.

Sports Injury Prevention, 1st edition. Edited by R. Bahr and L. Engebretsen Published 2009 by Blackwell Publishing
ISBN: 9781405162449

Table 9.1 Risk of shoulder pain in different sports. The numbers reported are estimates based on the studies available.

Sport	Competition incidence[1]	Training incidence[1]	Rank[2]	Comments
Team sports				
Water polo	3.40** ♂		# 1	College players
	8.09** ♀			
Volleyball	0.32* ♀	0.33* ♀	# 4	College players
	0.2 ♀/♂		# 5 overall	Dutch 2nd and 3rd divisions; did
			# 2 overuse injury	not report match versus practice shoulder injury rate
Baseball	0.81* ♂	0.37* ♂	# 1	College players
Softball	0.24* ♀	0.30* ♀	# 5	
American football	3.92* ♂	1.63* ♂	# 3	College athletes
Lacrosse	1.56* ♂	0.23* ♂	# 5	College athletes
Ice hockey	3.32* ♂	3.92* ♂	# 3	College athletes
	1.58* ♀	3.92* ♀		
Individual sports				
Tennis	5.18** ♀		# 4 in women's tennis,	College athletes
	7.22** ♂		# 1 in men's	
	3.89** ♀			
	1.56 ** ♂			High school athletes
	9.9 ** ♂		# 3	National championships for 15–18 years old
	18.4 ** ♂		# 1	National championships (girls 15–16 years old, boys 15–18 years old)
	19.0 ** ♀			
Swimming	6.55 ** ♂		# 1	College swimmers
	21.05** ♀			
Wrestling	3.73* ♂	0.47* ♂	# 3	College athletes

[1]Incidence is reported for adult, competitive athletes as the number of injuries per 1000 hours of training and competition or *per 1000 athletic exposures or **per 100 participant years.
[2]Rank indicates the relative rank of shoulder injuries within the sport in question.

Even more striking is the prevalence of shoulder pain, current or past, in these swimmers; 55% of male and 38% of female national age group swimmers (13–14 years old) had a current or past history of shoulder pain, whereas 67% of male and 64% of female competitive swimmers had a current or past history of shoulder pain that interfered with their swimming, and 71% of male and 75% of female national team swimmers had pain, currently or in the past, that interfered with their swimming. Collegiate and master swimmers have been reported to have a 50% prevalence of shoulder pain that lasted more than 3 weeks.

Water polo is a sport that combines swimming and throwing, particularly throwing without the benefit of the full kinetic chain, which may account for a high prevalence of shoulder pain.

Ice hockey and American football are the next two sports with very high incidences of shoulder injuries, and these tend to be traumatic in origin — contact with the ground (ice, turf, or grass) or boards (hockey) or opponent. In football, shoulder injury was the fourth most common injury at the National Football League combines (the preparticipation examinations), where 50% of the players had a history of shoulder injury and there was an average of 1.3 shoulder injuries reported per player. Acromioclavicular joint injury was most prevalent (41%), with anterior instability (20%), rotator cuff injury (12%), clavicle fracture (4%), and posterior shoulder instability (4%), being the other common injuries reported. In a 14-year study of the prevalence of injury at the NFL combines, acromioclavicular joint injury was the fifth most commonly reported injury (15.7 per 100 players) and shoulder instability was the ninth most prevalent injury (9.7 per 100 players).

Sports like body building and weightlifting may cause repetitive microtraumatic injury of the acromioclavicular joint, resulting in osteolysis of the distal clavicle (weight lifter's shoulder) with prevalence estimated at 27%.

Key risk factors: how to identify athletes at risk

Scientifically, little is known about the factors that lead to the majority of injuries in the shoulder. Consequently, the description of key risk factors is based, to some extent, on theoretical assumptions.

Intrinsic factors and extrinsic factors both contribute to overuse injuries, and to a limited extent, acute injuries. The intrinsic factors refer to growth and anatomic alignment, which are not very easy to control, but also include the muscle-tendon unit, balance, flexibility, ligamentous laxity, conditioning and anatomic variations (Table 9.2). The strength and flexibility of tissues and potential for adaptation to external loads are also dependent on age and probably gender. In terms of extrinsic factors: training errors, including throwing mechanics, overuse, environment, and equipment play a significant role (Table 9.2).

Age

Overload problems are more common with increasing age, for example, the incidence of shoulder pain in baseball players is 0.7% in youth, 12.7% in college players, and 13.9% in professionals. On the other hand young baseball players are more likely

Table 9.2 Internal and external factors for shoulder injury in different sports. The numbers reported are average estimates based on the studies available.

Risk factor	Relative risk[1]	Evidence[2]	Comments
Internal risk factors			
Previous injury	NA	0	
Age	NA	+	Overuse, such as length of time participating may be a confounding factor
Gender	NA	0	
Posterior capsular tightness	NA	+	Cadaveric, biomechanical data
Crowding of the coracoacromial arch	NA	+	
Weakness of scapular stabilizers and core	NA	0	(Su et al., 2004; Kibler & Safran, 2005; Laudner et al., 2006; Tripp et al., 2007)
Ligamentous laxity	NA	+	Conflicting results
External risk factors			
Mechanics of sports	NA	+	
bases	NA	+	Type of sliding Break-away bases
Position	1.2–1.52	++	
Overuse	NA		
Number of pitches thrown	1.77–3.29	++	
Type of pitch	1.52–1.77	+	
Years weight lifting	NA	+	
Hours swimming	NA	++	

[1]Relative risk indicates the increased risk of injury to an individual with this risk factor relative to an individual who does not have this characteristic. A relative risk of 1.2× means that the risk of injury is 20% higher for an individual with this characteristic. NA: Not available.

[2]Evidence indicates the level of scientific evidence for this factor being a risk factor for ankle sprains: ++ — convincing evidence from high-quality studies with consistent results; + — evidence from lesser quality studies or mixed results; 0 — expert opinion without scientific evidence. NA: Not available.

to have upper extremity injury. The length of time while participating may also be a confounding factor, as seen in weight lifting and swimming, where a cumulative effect over the years of overuse seems to be a reason for injury.

Some age-related anatomical variations are also risk factors. For example, growth-plate-related problems in the proximal humerus of young baseball players, also known as "Little Leaguers Shoulder," have been associated with the repetitive action of throwing. The forces caused by the repetitive throwing cause fragmentation and avulsion of the growth plate, resulting in shoulder pain. Improper pitching mechanics have also been identified as a concomitant risk factor for development of this condition. Thus, both intrinsic factors, such as the growth plate being the weakest link in the musculoskeletal system, combined with overuse and improper pitching mechanics, which are extrinsic forces, may coexist to produce injury.

Gender

There are no available data to identify gender as an independent risk factor for shoulder problems.

Anatomical factors

Overcrowding of the subacromial space, for example, if the acromion has a hooked shape or if the acromioclavicular joint is degenerated and hypertrophic, protruding into the subacromial space, is a risk factor for outlet impingement (pinching of the rotator cuff between the bones of the humerus and acromion). The precise contribution of this factor in athletes is difficult to weigh, as many competitive conditions that can cause impingement may be present. For instance, overhead athletes, such as those involved in baseball, swimming, water polo, and tennis, often suffer from not only tendinopathy or strains of the rotator cuff as a result of outlet impingement, but also because of cumulative tensile overload, instability, as well as with internal impingement (pinching of the rotator cuff between the greater tuberosity of the humerus and the postero-superior glenoid).

Overhead athletes, including volleyball players, baseball players, and tennis players not only have a relatively high risk of suprascapular nerve injury, which may be related to posterior capsular tightness of the shoulder, but also may be affected by a narrow suprascapular notch or bony change of the transverse scapular ligament. Posterior capsular tightness of the shoulder has also been implicated in other problems such as internal impingement and SLAP lesions (an injury to the **s**uperior **l**abrum, **a**nterior and **p**osterior to the biceps tendon anchor/attachment—essentially, an injury to the upper part of the fibrocartilage rim that surrounds the socket of the shoulder), as well as secondary impingement.

Passive stability

There is conflicting evidence regarding glenohumeral laxity as a risk factor for shoulder injury or pain. About 15% have an in born laxity (known as multidirectional), but anterior laxity is often seen in overhead athletes due to chronic overload. Excessive repetitive external rotation during the overhead motion places tremendous stress on the anterior capsular and ligamentous structures, causing microtrauma. Instability results when the dynamic stabilizers, such as the rotator cuff and periscapular muscles, fatigue with repeated activity. Hence anterior glenohumeral translation occurs, with subsequent development of instability. Some sports, like swimming, select for individuals who have inherent ligamentous laxity about the shoulder, as proper swimming mechanics require extreme range of shoulder motion. With repetitive motion, such as prolonged swimming, the muscles that provide dynamic stability to the shoulder may fatigue, resulting in microinstability. The rotator cuff fatigues as a result of having to work harder to maintain glenohumeral stability (due to the lax ligaments) and overuse from repeated activity (swim strokes). The rotator cuff fatigue leads to decreased ability to maintain the humeral head within the glenoid. As a result of this subtle instability, secondary impingement of the rotator cuff anterosuperiorly against the coracoacromial arch during forward flexion may occur, causing bursitis, tendinitis, or even undersurface tearing. Thus, in some sports, rotator cuff damage may be the result of overuse, pain from muscles fatiguing while trying to provide stability to a shoulder with ligamentous laxity as well as due to excessive translation of the humeral head resulting in impingement. This latter cause of impingement occurs, as the rotator cuff becomes pinched between the humeral head and coracoacromial arch as a result of the loss of containment of the humeral head in the center of the glenoid due to loss of strength with the fatigued rotator cuff muscles. Glenohumeral laxity may well be a risk factor for these conditions, but the development of clinical symptoms is also caused by other factors, such as fatigue of the rotator cuff muscles.

A condition known as "internal impingement" of the rotator cuff also occurs as a result of the altered kinematics in the injured shoulder of an overhead athlete. This occurs as the humeral head translates anteriorly with shoulder abduction and external rotation. There is internal impingement of the rotator cuff on the posterior superior region of the glenoid labrum. Concomitant posterior capsular contractures caused by repetitive stress may further exacerbate the impingement. This is also known as glenohumeral internal rotational deficit, or GIRD. Athletes typically present with decreased throwing effectiveness and pain, or a "dead arm."

Dynamic instability

It is well described that athletes with shoulder pain have weakness of the scapula stabilizing muscles (serratus anterior and trapezius) and bad core stability. It is generally assumed that scapulothoracic instability is a risk factor for shoulder pain, including dynamic (secondary) impingement. On the other hand it has been shown that pain causes significant changes in muscular coordination by inhibiting muscular activity, so it is still an open question which risk factor came first.

External factors: exposure to load

The total exposure to load (years of weight lifting, hours of swimming) is a risk factor for degenerative and inflammatory conditions. For example, weight lifter's shoulder is a problem of the distal clavicle, where there is osteolysis or bony resorption. The pathophysiology is unknown, but felt to be due to microtraumatic overuse, resulting in a stress reaction of the acromioclavicular joint. Weight lifting, such as doing the bench press or the clean and jerk, increases the load on the acromioclavicular joint. Whereas rest helps resolve the symptoms, return to weight lifting will result in recurrence of symptoms.

Also, a high number of pitches is associated with risk for shoulder symptoms. The relative risk in kids is 1.77 if more than 100 pitches are performed per game and 3.29 if more than 800 pitches are done within a season. The type of pitch is also a risk factor with a relative risk of 1.52 for curve ball and 1.77 for slider. The risk for shoulder problems is dependent on player position. In baseball, pitchers are at the highest risk, and in American football, quarterbacks have a relative risk of 1.52 and defensive backs of 1.2 for shoulder problems. Also, the injury pattern varies, as anterior shoulder instability is common in American football defensive players and posterior instability and rotator cuff injury is seen in linemen.

Mechanics of sports

There are well-described mechanical factors that are of significant importance for the risk of traumatic injury in baseball. Sliding with the head first as well as dive backs cause more shoulder injuries than other techniques. The power in the collision with the base is correlated to the severity of injury, and the use of breakaway bases instead of traditional solid bases reduces this power and the risk for injury.

Identifying athletes at risk of injury

Screening athletes for risk of shoulder problems can be done at the beginning of or at any time during the season. The reason to repeat the screening at intervals is that mismatch in muscle coordination may develop during training, even though it was not present at the start of the season. For instance, it has been shown there is a slowing in conduction velocity of the suprascapular nerve in baseball pitchers as the season progresses, though the players remained asymptomatic. Further, it has been shown, that volleyball players with shoulder pain have a depressed and lateralized scapula and tightness of the posterior capsule and posterior muscles (Kugler et al., 1996). It can, of course, be questioned whether these changes are the cause of pain or the result of pain.

Table 9.3 Screening tests to identify risk factors for shoulder symptoms in athletes.

Test	Comments
Inspection of stature	An increased thoracic kyphosis leads to a downward-anterior position of the acromion, which reduces the subacromial space and increases risk of impingement. Cervical lordosis increases posterior compression and the risk of compression to the C5 and C6 nerve roots, and may lead to referred pain in the shoulder region (Figure 9.6).
Inspection of resting position of the arm	Protrusion of more than 1/3rd of the humeral head anterior to the acromion stresses the anterior shoulder capsule and may be caused by a tight posterior capsule or contract outward rotating muscles. Inward rotation of the arm is caused by dominant pectoralis major and minor and latissimus dorsi muscles and reduces the subacromial space, increasing risk of impingement.
Inspection of the resting scapula	Winging as well as when the superior, medial corner is more lateral than the inferior, reduces the subacromial space, increasing risk of impingement.
Inspection of the moving scapula	If the inferior corner of scapula does not reach the mid-axillary line during full flexion of the arm, the acromion is not elevated sufficiently during motion, increasing the risk of impingement. If winging occurs early during arm push-ups there is mismatch in muscular coordination. If it occurs late during repeated push-ups, there is weakness of some of the scapular stabilizing muscles.
Testing glenohumeral laxity	Objective laxity is tested by the sulcus test, the load and shift test, and the posterior stability test. Subjective laxity is tested by the apprehension and relocation tests. Difference in laxity between the two sides indicate pathology and risk of secondary impingement.
Testing scapular dynamic stability (Box 9.1)	Weakness increases risk of overuse problems.
Testing functional shoulder stability with the arm in various, relevant positions. Investigator tries to break the position to identify weakness	Weakness increases risk of impingement and overuse problems.

Even though there are no good data available regarding which conditions that increase the risk for shoulder problems, previous injury and symptoms at present are probably high ranking risk factors that call for a thorough test of possible dysfunctions, as described in Table 9.3. Athletes with an increased laxity in the glenohumeral joint (demonstrated by a sulcus sign) are theoretically at risk of injury and should also be tested for dysfunctions, but there is no proof that laxity per se in a well-trained individual without dysfunctions or "black holes" is a risk factor.

In players without symptoms or recent injury, the screening concentrates on identifying traditional dysfunctions, as described by Caldwell et al. (2007). In one-arm dominant sports these dysfunctions usually appear in the dominant arm, and the two shoulders should always be compared. Even though there is only little scientific evidence on whether dysfunctions cause shoulder symptoms and overload injuries or that identification and correction of dysfunctions can prevent overload problems, this strategy is generally accepted.

The contents of a *screening* examination are listed in Table 9.3. A description of the various tests can be found in other textbooks. Tests for scapular stability are shown in Box 9.1.

Take-home message

Though, as of yet there is not much scientific proof that injuries can be predicted based on physical examination or prevented by correcting problems identified on examination, there is hope that correcting some of the above physical examination findings may prevent overuse injuries and may enable the shoulder to sustain traumatic incidents. Athletes should be screened for dysfunctions, as well at the beginning of the season as during the season. Athletes with symptoms or earlier injury are probably at special risk. Abnormalities that are identified during screening should be corrected

> **Box 9.1 Low and high load tests for assessment of scapular stability**
>
> **Low load test for scapular stability**
> The athlete is standing on all four extremities with the scapula held stable, while rocking forward and backward, as well as from side to side without winging of the scapula.
>
> **Side bridge as a dynamic stability test of the scapula muscles**
> The athlete is lying on one side on his elbow, while holding his shoulder, hip, knee, and ankle in line (= maintaining core stability). He lifts his body from the floor and keeps his scapula stable without any winging.
>
> **Wall-press test for scapular stability**
> The feet are pressed against the wall. The lumbar spine must be kept neutral. Bend one knee and flex the hip to 120°, followed by a 15° extension of the hip. The feet can be positioned at various heights on the wall. Progression is pictured from upper left to lower right.

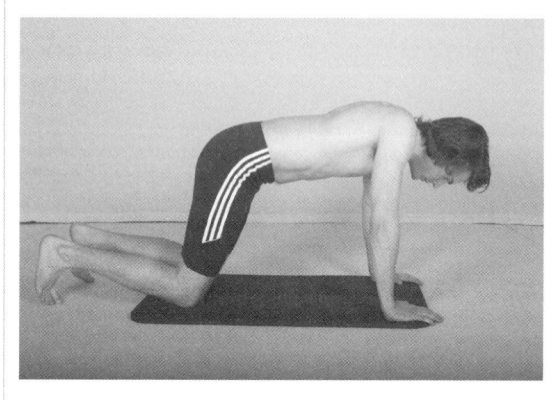

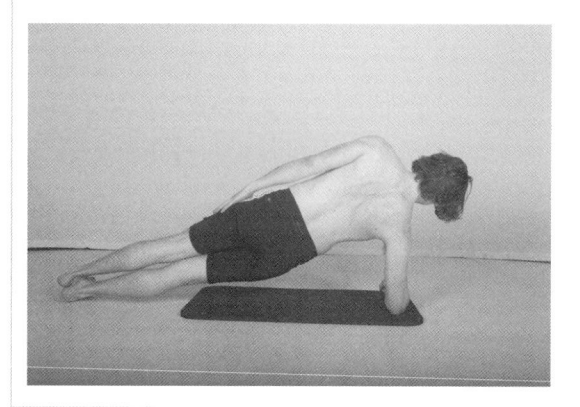

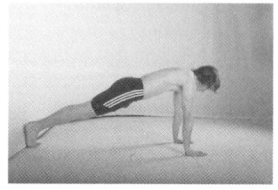

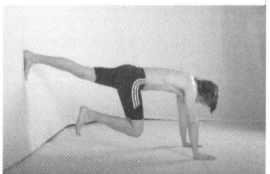

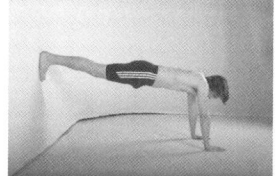

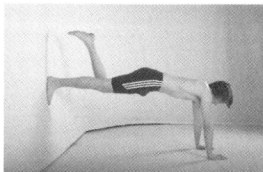

prior to participation with the intention of preventing injury and shoulder symptoms.

Injury mechanisms

Because the shoulder has more motion than any other joint in the body, it has little bony constraint to allow for this motion, and the stability and motion is primarily controlled by muscles and soft tissues. Traumatic and overuse injuries to the shoulder can therefore damage a large number of different structures in and around the shoulder. Traumatic injuries can be divided into direct and indirect injuries, depending on according to the position of the arm and the applied force.

Direct traumatic injuries

Direct injuries are falls or blows directly on the shoulder, most often on the lateral side or the front. In most cases, there is a contusion of the soft tissues

enormous compression force between the opponent and the fence. A similar compression occurs in American football when being tackled.

The resulting injury depends on the exact direction of the force and the anatomical structure that is subject to the trauma. If the acromion is hit in a skeletally mature athlete, an injury to the acromioclavicular joint is most likely, if the clavicle is hit a clavicular fracture is likely, and if the upper arm is hit, a proximal humerus fracture is likely to occur. In the older athlete, fracture of the clavicle or the humerus is more likely to happen than dislocation of the acromioclavicular joint, as the bone becomes weaker with age. Acromioclavicular and sternoclavicular joint injury is the result of a lateral force. The brachial nerve plexus can be stretched by a direct blow to the superior side of the shoulder, anterior or posterior sudden, forceful pushes to the shoulder or pulls of the arm, and may lead to a "burner," that is, diffuse pain of the shoulder and arm, caused by injury of one or several nerves, though usually the upper trunk (Figure 9.2). This typically happens if a player uses the shoulder to butt other players.

Indirect traumatic injuries

Indirect injuries are caused by transmission of force through the arm. Fall on an outstretched, flexed arm may result in a Bankart-like lesion of the posterior capsule, but most often in acromioclavicular joint damage, as the posterior shoulder capsule is very tight and transmits the force to the scapula. The injury after fall on an outstretched, abducted arm depends on the amount of abduction: below horizontal a SLAP lesion can occur, above horizontal a Bankart lesion/dislocation is more likely (where the labral or cartilage rim injury is in the anterior lower quarter of the socket). Fall on extended arm results in a SLAP or Bankart lesion or an acromioclavicular-joint lesion. A force that involves rotation of the arm, that is, blocking a throw or falling on a slightly abducted/outwardly rotated arm with flexed elbow applies tremendous force on the rotator cuff and the accelerating muscles. This can be an eccentric or a concentric type of load and result in a muscle/tendon sprain, rupture of a tendon, avulsion of a tendon, or fracture

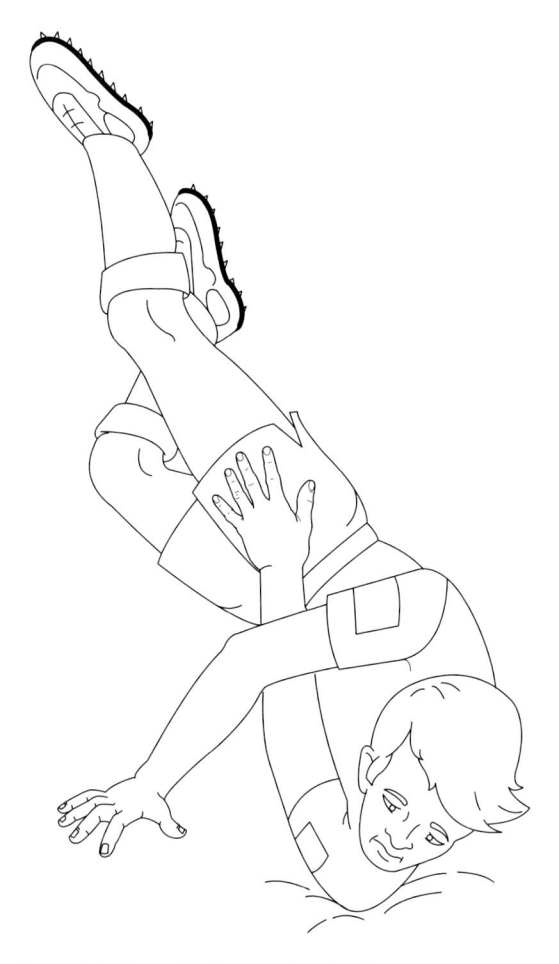

Figure 9.1. Typical injury mechanism for acromioclavicular joint dislocation: fall directly on the lateral side of the shoulder

around the shoulder or a hematoma. More severe trauma may result in a clavicle fracture, a contusion or dislocation of the acromioclavicular joint (Figure 9.1) or fractures of the upper humerus or (rarely) the glenoid. Falls are common in cycling (when going over the handle bars) and skiing. Blows are common in American football (i.e., when a player gets low and uses the shoulder to take an opponent or gets tackled and lands on their shoulder) and ice hockey (when the player hits an opponent or the boards with the shoulder). Compression happens in ice hockey, when the player skates alongside the boards and is hit by an opponent. Because of the high velocity, the player is subjected to an

142 Chapter 9

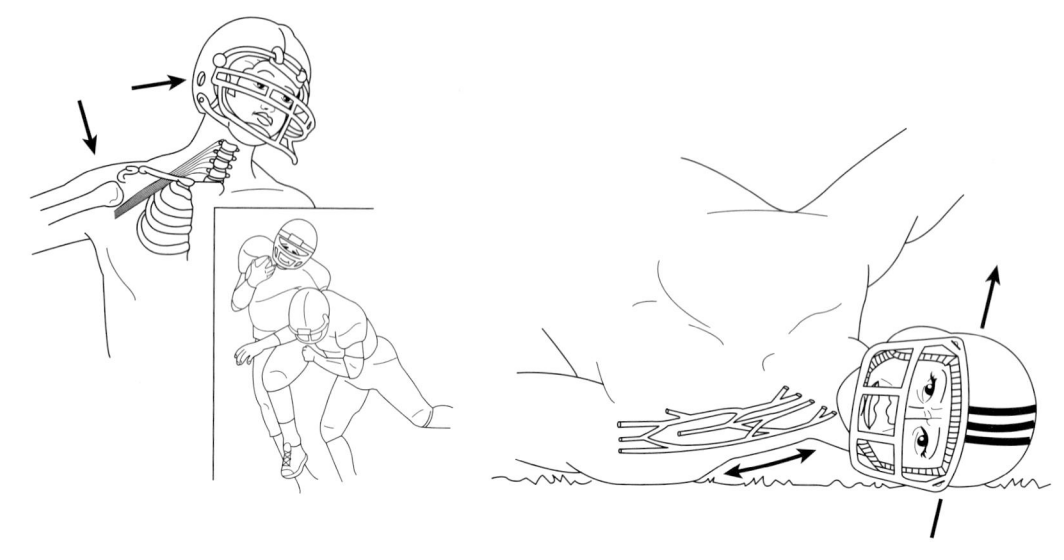

Figure 9.2. Typical injury mechanisms for "burners:" stretching of the brachial nerve plexus

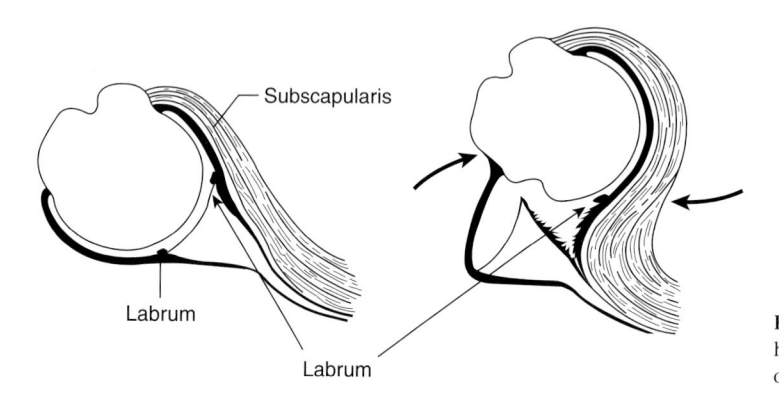

Figure 9.3. Dislocation of the humeral head results in a Bankart lesion (avulsion of the labrum and the glenohumeral ligaments from the anterior glenoid)

at the site of insertion. If the arm is positioned behind the shoulder joint, blocking can result in an anterior translation of the humeral head and an injury of the anterior structures of the glenohumeral joint, typically a Bankart lesion (Figure 9.3). This injury mechanism is quite common in body building/strength training as a result of an extreme extension of the arms during bench press or downward pulls. If the arms are extended to more than 0° during these exercises (i.e., if the arms are moved behind the shoulder joint), there is extreme tension on the anterior structures of the glenohumeral joint, in particular the labrum and glenohumeral ligaments. If the internal rotators of the arm fail to resist the load, this may cause a Bankart or SLAP lesion or stretching of the anterior capsule. Incidents that make a sudden, powerful inward rotation of the arm combined with flexion of the elbow necessary, if to avoid an object from hitting the head, can rupture the lateral portion of the coracohumeral ligament (which covers the biceps groove between the lesser and greater tubercles and holds the biceps tendon in the groove) as well as the upper part of the subscapularis tendon insertion on the lesser tubercle. This results in a biceps tendon dislocation or subluxation.

It is the least strong tissue that is damaged during trauma. In children, the epiphyseal growth plates and bones are soft, and avulsions of the bony attachment of a ligament or capsule rather than rupture of the soft tissue is more likely to happen than in adults with stronger bones. Also epiphysiolysis of the greater tubercle or the neck of the humerus can happen. In young and middle-aged athletes, the soft tissue is usually the weakest. In athletes above 60 years the natural decrease in bone mineral content makes fractures and avulsions more likely to happen, but tendons—in particular the rotator cuff tendons and the long head of biceps—also weaken with age, and ruptures can happen after minor trauma or almost spontaneously, such as during tennis or badminton.

Overuse injuries

Overuse injuries can be caused by a repeated, powerful force to a structure through sports (*extrinsic factors*). In most cases this is the result of an increase in training intensity, introduction of a new technique, or new equipment, etc. The load on soft tissue structures exceeds capacity of the tissue, leading to inflammation and pain. This acute condition is easily reversible, if the load is adjusted to the capacity.

Weight lifting applies enormous forces through the acromioclavicular joint, and swimming applies a huge number of rotations in the acromioclavicular joint, both mechanisms resulting in inflammation and gradually degenerative disease in the acromioclavicular joint.

A very specific injury develops because the best performance in throwing is achieved if the shoulder is cocked, that is, positioned in full abduction and external rotation (Figure 9.4). This motion is naturally stopped by collision between the under-surface of the supra- and infraspinatus tendons and the superior labrum. Repeated collisions with large force result in fraying of both structures and stretching of the inferior glenohumeral ligaments (resulting in glenohumeral instability and secondary impingement) (Figure 9.5).

It is not obvious that repeated use of the rotator cuff in forceful tasks during sports results in wear of the rotator cuff/long head of biceps. Such changes may more likely be caused by repeated minor traumas with smaller, partial ruptures.

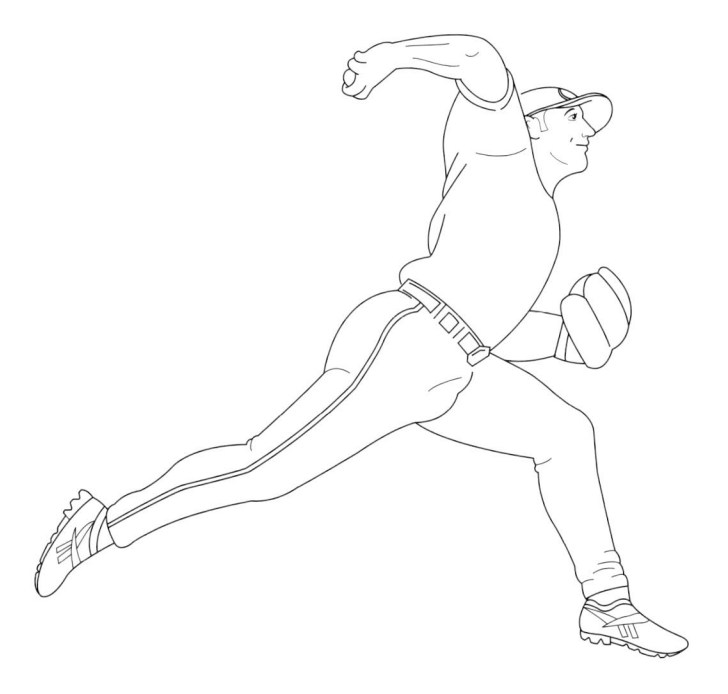

Figure 9.4. In throwing the arm is taken into full abduction and outwards rotation, which result in internal impingement and applies enormous stress to the anterior shoulder capsule

(a) (b) (c)

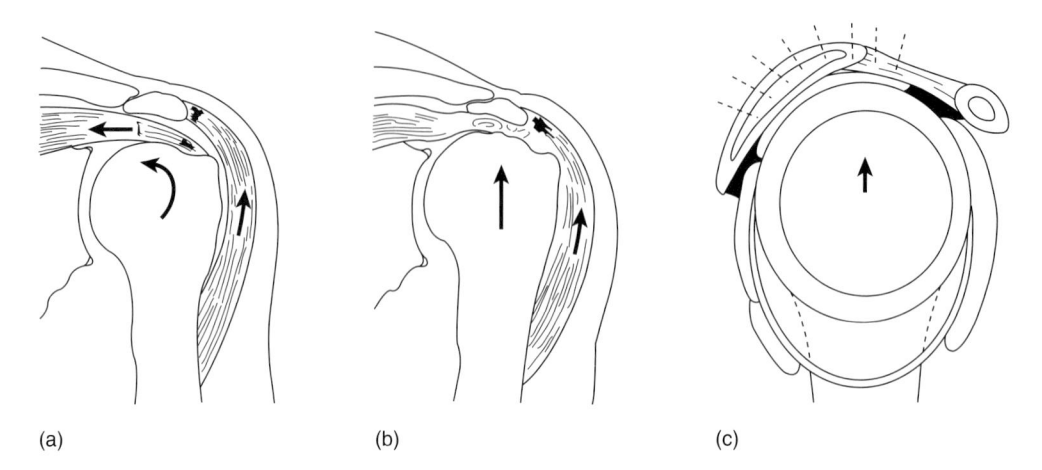

Figure 9.5. Mechanism of secondary impingement: the humeral head is elevated and the supraspinatus tendon is compressed (a) Natural situation where the rotator cuff muscles and the passive stabilizers keep the humeral head centered in the glenoid during motion and counteract the proximal pull of the deltoid muscle, allowing for shoulder rotation. (b) and (c) If the dynamic and passive stabilizers of the humeral head fails (due to rotator cuff fatigue), the deltoid muscle pulls the humeral head proximally, resulting in impingement of the rotator cuff between the humeral head and acromion.

Overuse injuries can also be caused by preexisting, less optimal conditions, or by dyscoordination/lack of dynamic stability in the shoulder and thoracoscapular junction (*intrinsic factors*). Laxity of the glenohumeral joint (which is seen in 10% of the population, represented as a large sulcus sign) is compensated for by activation of the rotator cuff muscles, when the athlete is using the arm in activities, which are dependent on stability. If these muscles are not strong enough for this work, then either the muscles are overused (resulting in tendonitis and tendinosis of the tendons and muscle pain) or the humeral head is not positioned correctly during the activity (resulting in painful stretching of the glenohumeral ligaments and the capsule). The thoracoscapular junction is the base of the arm. Insufficient stability of this is caused by relative weakness of the rhomboids and serratus anterior (pressing the scapula against the thoracic wall), resulting in compensating, painful dysfunctions in other muscles. Dyscoordination of the scapula in throwing or overhead activities is most often caused by weakness or fatigue of serratus anterior and trapezius—both muscles are responsible for the elevation of acromion during overhead activities, and if this motion is delayed or insufficient, the acromion presses against the humeral head, resulting in impingement of the supraspinatus tendon and inflammation of the subacromial bursa (Figure 9.5). Overuse injuries caused by these preexisting conditions are seen in throwing sports (repeated powerful activities to the extreme ranges of motion), swimming (repeated activities), weight lifting (powerful activities), and body building (powerful activities and a risk that only the accelerating muscles are body built).

Pain

Pain in the shoulder has great influence on the function of muscles. The activity of the agonist for the painful motion is reduced under dynamic conditions, probably as a reflex-like reaction, and in some cases the antagonist activity is increased. Also, motion patterns are changed to avoid pain. This happens in any painful condition, either after a trauma or during overload, leading in itself to dyscoordination. In this way, a self-perpetuating process may be initiated.

Protective equipment

The use of protective equipment can in some cases cause injury. It is obvious that if a hard shoulder protector is used by a player to butt others, it may give rise to traumatic injuries on other players. Protective devices may also give the athlete a sense of security, prompting them to play more aggressively, leading to injury to themselves and others.

Strangely, the use of wrist guards by snowboarders is connected to an (insignificant) increase of injury in elbow and shoulder (Hagel et al., 2005), but the injury mechanism is unknown.

Identifying risks in the training and competition program

In sports with a season, the athletes may be less fit at the beginning of the season. The smaller muscles (including the rotator cuff muscles) are at higher risk than the larger muscles to lose strength. A mismatch between the shoulder muscles can often be identified as described earlier, but smaller changes, that become important with 50 or 100 repetitions, may be difficult to demonstrate clinically. For example, the rotator cuff muscles may fatigue after 25 hard throws, whereas the larger muscles can easily do 100. This mismatch may also occur later during the season, because the larger muscles adapt more easily to increasing load. Thoracic kyphosis may increase as the shoulders rotate anterior and inward due to strong latissimus and pectoralis major muscles, and the scapula is rotated downward due to the pectoralis minor muscle, both decreasing the subacromial space and increasing the risk of impingement.

It is therefore essential that the training program contains a balanced amount of exercises all through the season. It is not uncommon to concentrate on maximum efforts in function (strength) and coordination, and only do very demanding training. This will leave the weaker and smaller muscles behind. Warm-up, which should start every training session, activates all structures (muscles, tendons, ligaments, joints) as well as the psyche (concentration and awareness, which should not be neglected). The structures become ready for maximum work, and the maximum effort training is suitable after warm-up. All athletes know that after having performed maximum training for a while, either some structures fatigue or the athlete loses concentration and awareness. Instead of ending training abruptly from the heavy exercises, lighter and easier activities, that all structures and the psyche can participate in, should complete the training session. In this way, no structure is lost

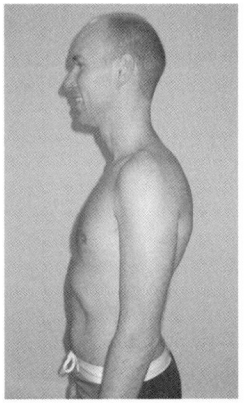

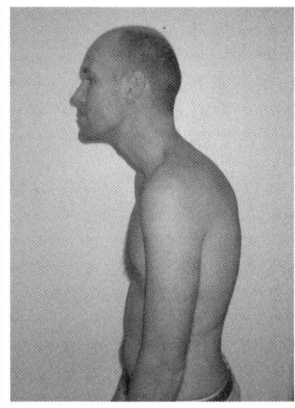

Figure 9.6. Different statures. Left: Normal stature. Right: Extended thoracic kyphosis and protracted shoulder, increased lordosis of the cervical spine

due to fatigue. Also, if just one structure is not participating, the heavy exercises should not be continued. It is common to continue until complete fatigue, but this leads to a high risk of losing the weaker structures.

That mismatch between muscle groups is common was shown in a project, where 2000 m swimmers were tested for scapular stability by wall-push ups at several swimming distances. After 500 m 36% had winging of scapula, after 1000 m this was seen in 79%, and after 1500 m in 93%.

Even though we do not walk on our shoulders, turf changes may affect the risk for shoulder injury. In tennis, the speed and force of the ball changes from slow and weak on the relatively soft outdoor ground, particularly clay surface, to fast and forceful on hard indoor courts. This increases the need for strength, fast reaction, precision, and coordination markedly, and if the player has not prepared for this through training, overuse injury and traumatic lesions to muscles, tendons, etc. may occur. This is naturally also the case if equipment is changed, for instance, if tension of the strings in the racket is changed or another type of tennis ball is used.

Preventive measures

In theory, there are many ways to prevent traumatic and non-traumatic shoulder injuries. Some

Table 9.4 Injury prevention matrix applied to shoulder injury prevention: potential measures to prevent injuries.

	Pretrauma	Trauma	Post-trauma
Athlete	Assure glenohumeral and thoracoscapular stability Avoid "black holes" in muscular performance Throwing technique Caution if shoulder is painful Prevent falls: only sport within your own limitations, avoid risks (off piste, skiing in bad snow/weather conditions) Prevent huddling (bicycling)	Training status Falling techniques Reduce and restructure training if shoulder is symptomatic Avoid loading of the arm, while it is behind the shoulder	Rehabilitation
Surroundings	Playing rules (forbid body checking, tearing, or blocking of arm)	Breakaway bases Soft fences	Emergency medical coverage Physiotherapist instruction
Equipment	Caution if equipment is changed (other characteristics)	Shoulder pads Neck roll	First aid equipment

of these are listed in Table 9.4. Unfortunately, only one of these methods has been investigated for effectiveness.

Preventing traumatic injury

Shoulder pads can theoretically spread the force from an impact over a large area of the body and absorb energy (just like a bicycle helmet). There are no studies that prove that this can actually reduce the number or severity of shoulder injuries caused by direct blows, and hard shoulder pads have the drawback that they can hurt other players, particularly if they are used to butt others. In American football, shoulder pads protect the shoulder, dissipating the forces that would otherwise be placed on the acromioclavicular joint or the sternoclavicular joint during an axial load. Proper falling mechanics can also be taught to potentially lessen the direct impact placed across the shoulder joint by learning to roll when landing from a fall, rather than landing directly on the shoulder. Cervical orthoses are used to prevent injury to the neck and the brachial plexus ("burners"). In a laboratory setting they can be shown to reduce hyperextension of the neck, but lateral bending—which is assumed to be a major cause of nerve injury—is not consistently reduced, and the clinical relevance remains to be proven.

Head-first and diveback sliding techniques in baseball and softball can result in upper extremity injuries. But changing of techniques (e.g., banning sliding or forbidding head-first/diveback sliding) is impractical and unsatisfactory to players, and instructional courses regarding injury prevention have proved ineffective (players did not attend) (Janda, 2003). The only studies on injury prevention in softball are the breakaway base studies (Janda et al., 1988; Pollack et al., 2005).

Injury prevention strategies like protective equipment, rule changes, preseason and season prevention interventions, safety measures, better coaching, education and a social awareness have been recommended to reduce sports injuries in children (Demorest & Landry, 2003), but none of these strategies have been shown to be effective.

It has been suggested that extrinsic factors may be positively modified to reduce collision injuries and falls by using deformable walls and padded back stops as well as maintaining fields appropriately, however this has not been supported in the literature. Another statement modifying intrinsic risk factors, such as better coaching techniques as well as stretching and conditioning programs have been purported to benefit players in the prevention of their injuries, though again, this has not been objectively supported in the literature.

It has been suggested, that injuries from skiing and snowboarding can be prevented by "interventions in education and technique, conditioning and equipment and environment" (Kocher et al., 1998), but this remains to be proven. Koehle et al. (2002) states that skiing injuries to the upper extremity can be prevented by proper poling techniques and avoidance of non-detachable ski pole retention devices, as well as through specific programs focused on techniques to prevent falls. A positive effect of these interventions on injury risk remains to be proven, though. Neither traditional ski instruction nor preseason conditioning has demonstrated any positive effect (Koehle et al., 2002).

Theoretically it would to prevent some traumatic injuries if the athlete only did sports within the limits of his/her personal qualifications or physical condition, and avoided risky situations (like skiing off piste, skiing in bad weather conditions, huddling in bicycling, etc.). Also the rules can be used to prevent injury, for example, by forbidding body checking, tearing, or blocking of the arm.

Preventing overuse injuries

The thrower's paradox is that functional stability is a key basis for performance, while at the same time performance is dependent of full mobility. Therefore stability cannot be achieved by tightness, but relies mainly on muscular coordination and strength.

To some extent the training programs are the same for preventing overuse shoulder injuries and for treating symptomatic shoulders. The strategy is also the same: training should always address all structures and all functions (strength, stability, flexibility, coordination, core stability). In addition, the athlete is tested for possible risk factors (as described earlier) and the standard training program is adapted individually to compensate for "black holes." In addition, when treating symptomatic shoulders, the physiotherapist has knowledge of the condition of the tissues that suffer, and must modify the programs further in relation to this.

The standard training program will typically contain the elements listed in Table 9.5. Traditional body building of muscles that are used to create power is often not necessary, as strengthening of these muscles often follows from the specific sports activities.

The strength of the rotator cuff muscles is trained either with a rubber band (which is very handy, as it can be brought everywhere) or weights. The athlete should mix power training (with sufficient weight, that only 6–10 repetitions leads to fatigue)

Table 9.5 Standard shoulder training program.

Prophylactic training of stabilizing muscles:

- Glenohumeral stability: the rotator cuff muscles
- Thoracoscapular stability: the serratus anterior and trapezius musles
- Training of coordination
- Training of thoracic extension
- Training of the rest of the kinetic chain (core stability, knee placing training, etc.)

Stretching to prevent tightness of:
- The posterior capsule
- The rhomboid muscles
- The latissimus dorsi muscle
- The pectoralis minor muscle

and endurance training (less load, where the athlete can perform 20–25 repetitions). The specific exercises are shown in Box 9.2.

Serratus anterior and trapezius are the muscles that lift scapula during abduction, flexion, and throwing, and they are often overruled by, for example, the levator scapula muscle. The trapezius should be trained in order to maintain scapular stability and mid-thoracic stability of the spine. The serratus anterior muscle can be trained with side bridge and wall-press exercises as well. The serratus anterior and trapezius muscles in addition to the other scapular stabilizers are trained with side bridge exercises.

Balancing a fit-ball or a racket are two of the most demanding exercises for coordination. Thoracic extension is trained by leaning back over the back of a chair or laying on the back on a fit-ball. Just like it is much more difficult to manipulate a heavy load if you are standing in loose sand, it is difficult to make a powerful throw, if the body is not a strong, supportive basis. Therefore core stability training is also a part of basic shoulder training.

Core stability training is part of many of the exercises previously described and trains the transversus abdominis muscles, the other abdominal muscles (including diaphragm), the multifides, and a number of other spinal muscles. Core stability is obtained by pulling the umbilicus toward the third lumbar segment, flattening the abdominal wall.

Strong muscles tend to shorten and change the resting position of the shoulder. This is also the case with the posterior capsule. To avoid this, stretching should end all training sessions.

Box 9.2 Training program to prevent shoulder problems

Rotator cuff strengthening exercises
Use a rubber band. The athlete in standing position (keeping core stability) holding a rubber band in his right hand doing lateral and medial rotation. The scapula must be held stable and the humeral head must be kept from gliding anterior. The elbow must be kept in the scapular plane during exercises. When doing lateral rotation the rubber band comes from inferior and when doing medial rotation from behind the athlete at shoulder level. The exercise can be progressed by using a harder rubber band.

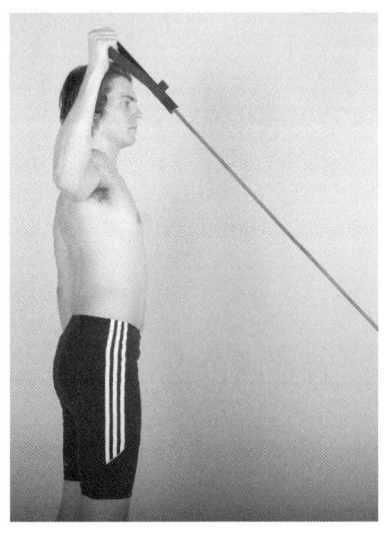

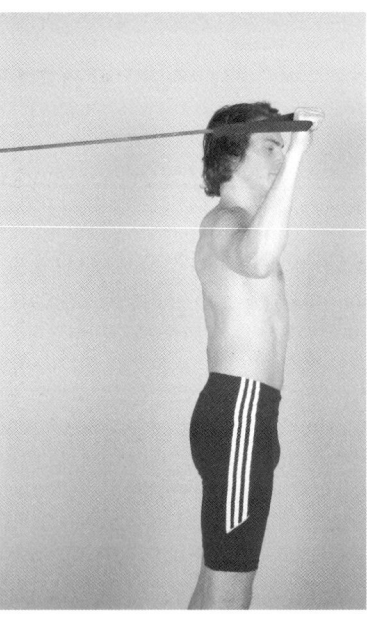

Training of the trapezius and the opposite serratus anterior muscles
In the standing position the athlete ties a rubber band around the left foot and holds the other end in the right hand. By elevating his right shoulder, he is training the upper part of trapezius (also called Trapezius 1). When flexing the right arm further posterior, he is training the middle and lower parts of trapezius (also called Trapezius 2 and 3). At the same time the left arm and shoulder can grab the rubber band and be pushed forward, in order to train the left serratus anterior muscle.

During these exercises the thoracic extension can also be trained by lifting the sternum. The lumbar spine must be kept stable.

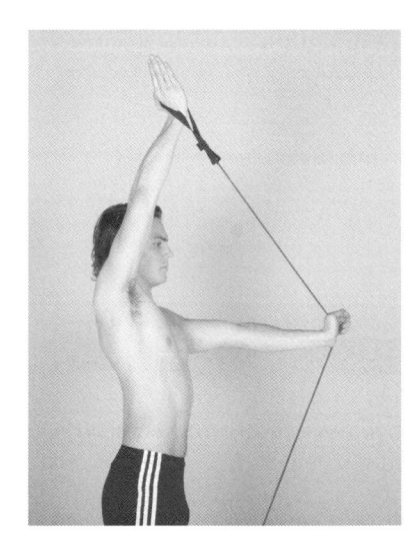

Training of the serratus anterior and trapezius muscles
The athlete is sidelying on his right elbow maintaining core and scapular stability, holding his left arm in 90° of flexion/abduction while rotating his body and reaching as far as possible. The exercise can be progressed by holding a weight in the left hand.

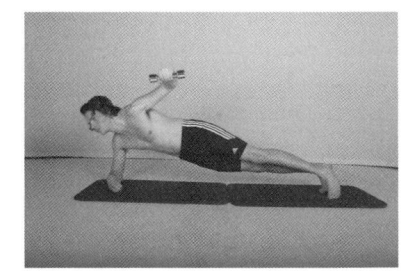

(Continued)

Box 9.2 (Continued)

Training of coordination with a racket
The athlete in standing position is balancing a racket on one finger without moving his feet and constantly changing the position of the arm. Exercise should be performed for 3 min.

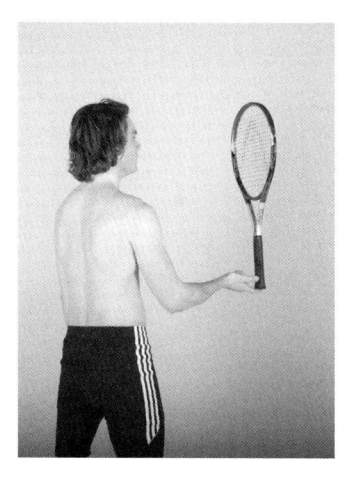

Training of coordination with a fit-ball
The athlete laying on the floor balancing a fit-ball on his hand while changing position of the arm into flexion/extension and abduction/adduction. Exercise should be performed for 3 min.

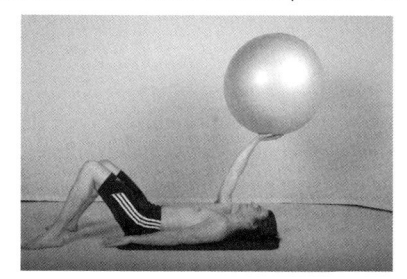

Training of thoracic extension I
Athlete standing with his elbows against a wall with his hands fingers placed around a segment of the thoracic spine making extension of the thoracic spine while the lower back is kept stable.

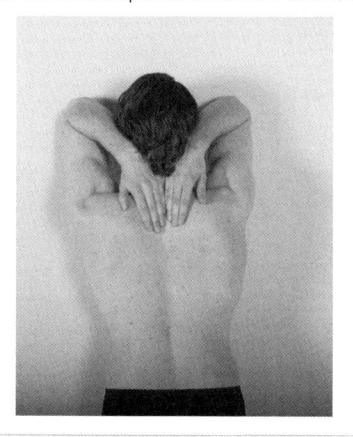

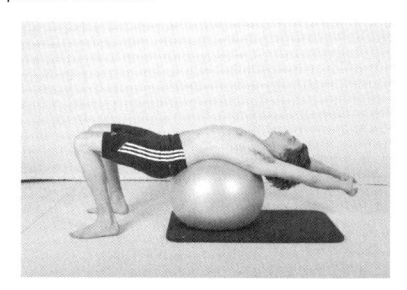

Training of thoracic extension II
The athlete is lying on his back on a fit-ball with his arms over the head rocking forward and backward, mobilizing the thoracic spine in passive extension.

Training of thoracic extension III
Athlete sitting on a chair leaning backward over the back of the chair mobilizing the thoracic spine into extension.

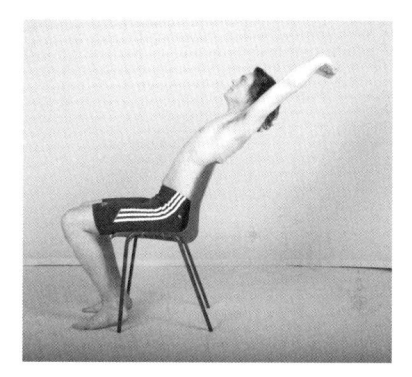

Stretching of the posterior capsule and outward (lateral) rotators
The athlete is side-laying with his right arm in 90° of flexion. The left arm presses the humeral head posterior and inwardly (medial) rotates the right arm at the same time. Each position should be kept for 40 s.

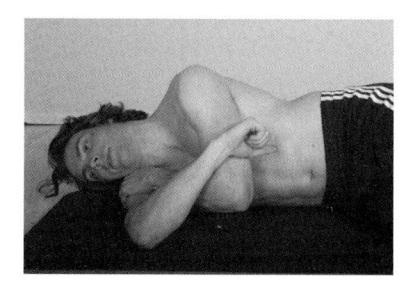

(Continued)

Box 9.2 (Continued)

Stretching of latissimus dorsi, the rhomboids muscles, and other inward rotating muscles
The athlete is standing in a corner doing wall-slide. By elevating the arms while keeping the scapula stable and not allowing any inward rotation of the arms, the muscles are stretched. Each position should be kept for 40 s.

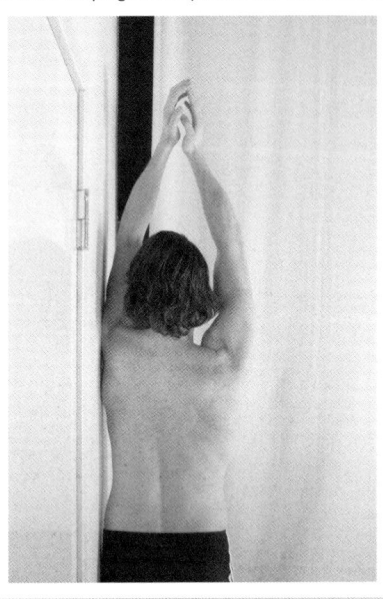

Stretching of the pectoralis minor muscle
The athlete standing in a doorway with his right arm in 180° of flexion and his elbow against the door-frame, leaning his body forward to stretch the pectoralis minor muscle. Each position should be kept for 40 s.

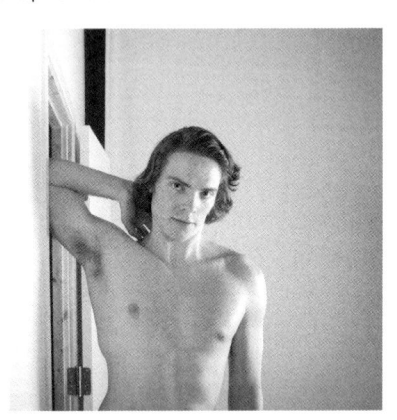

The elements of this basic, prophylactic training program can be adjusted depending on the finding of "black holes" in the screening of the athletes.

Proper throwing mechanics and limiting the number of pitches and innings thrown are crucial for prevention of injury, particularly in the growing athlete. Control, not speed, should be emphasized in training regimens. In addition, educating coaches and players about appropriate stretching, strengthening, conditioning, and proper throwing mechanics is vital. The literature on this topic has fortunately resulted in published guidelines that limit the number of innings that young pitchers are allowed to pitch per week. The American Academy of Orthopedic Surgeons recommends limiting pitches to about 4 to 10 innings per week, 80–100 pitches maximum per game, and 30–40 pitches per practice session (Tables 10.7 and 10.8).

It has been suggested that certain pitching, batting, and fielding techniques might be related to injury, in particular the underarm technique during softball pitching (Flyger et al., 2006). This is based on biomechanical and not clinical studies.

Shoulder problems caused by overloading during the golf swing can theoretically be prevented by a warm-up program. Overuse injuries are more common in golfers that do not perform a warm-up program, but the effect of the program has never been studied in a regular trial (Fradkin et al., 2005).

Cushion grip bands have been proven to reduce impact shock and vibration transfer in tennis racquets. This could reduce the load on elbow and shoulder and positively influence the risk for overload injuries, but the effect remains to be proven.

Strength training

In athletes, strength training of the shoulders should not be performed without the basic shoulder training program, which is described earlier. Without the basic program, there is an obvious risk of creating mismatch between muscles.

Strength training can be performed after standard principles as high load (maximum 10 repetitions possible) to increase power or as low load (many repetitions) to increase endurance and flexibility.

Moving the arm posterior to the shoulder joint (shoulder extension) should always be avoided, as this is unnecessary to achieve the full effect of strength training and results in potentially injurious large stresses the anterior structures of the glenohumeral joint. Bench press is typically an exercise in which the arms are quite often moved behind the shoulders, creating anterior pain in the shoulder.

Getting back after shoulder injury

The aim of physical therapy after shoulder injury is to relieve pain, expedite the return of the athlete to play, and most importantly, to prevent new injuries before they develop. Stretching is important to establish and maintain full range of motion, especially in patients with tight posterior capsules with limited internal rotation. "Sleeper stretches" are stretching maneuvers which are effective in stretching the posterior capsule, and prevent internal impingement associated with GIRD. They are performed with the athlete lying on the affected side, with the shoulder abducted 90°. Gentle constant pressure is applied by the opposite arm, pushing the affected shoulder into internal rotation.

During the acute phase of tendinitis, exercises should be performed below shoulder level to avoid rotator cuff outlet impingement, with gradual progression as symptoms decrease. In the majority of cases, non-surgical treatment allows gradual return to sport.

A strengthening program is instituted to increase strength in the rotator cuff as well as in the scapular stabilizers to provide dynamic glenohumeral stability. Both concentric and eccentric exercises are included. Improper throwing mechanics also must be corrected. Throwing athletes are allowed to return gradually to throwing once stability, strength, and endurance have improved (usually within 3 months). Most will be able to return to their prior level of activity in 6 months.

Swimmers tend to develop tightness in the pectoralis minor, which leads to a protracted shoulder posture. This decreases the subacromial space and contributes to outlet impingement syndrome. This may be prevented by stretching the pectoralis minor.

Wrestlers tend to strengthen their anterior shoulder and chest muscles disproportionately in relation to their periscapular and back muscles, resulting in a protracted shoulder posture. This also decreases the subacromial space and contributes to outlet impingement syndrome. This may be prevented by strengthening the rhomboids and scapular retractor muscles.

Take-home message

The only intervention that has been proven effective in preventing traumatic shoulder injury is the introduction of break-away bases in softball. Theoretical preventative measures like shoulder pads, collars, learning falling techniques, forbidding risky playing habits, and softening walls, and back stops have yet to be proven effective.

The risk for overload injuries, which are very common in shoulders, can theoretically be reduced if all athletes are screened regularly for weakness in glenohumeral and scapulothoracic stability and for lack of balance between muscles (identifying dominance of muscles, most often inward rotators of the arm and downward rotators of the acromion). It is recommended that weaknesses and dysfunctions are treated by exercise programs, but the effect of this on injury prevention remains to be proven. Learning the proper techniques in the individual sports is thought to be important for prevention of overload.

The growing athlete is at particular risk for overload injury, for example, at the growth plates, and repeated, forceful activities should be reduced, for example, the number of pitches per game.

References

Caldwell, C., Sahrmann, S., Van Dillen, L. (2007) Use of a movement system impairment diagnosis for physical therapy in the management of a patient with shoulder pain. *The Journal of Orthopaedic and Sports Physical Therapy* **37**, 551–563.

Demorest, R.A., Landry, G.L. (2003) Prevention of pediatric sports injuries. *Current Sports Medicine Reports* **2**, 337–343.

Flyger, N., Button, C., Rishiraj, N. (2006) The science of softball: implications for performance and injury prevention. *Sports Medicine* **36**, 797–816.

Fradkin, A.J., Cameron, P.A., Gabbe, B.J. (2005) Golf injuries—common and potentially avoidable. *Journal of Science and Medicine in Sports* **8**, 163–170.

Hagel, B., Pless, I.B., Goulet, C. (2005) The effect of wrist guard use on upper-extremity injuries in snowboarders. *American Journal of Epidemiology* **162**, 149–156.

Janda, D.H. (2003) The prevention of baseball and softball injuries. *Clinical Orthopaedics and Related Research* **409**, 20–28.

Janda, D.H., Wojtys, E.M., Hankin, F.M., Benedict, M. (1988) Softball sliding injuries: a prospective study comparing standard and modified bases. *Journal of the American Medical Association* **259**, 1848–1850.

Kibler, W.B., Safran, M.R. (2005) Tennis injuries. *Medicine and Sports Science* **48**, 120–137.

Kocher, M.S., Dupre, M.M., Feagin Jr., J.A. (1998) Shoulder injuries from alpine skiing and snowboarding. Aetiology, treatment and prevention. *Sports Medicine* **25**, 201–211.

Koehle, M.S., Lloyd-Smith, R., Taunton, J.E. (2002) Alpine ski injuries and their prevention. *Sports Medicine* **32**, 785–793.

Kugler, A., Krüger-Franke, M., Reininger, S., Trouillier, H.H., Rosemeyer, B. (1996) Muscular imbalance and shoulder pain in volleyball attackers. *British Journal of Sports Medicine* **30**, 256–259.

Laudner, K.G., Myers, J.B., Pasquale, M.R., Bradley, J.P., Lephart, S.M. (2006) Scapular dysfunction in throwers with pathologic internal impingement. *The Journal of Orthopaedic and Sports Physical Therapy* **36**, 485–494.

Pollack, K.M., Canham-Chervak, M., Gazal-Carvalho, C., Jones, B.H., Baker, S.P. (2005) Interventions to prevent softball related injuries: a review of the literature. *Injury Prevention* **11**, 277–281.

Su, K.P., Johnson, M.P., Gracely, E.J., Carduna, A.R. (2004) Scapular rotation in swimmers with and without impingement syndrome. Practice effects. *Medicine and Science in Sports and Exercise* **36**, 1117–1123.

Tripp, B.L., Yochem, E.M., Uhl, T.L. (2007) Functional fatigue and upper extremity sensorimotor system acuity in baseball athletes. *Journal of Athletic Training* **42**, 90–98.

Further reading

Andrews, J.R., Wilk, K.E. (eds.) (1994) *The Athlete's Shoulder*. Churchill Livingstone, New York.

Burkhart, S.S., Morgan, C.D., Kibler, W.B. (2003) The disabled throwing shoulder: spectrum of pathology Part I: Pathoanatomy and biomechanics. *Arthroscopy* **19**, 404–420.

Burkhart, S.S., Morgan, C.D., Kibler, W.B. (2003) The disabled throwing shoulder: spectrum of pathology. Part II: Evaluation and treatment of SLAP lesions in throwers. *Arthroscopy* **19**, 531–539.

Burkhart, S.S., Morgan, C.D., Kibler, W.B. (2003) The disabled throwing shoulder: spectrum of pathology Part III: The SICK scapula, scapular dyskinesis, the kinetic chain, and rehabilitation. *Arthroscopy* **19**, 641–661.

Harries, M., Williams, C., Stanish, W.D., Micheli, L.J. (eds.) (1998) *Oxford Textbook of Sports Medicine*. Oxford Medical Publications, New York.

Hawkins, R.J., Misamore, G.W., Huff, T.G. (eds.) (1996) *Shoulder Injuries in the Athlete: Surgical Repair and Rehabilitation*. Churchill Livingstone, New York.

Jobe, F.W., Tibone, J.E., Pink, M.M., Jobe, C.M., Kvitne, R.S. (1998) The shoulder in sports. In C.A. Rockwood, F.A. Matsen, M.A. Wirth, & D.T. Harryman (eds.) *The Shoulder*, pp. 1214–1238. Saunders, Philadelphia, PA.

Krogsgaard, M.R., Debski, R.E., Norlin, R., Rydqvist, L. (2003) Shoulder. In M. Kjær, M. Krogsgaard, P. Magnusson, L. Engebretsen, H. Roos, T. Takala, & S.L.-Y. Woo (eds.) *Textbook of Sports Medicine: Basic Science and Clinical Aspects of Sports Injury and Physical Activity*, pp. 684–738. Blackwell Science, London.

Sahrmann, S.A. (2002) *Diagnosis and Treatment of Movement Impairment Syndromes*. Mosby Inc, St. Louis, MO.

Warren, R.F., Craig, E.V., Altchek, D.W. (eds.) (1999) *The Unstable Shoulder*. Lippincott–Raven Publishers, Philadelphia, PA.

Chapter 10
Preventing elbow injuries

Mark R. Hutchinson[1] and James R. Andrews[2]

[1]Department of Orthopaedics, University of Illinois at Chicago, IL, USA
[2]Medical director, American Sports Medicine Institute, Birmingham, Alabama, USA, Andrews Sports, Medicine Institute, Gulf Breeze, FL, USA

Epidemiology of elbow injuries in sports

The elbow is a complex hinge joint that joins the distal humerus to the proximal radius and ulna. The joint has two degrees of freedom, flexion/extension and pronation/supination, which play important roles in most sports by transferring forces between the body core and shoulder to the hand. In addition, the elbow allows the athlete to specifically, repetitively, and with a great deal of finesse position their hand in space. Excessive forces leading to injury can come from acute loads as seen in direct trauma and falls or chronic loads as seen in overuse and repetitive microtrauma.

High demand versus low demand sports

Sports with relatively low upper extremity demand would be expected to have low risk of elbow injuries; and, indeed, this is true. Soccer (other than the goalie), track and cross-country, as well as the purely jumping sports such as long jump, high jump, and triple jump have a low risk of elbow injuries. Other sports such as Nordic or Alpine skiing, equestrian, cycling, speed skating, and figure skating have relatively low risk until high energy falls are considered. When all sports are considered in adolescent athletes, the elbow accounts for only 2–5% of all injuries (Table 10.1). In sports that have a higher throwing demand such as baseball the incidence jumps up to 17–70% depending on the position, age, and definition of injury (Table 10.1).

High energy injuries

The transfer of large, acute loads risks catastrophic failure of ligaments, tendons, or bone. The most common acute traumatic mechanism is a fall on an outstretched hand. Acute traumatic injuries are most common in contact and collision sports (American football, rugby, martial arts, etc.), sports that place an athlete at elevated heights (high jump, ski jumping, gymnastics, etc.), and high energy sports in which the athlete is at a great rate of speed (alpine skiing, speed skating, cycling, etc.). Eight percent of judo injuries, 4% in wrestling, and 3–4% in ice hockey involve the elbow (Table 10.1). In addition, sports such as weight-lifting, boxing, shot put, and gymnastics place acute and heavy loads across the elbow joint during the course of participation. In some cases, the force across the elbow can far exceed the body weight of the gymnast, the weight being lifted, or the weight being thrown. If the loads aren't balanced appropriately across the joint, catastrophic failure occurs. The differential diagnosis of traumatic injury of the elbow includes: elbow dislocation, radial head dislocation; intra- and extra-articular distal humerus

Sports Injury Prevention, 1st edition. Edited by R. Bahr and L. Engebretsen Published 2009 by Blackwell Publishing ISBN: 9781405162449

Table 10.1 Risk of elbow injury in different sports. The numbers reported are average estimates based on the studies available.

Sport	Competition incidence[1]	Training incidence[1]	% of all injuries Rank	Comments
Team sports				
Baseball	0.29*		8.60%	
Softball	0.17*		4.70%	
Ice Hockey	0.14*		2.8–4.6%	
Basketball (♀)	0.06*		1.20%	
Basketball (♂)	0.06*		1.10%	
Football (American)	0.08*		1%	
Lacrosse (♂)	0.04*		0.70%	
Lacrosse (♀)	0.03*		0.60%	
Volleyball (♀)	0.01*		<0.5–1.6%	
Beach volleyball	0.01		<1% (14th out of 17)	Competition 3× more common than training
Soccer (♂)	0.01*		<0.5–1.3%	
Soccer (♀)	0.01*		<0.5%	
Field hockey	0.01*		<0.5%	
Waterpolo	0.02		<1%	
Individual sports				
Sailing	0.04		13% (3rd most common)	
Javelin	0.11	0.03	1.4–6%	High risk of DJD at long term follow up
Tennis				
– Club level	2.4		35%	
– Elite <18 year	1.2		5%	
Golf				
– professional	0.06–0.12		5% ♀/7% ♂ (2nd most common)	Overuse most common
– amateur	3× more common than pros		35.5% ♀/32.5% ♂	
Judo	1.2		7.70%	
Wrestling	0.39*		4.30%	
Gymnastics (♀)	0.38*		4.10%	
Gymnastics (♂)	0.10*		1.90%	
Karate	0.10		3.80%	
Weight-lifting (Olympic)			2.50%	
Boxing	0.5*		1.00%	↑ DJD when retired
Mixed martial arts	0.06*		2.10%	
Paralympic sport				
– Wheelchair sports	1.5		12%	30–60% related to training
– Sled hockey	1		5%	
Luge	0.39		6–13%	

[1] Incidence is reported for adult, competitive athletes as the number of injuries per 1000 hours of training and competition or *per 1000 athletic exposures.

fracture; physeal injury in the skeletally immature, radial head or neck fracture; avulsion injury of the epicondyle, olecranon, or coronoid; distal biceps tendon rupture; triceps rupture; nerve contusions; ulnar nerve subluxation; or neurovascular injury. In some instances, the rules of participation may reduce the risk of catastrophic injuries; nonetheless, traumatic injuries are the most difficult to target with prevention. They also have the greatest risk of leaving residual deformity, loss of function or restrictions in motion, or arthritis, which can lead to permanent disability.

Low energy/overuse injuries

Repetitive subcatastrophic load may cause chronic overuse or repetitive microtraumatic injury such as tendinopathy, stress fracture, and ligament sprain. Chronic overuse can weaken the native structural elements to the extent that normally submaximal loads exceed the ultimate strength of the structure and lead to catastrophic failure. Repetitive overuse injuries are more common in upper extremity demanding sports that use a racquet or stick (tennis, racquetball, golf, lacrosse, etc.) or throw an object (javelin, baseball, softball, etc.). Nearly 9% of baseball injuries, 7% of javelin injuries, 5% of softball injuries, and 3% of tennis injuries involve the elbow (Table 10.1). It is in these sports that the elbow's functional demand of repetitively placing the hand in space is particularly important. With subtle variations of hand positions the ball or object to be delivered may end up in a completely unintended location. Failure or dysfunction at the elbow will lead to poor performance and potentially further injury at the elbow or adjacent structures. Chronic overuse injuries about the elbow include: tendinopathy of the extensor carpi radialis brevis (tennis elbow), tendinopathy of the flexor muscle insertions (golfer's elbow), bicipital tendinopathy, cubital tunnel syndrome (ulnar neuritis), ulnar nerve instability, pronator teres syndrome (median nerve entrapment), stress fractures, osteochondritis dissecans, or valgus extension overload syndrome with associated spurring or loose body formation from the olecranon or capitellum. Overuse injuries are more common than acute traumatic injuries, and are easier to target regarding injury prevention. In one study of 21 javelin throwers 19 years after sports participation, all had degenerative changes in their elbow and 50% had loss of extension.

Key risk factors: how to identify athletes at risk

When making an effort to prevent injuries, it is important to recognize not only the overall risk in a specific sport but also any key risk factors relative to the athlete. Is it possible to identify athletes at risk to be able to target prevention programs? These factors may be categorized as either internal or external influences. Internal factors include the unique anatomy of the elbow, age of the participant relative to physeal closure, articular alignment, physical strength, and coordination of the kinetic chain (Table 10.2). Gender may play a small role; however, it is more likely that how intensely and how often the athlete uses his elbow is the greatest risk factor. External factors include such things as the level of play, number or repetitions or throws, amount of rest between competitions, risk of contact and collision in a specific sport, equipment, environment, and the technical style (form, overhead motion versus side-arm motion, or coordinated progression of the kinetic chain).

Young athletes and growing bones

The skeletally immature elbow has numerous ossification centers and growth plates which, regarding injuries, are the "weak link." The ossification center of the capitellum is at risk of vascular injury secondary to repeated compression associated with weight-lifting and boxing, the weight-bearing demands of gymnastics, or the valgus stresses associated with throwing (Figure 10.1). On the medial aspect of the skeletally immature elbow, the medial epicondylar ossification center serves as the insertion of the medial collateral ligament and flexor muscles of the forearm. It is at risk of avulsion secondary to the tension forces when the elbow perceives valgus loads such as in weight-bearing, weight-lifting, or throwing. Isolated ulnar collateral ligament injuries are uncommon in the skeletally immature thrower; however, a growing field of literature has reported this injury as well as surgical reconstruction in this population.

Mature and masters athletes

For the skeletally mature athlete, chronic changes can occur on the lateral side of the elbow including the creation of bone spurs, radial head hypertrophy, flattening and fragmentation of the capitellum which in turn leads to loose bodies. On the medial side of the mature elbow, the ulnar collateral

Table 10.2 Internal and external factors for elbow injuries in different sports. The numbers reported are average estimates based on the studies available.

Risk factor	Relative risk[1]	Evidence[2]	Comments
Internal Risk Factors			
Prior injury	2×	++	
Prior osteochondrosis	2×	+	Increased risk of OCD of the elbow in athletes with prior osteochondrosis
Alignment			
– Elbow carrying angle	1×	+	
– Developmental glenohumeral external rotation deficit (GERD)	?	+	Unknown correlation with elbow injuries
Skeletally immature	2×	++	
Gender (male vs female)	1×	+	Males > Female likely related to # of participants & sport demands, not gender
External Risk Factors			
Court surface	1×	+	No effect on elbow injury rates
Number of throws	3×	++	
Number of years of throwing	2×	+	Cumulative effect ↑risk over time
Throwing style	1×	+	Overhand vs sidearm styles
– Softball	0.5×	+	Windmill style reduces elbow risk
Backhand style in tennis	0.5×	++	Two fisted ↓elbow injury risk
Type of pitch	X	+	Little effect but poorly thrown curveball, ↑ risk of injury in the youth
– Fast ball vs curveball			
Elbow pads	0.5×	+	
Tightly strung racquets	2×	+	
Oversized racquet heads	0.5×	+	
Oversized grips	0.5×	+	Some debate. Probably reduces the tension over the extensor muscle mass which reduces the risk of tennis elbow
	2×	+	
Wet or heavy balls			

[1]Relative risk indicates the increased risk of injury to an individual with this risk factor relative to an individual who does not have this characteristic. In this chart, standard risk would be 1×. The magnification estimates are based on considering a mild increased risk to be 2× and a moderate to significant increased risk to be 3×. A mild estimate of reduction of risk would be 0.5× and a moderate to significant risk reduction to be 0.25×.
[2]Evidence indicates the level of scientific evidence for this factor being a risk factor for ligament sprains: ++ — convincing evidence from high-quality studies with consistent results; + — evidence from lesser quality studies or mixed results; 0 — expert opinion or hypothesis without scientific evidence.
* Odds ratio and not relative risk.
NA: Not available.

ligament and not the medial epicondyle is the weak link. Weight bearing on the upper extremity or the throwing motion places a tension load across the ulnar collateral ligament which can lead to injury or failure (Figure 10.2). Masters athletes (older athletes) have placed a life-time of wear and tear on their joints and are at greater risk of degenerative and overuse problems than the young athlete. The elevated risk of tennis elbow (extensor carpi radialis tendinopathy) in the master's athlete compared to the younger athlete is well recognized. Chronic degenerative changes including joint space narrowing and peri-articular spurring are more commonly seen in older throwers, gymnasts, weight-lifters, and martial artists.

Injury risk builds from the ground up

Recent focus on elbow injury prevention has looked beyond specific anatomic structures of the elbow and targeted the efficient transfer of forces from the ground through the body core and shoulder to the elbow in throwing athletes; that is, the kinetic chain (Figure 10.3). The health

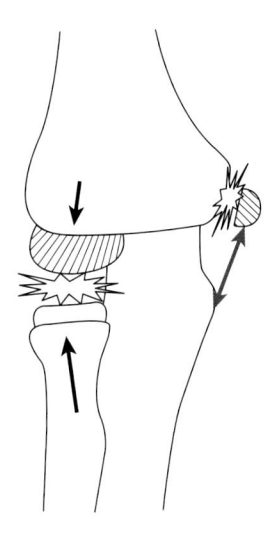

Figure 10.1. Valgus load on the skeletally immature elbow risk compression of the capitellum and development of osteochondritis dissecans (solid black arrows) and/or traction of the medial epicondyle apophysis with possible avulsion (solid grey arrows)

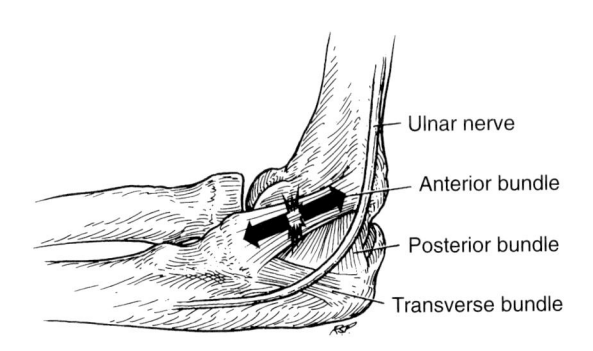

Figure 10.2. Anatomic drawing of the medial elbow ligaments. Anterior bundle is loaded during the throwing motion and is at risk of failure due to tension loads. Reproduced with permission @ Mary Lloyd Ireland M.D., Kentucky Sports Medicine

of the elbow is dependent on coordinated movement, transfer of forces, and health proximally in the kinetic chain. This is particularly true in the throwing athlete where poor coordination of the scapular stabilization muscles (scapular dyskinesia) has been directly correlated with an increased risk of elbow injuries. Similarly poor coordination of core muscles including the lumbar spine, abdominals, and gluteal muscles has been associated with poor transfer of kinetic forces and overuse of the structures about the elbow. The throwing athlete with poor core mechanics tends to alter their throwing style in an effort to maintain the same throwing velocity. This is often at the expense of ideal shoulder and elbow positioning which places the elbow at an increased risk of injury. A history of shoulder injuries, indeed a history of any injury along the kinetic chain, has been directly correlated to an increased risk of elbow injuries (Table 10.2).

Identifying external risk factors

In addition, a number of external factors play key roles in the incidence of elbow injuries. These external influences include how frequently the athlete is asked to use or load the elbow, how much rest is allowed between events to allow the elbow to recover, certain styles of performance, as well as the effect of equipment modifications including grips, braces, string tension of racquets, and weight or size of a projectile being thrown (Table 10.2). Baseball, a classic throwing sport, and tennis, a classic racquet sport, have been the two sports subjected to the greatest scientific scrutiny.

In baseball, a ball is delivered in an overhand throwing style at speeds approaching 160 km/h over 100 times in a game. As the athlete fatigues, he may develop a poor throwing style that does not take advantage of an efficient kinetic chain and leads to an increased risk of overuse and injury. Excellent studies are available in the skeletally immature thrower that show that elbow injuries including medial epicondyle epiphysitis and osteochondritis dissecans are directly associated with the total number of pitches delivered per game, per week, and per season (Table 10.2). The same studies reveal that limiting young throwers to a certain number of pitches can reduce the overall incidence of injury. In addition, when the young athlete is allowed a period of rest between outings, his elbow is allowed to recover and the incidence of injury is further reduced.

Throwing mechanics including specific pitch type have also been carefully studied in baseball regarding their relationship to injury risk (Figure 10.4). Fast balls and change-ups are thrown with

Push off and cocking
energy storage

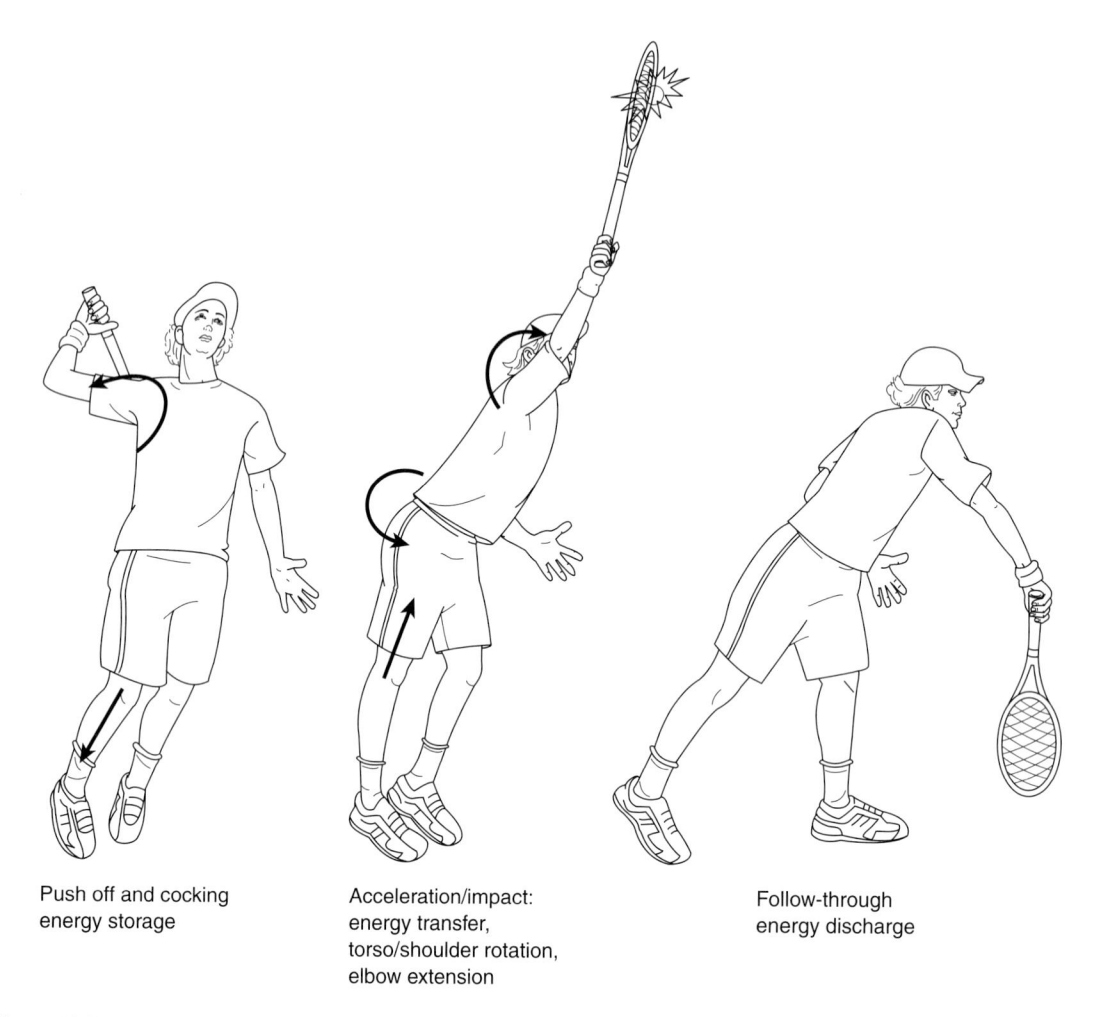

Acceleration/impact:
energy transfer,
torso/shoulder rotation,
elbow extension

Follow-through
energy discharge

Figure 10.3. Optimal throwing or serving technique requires a sequential force transfer from the floor up the leg, thru the torso and shoulder to the elbow and hand at delivery; that is, the kinetic chain

the most natural of mechanics and are the pitches by which all others are compared. The fast ball has been shown to create the greatest forces across the elbow joint followed by the slider, curveball, and change-up. A curveball is thrown by altering the pitcher's grip on the seams and by repositioning their wrist during the delivery. In a well-thrown curveball, very little mechanical change is perceived across the elbow. However, in a young thrower learning to throw the pitch, they tend to drop their hand delivering the ball in a more side-arm motion, they tend to lead with their elbow throwing the ball more like a dart. Alternatively, the young thrower may try to explosively supinate their forearm with delivery. These mechanical alterations increase the load across the elbow and increase the risk of injury. For this reason, throwing the curveball is discouraged in the skeletally immature thrower until nearing skeletal maturity when they can perform it with proper technique and do not risk their open growth plates.

In elite level pitchers the side-arm motion has been studied and shown to have very little correlation with elbow injuries. In a well-thrown side-arm pitch, the angles and forces across the

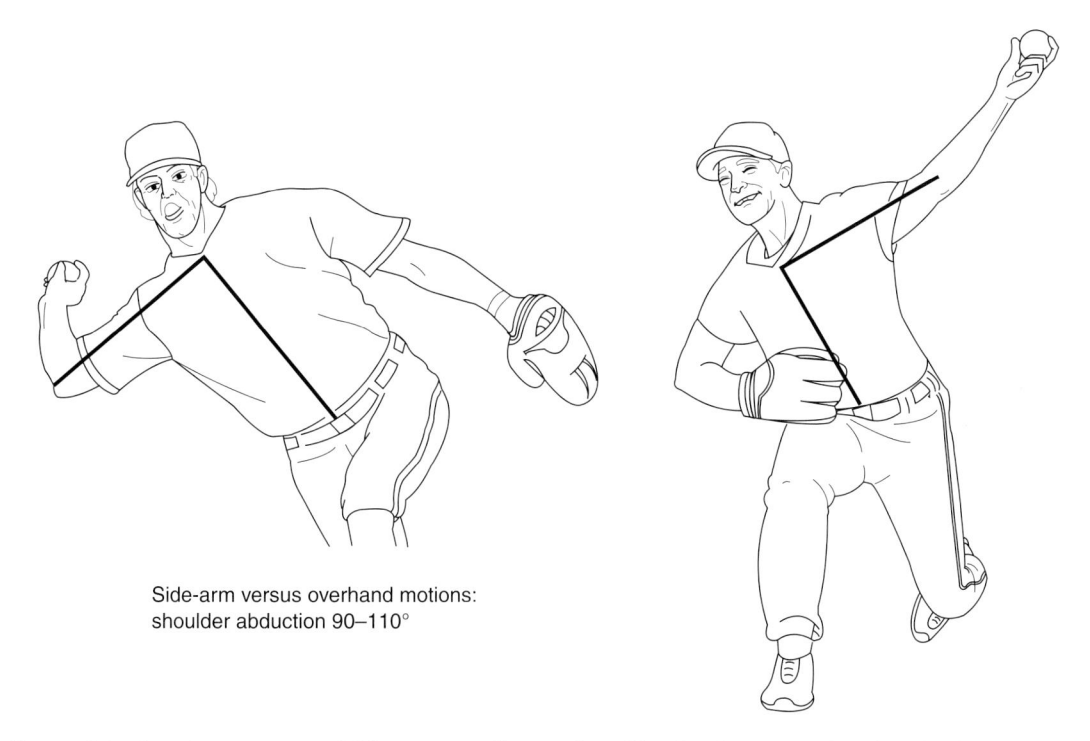

Side-arm versus overhand motions:
shoulder abduction 90–110°

Figure 10.4. The side-arm motion of delivery is actually just a lateral bend at the torso and not less shoulder adduction

shoulder and elbow are nearly identical to the overhead motion. The difference occurs in the lateral tilt of the torso in the side-arm thrower. While this may increase the risk of low back problems, there does not appear to be increased loads across the elbow (Table 10.2, Figure 10.4). Windmill style of pitching seen in softball has very little risk of elbow injury.

Risk factors in racquet sports

During service, tennis and many racquet sports mimic the overhead throwing motion. Therefore, athletes in racquet sports can be equally susceptible to repetitive overuse injuries and failures in the kinetic chain as are athletes participating in predominantly throwing sports. The racquet provides an increased extension moment that can further load all units of the kinetic chain including the elbow (Figure 10.5). Longer racquets increase the load. Tighter strung racquets or more rigid racquets absorb less shock and transfer the loads directly up the kinetic chain with the first stop being the wrist and elbow. It is, therefore, not surprising that longer, rigid racquets with tight strings increase the risk of tennis elbow in the athletes that use them (Table 10.2). Increased forces are also seen when players play with wet or heavy tennis balls. Large headed racquets increase the size of the "sweet spot" which reduces the chance of a miss hit that might cause rotational torque in the forearm. Theoretically this will reduce the risk of injury. Grip size has also been associated with injury risk and particularly increased risk of tennis elbow. A small grip forces the athlete to shorten their flexors and places the finger and wrist extensors at greater length. This increases the forces at the elbow during a backhand or wrist extension maneuver. Larger grips have been used to reduce this risk or treat the athlete with an early onset of lateral tendinopathy. Recent studies have suggested that grip size changes of less than ¼ of an inch have no effect on forearm muscle firing patterns. Reduction of the forces along the elbow extensors has also been targeted through biomechanical adjustments in technical style. Two-fisted

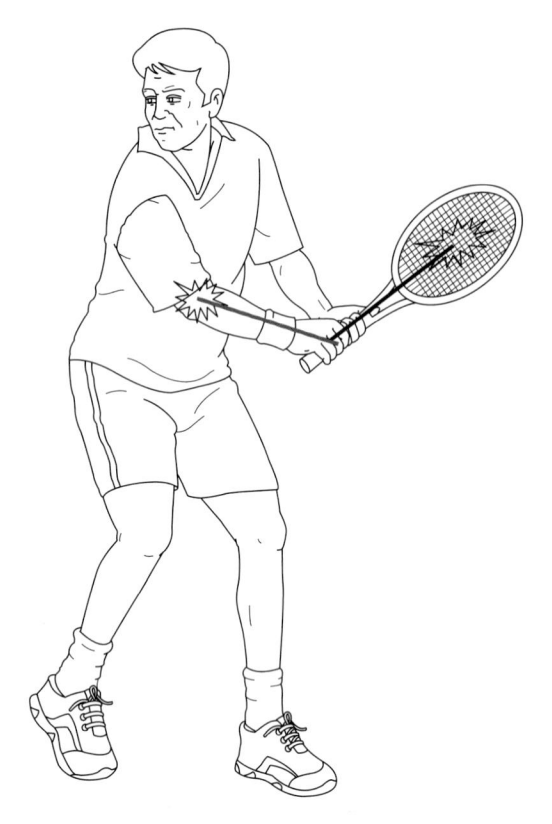

Figure 10.5. The racquet increases the distance of the impact of the ball from the elbow. This increased moment magnifies the forces felt at the elbow

back-hands have been shown to reduce the forces across the lateral elbow when compared to single-fisted backhands.

The training location and court surface may play a minimal role. Court surface in tennis, clay versus grass versus synthetic, does alter ball speeds but has not been directly related to elbow injuries. Likewise ball players on grass versus synthetic turf have not been correlated with an increased risk of elbow injuries although falls on synthetic turf lead to more skin abrasions than on natural grass.

Sports with compressive loads across the elbow

Repetitive compressive loads across the elbow such as seen in weight-lifting, boxing, and gymnastics are another key risk factor for the development of chronic elbow problems. In the skeletally immature elbow these repetitive compressive loads have been directly associated with osteochondritis dissecans of the capitellum, olecranon impingement, and medial epicondylitis (Figure 10.1). The intensity and frequency of loading may place the skeletally mature elbow at risk of degenerative changes of the articular surface or the creation of osteochondral loose bodies. Many master athletes who have participated for many years develop secondary changes and degenerative changes in the lateral and posterior compartments of the elbow. Identifying the athlete at risk of elbow injuries from compressive loading begins with early recognition of complaints and an immediate period of rest. Loading and weight-bearing are inherent to the sports of boxing, gymnastics, and weight-lifting and cannot be eliminated completely.

Take-home message

So which athlete should you keep the closest eye on and plan an early intervention? Surprisingly, the answer is usually the best athlete. He/she is the one who has the most repetitions, creates the highest forces across the elbow, and is likely to be the most intense in training taking minimal periods of rest. Be attentive to faulty mechanics in not only sport-specific techniques but also of core strength and stability. Young athletes should be progressive in their skill-building. If performance begins to decline, it may be the first sign in the development of an overuse injury which should indicate initiating a period of rest and recovery.

Injury mechanisms

As noted earlier, elbow injuries can be classified as acute or chronic. Acute injuries are more common in contact and collision sports (American football, rugby, ice hockey, and martial arts) or in any sport at risk of high energy falls (skiing, snowboarding, gymnastics, and equestrian). There may be direct (impact directly onto the elbow) or indirect (fall on an outstretched hand or torques across

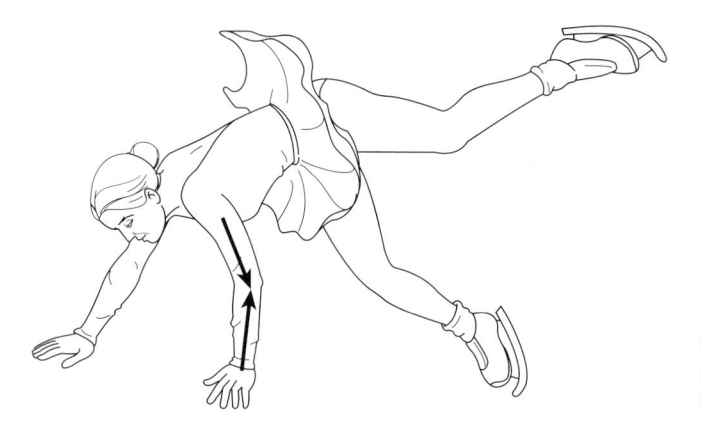

Figure 10.6. Fall on an outstretched hand (FOOSH) is a common cause of elbow injury and dislocation

the elbow. Most acute injuries are hazards of the sport and therefore difficult to prevent. Educating athletes on how to fall and the use of protective equipment like elbow pads in certain sports may provide some prevention effect.

FOOSH: fall on an outstretched hand

The classic description is a fall on an outstretched hand (FOOSH) (Figure 10.6). When the forces are excessive, the elbow is hyper-extended leading first to rupture of the collateral ligaments (medial before lateral) and anterior capsule. If the force continues, the elbow will dislocate. In some cases, bony avulsions of ligaments or apophyses will occur instead of pure ligamentous injury. In severe injuries, neurovascular structures will be injured with severe displacement. Urgent reduction is essential. In athletes who fall on extended elbow with the hand in full supination, there is a risk of an isolated injury to the posterolateral corner of the elbow. In this case, the lateral collateral ligament and annular ligament at the radial neck are injured and lead to posterior subluxation or instability of the radial head.

In children who fall on an outstretched arm, the weak link is the growth plate. Injuries that appear as elbow dislocations frequently have associated epiphyseal or apophyseal injuries. It is strongly recommended to obtain bilateral radiographs in the skeletally immature for comparison. The appearance and position of each growth center should be symmetric to the opposite side. Anatomic reduction of any displaced intra-articular fracture or a supracondylar fracture is essential to avoid long-term complications of malalignment or arthritis. Admittedly, this does not prevent the initial injury but early recognition and treatment can prevent later problems and disability.

Direct impact injuries

Direct impact onto the elbow by an object, impact onto the court surface, or collision into a barrier wall can lead to elbow injuries including bone bruises, ligament strains, muscle contusions, and skin abrasions. The ulnar nerve is relatively subcutaneous on the posterior medial aspect of the elbow. Direct impact can lead to a temporary neuropraxia or chronic ulnar neuritis. Direct impact onto the olecranon can lead to an inflamed or blood-filled olecranon bursa. Prevention of these direct impact injuries can usually be accomplished through protective padding. Unfortunately, many acute injuries are simply accidents which occur during the usual performance of a high risk sport. One potential exception is the risk of elbow dislocation in the sport of judo. In judo, a competitor is allowed to place his opponent's elbow in an elbow lock, a position of hyperextension. Indeed, if the athlete on the receiving end of this maneuver does not "tap-out" to concede defeat continued force may lead to an elbow dislocation.

Overuse injuries

While traumatic injuries can occur across sports, the most elbow problems in athletes are secondary to chronic repetitive stresses. Fortunately, it is this overuse that gives us our best target to prevent elbow injuries. Repetitive varus loading as seen in the lead hand in golf and in the backhand during tennis leads to strain of the lateral collateral ligament as well as the wrist extensor muscles. Repetitive valgus stress seen in throwing and racquet sports leads to an increased strain of the medial collateral ligament, overuse of the flexor muscles, and compression of the radiocapitellar articulation (Figure 10.7). Repetitive extension loads seen in the follow-through phase of throwers or when weightlifters lock their elbow in full extension can lead to impingement of the olecranon posteriorly, traction of the triceps muscle, and tension the capsule anteriorly. Repetitive compressive loads seen in gymnastics and weight-lifting serve to load the articular surface directly. In each case the ligaments and bones feel the direct force of the loading, however, the muscles that cross the joint serve as dynamic stabilizers that are at risk of injury with repetitive overuse.

To resist varus loading, the lateral muscles fire to assist in stabilizing the joint. Unfortunately due to the relative proximity to the joint surface they are at a mechanical disadvantage to overcome these repetitive loads. The classic example of this occurs with the tennis backhand. Energy is transferred at ball impact through the racquet to the wrist extensors which insert on the lateral aspect of the elbow. Chronic repetitive overuse with inadequate opportunity to recover leads to tendon failure or tendinopathy of the wrist extensors, most commonly the extensor carpi radialis brevis. Indeed a similar phenomenon is seen on the medial aspect of the elbow in golfers (Figure 10.8). As ball impact occurs or a divot is taken, forces are transferred up the shaft to the wrist flexors as the insert on the medial aspect of the elbow. Golfer's elbow is a tendinopathy on the medial aspect of the elbow secondary to overuse or injury the flexor muscle insertions onto the medial epicondyle. It is possible that the strong supination of the lead hand/pronation of the trailing hand that occurs during the golf swing could

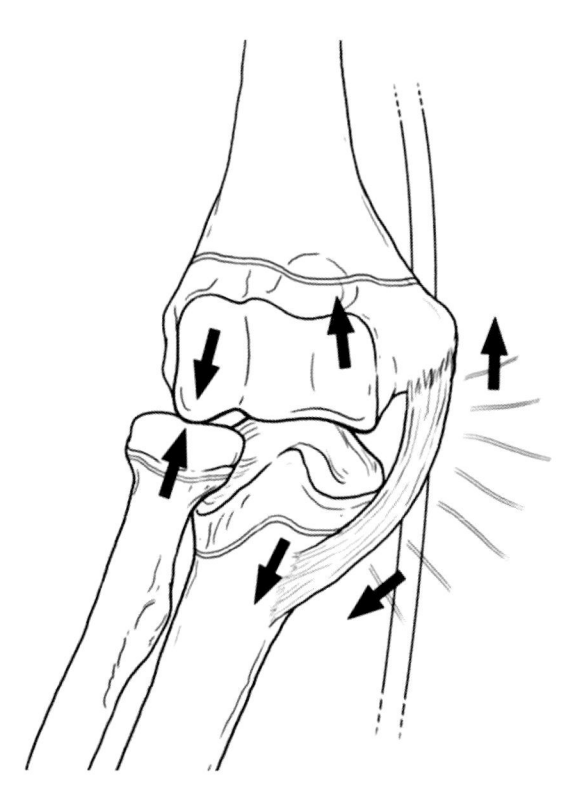

Figure 10.7. Valgus-extension overload is the most common mechanism of overuse injuries about the throwing elbow. It is made up of medial tension, lateral compression and posterior olecranon impingement. Reproduced with permission @ Mark R. Hutchinson, UIC Sports Medicine

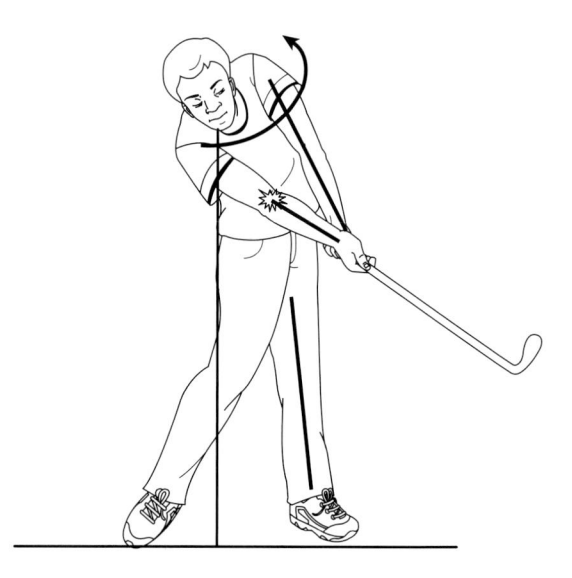

Figure 10.8. Golfer's elbow is an overload of the medial structures of the elbow which can be caused by acutely taking a deep divot

contribute to this problem; however, this would not explain the increased incidence in the amateur population compared to the professional ranks. The more likely mechanism of injury is that the injury occurs when the golfer hits down on the ball too forcefully and takes too large a divot. This would lead to acute loads of the flexor muscles of the trailing hand at impact. Indeed this occurs much more frequently in amateur golfers than professional golfers who have honed their swing.

Injuries in throwing sports

Perhaps the greatest focus of study on injury mechanisms about the elbow has occurred in throwing sports. As the ball or javelin is delivered, the elbow goes through a sequence of muscle activity, loading, and mobility that stresses different aspects of the joint through the range of motion. In the early cocking phase, the elbow is usually in slight to moderate flexion and is relatively at a low stressful position as the arm is being positioned to begin transferring loads up the kinetic chain with the goal of ultimately delivering the projectile from the hand. In late cocking and early acceleration the medial collateral ligament and radiocapitellar articulation are loaded with valgus stress that continues to increase as acceleration occurs (Figure 10.9). Throwers usually pronate their arms to some degree in this phase to reduce the intense valgus loads. As the projectile is delivered, the elbow comes into full extension and the periarticular muscles (especially elbow flexors) fire to resist the large extension moment. The extension moment is also resisted by the bony architecture posteriorly as the olecronon falls into the olecranon fossa posteriorly. This repetitive valgus loading and extension moment can lead to specific group overuse injuries and, therefore, this pathomechanic has been coined valgus-extension overload. The valgus component can lead to ulnar collateral instability, avulsions of medial epicondyle, medial epicondyle epiphysitis, secondary ulnar nerve neuropraxia. In addition the valgus loads apply compressive loads to the radio-capitellar articulation which can lead to radial head fractures, radial head hypertrophy, osteochondral lesions, degeneration of the capitellum, or osteochondritis dissecans. The extension component leads to posterior olecranon impingement. In association with valgus instability, this extension component leads to specific spurs on the posterior medial aspect of the olecranon that engage during the throwing motion and can lead to pain or create loose bodies. This valgus extension overload mechanism is exactly the same during the overhead service in racquet sports.

Another common mechanism of chronic elbow injury is the repetitive compressive loading as seen in sports such as gymnastics, boxing, and weightlifting. The anatomic structures at risk are the same as those with throwing athletes; however, the compressive loads are greater. This places the articular surface at a relatively greater risk of overuse failure compared to throwers with similar number of loads events. This may explain why gymnasts

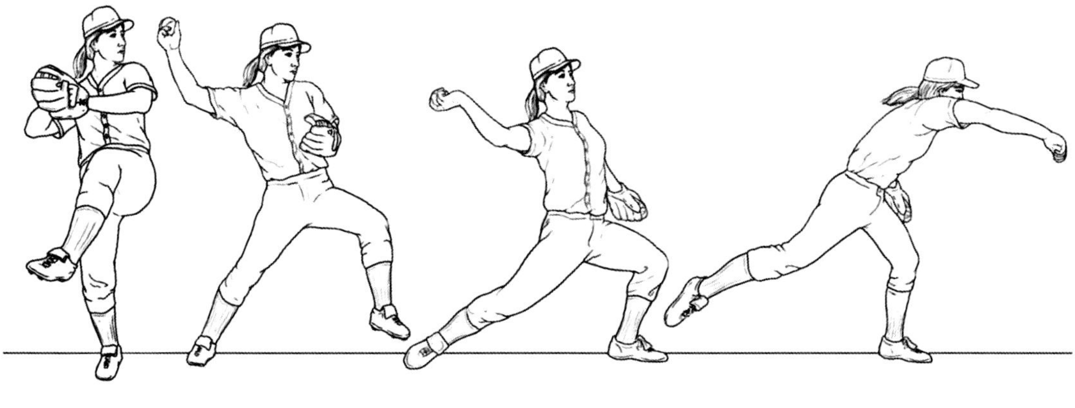

Figure 10.9. The normal throwing sequence consists of wind-up, cocking, acceleration, and follow-thru phases. With approval @ Mark R. Hutchinson, UIC Sports Medicine

who suffer osteochondritis dissecans have a miserable prognosis regarding return to sport compared to their young baseball counterparts who seem to have a better prognosis.

Identifying risks in the training and competition program

As we have seen, multiple factors contribute to the incidence and prevalence of elbow injuries in athletes. The relationship of training, practice, or competition to injury incidence has been well studied regarding injuries in general but less well evaluated for elbows in particular. The key issues for elbow injuries are the number of repetitions or exposure to traumatic events in training versus competitive situations. In contact and collisions sports, the athlete is at greater risk of acute trauma during competition where their opponent is trying to overwhelm their strength or position. In practice situations, players more frequently are less "all out" as compared to a competition. An exception to this rule is spring football in American rules football in which teams play competitively amongst their own team vying for positions on the next years teams. Injury rates are greater at this time than the regular season. For gymnasts, they are at risk of traumatic injuries at any time they are at competition height on apparatus regardless practice or competition.

Training versus competition seems to have a major effect on overuse injuries. Overuse injuries are always more common when an athlete begins to train intensely after an extended period of rest or when they are asked to significantly ramp up their training immediately prior to a major competition or event. This is true for the elbow as it is for most body parts. Prevention usually targets a gradual increase in stresses and intensity rather than these acute changes in training patterns to avoid the risk of overuse injuries.

Skeletal maturity and training

For the skeletally immature thrower, the injury risk appears to be less related to training or competition compared to the actual number of full speed tosses they perform in a given time period. Too many throws on too little rest is directly related to an increased injury incidence. Likewise for the mature thrower, overuse elbow injuries have been related to the total number of pitches and amount of rest between outings.

For the mature athlete, core strength and a coordinated kinetic chain have a central role in injury prevention. Coaches and trainers should carefully evaluate the throwing mechanic of their athletes early in the training season to assure that there are no deficits in the kinetic chain that might predict future injury. During competition, the kinetic chain may also play a key role in the risk of elbow injury. As the athlete fatigues later in competition, he is more likely to overuse single components of the kinetic chain leading to a failure of the coordinated sequence of movement and placing any link at risk of injury. Based on this knowledge, coaches should be astute observers of athletic performance and biomechanics during competition. The athlete should be removed from play when proximal links of the kinetic chain reveal weakness, poor coordination, or failure because the elbow may be the next link to fail.

Preventive measures

The foundation of a targeted prevention plan to reduce elbow injuries should be based on available science and our historical knowledge regarding incidence and mechanism. The ideal of eliminating all injuries is not reasonable as athletic participation carries some inherent risk. Nonetheless, minimizing risk and preventing the progression of a minor deficit or problem to a more significant injury is clearly our best option. A valid prevention plan should target the injury patterns that are most common, most potentially disabling, and in which intervention can be the most effective.

Targeting acute injuries

For acute and traumatic injuries of the elbow, prevention should target minimizing risk exposures and energy level when such an exposure would not affect the routine and legal performance of

Table 10.3 Injury prevention matrix for elbow injuries: potential measures to prevent injuries.

	Precrash	Crash	Postcrash
Athlete	Hand dominance Throwing technique Backhand technique in tennis Core strength and stability Optimal shoulder function Pitch counts	Falling techniques	Comparative radiographs in children to avoid missing complex injuries Regain motion ASAP to avoid contractures
Rules	Restrictions of repetitions in underage throwers Regulations versus at risk techniques in martial arts		
Material	String tension in racquet sports Racquet rigidity Length of racquets Decrease weight of projectiles	Elbow pads in collision sports	Therapeutic taping to avoid recurrent hyperextension Pads to avoid recurrent bursitis
Environment	Rainy weather increases ball weight	Padded surfaces absorb fall energy	First aid readily available Only qualified professional to perform reduction of dislocation

the sport. This may be accomplished via rigid rule enforcement, more severe penalties for violations, or rules changes. An example that has been effective was limiting the height of cheerleader towers which, in turn, reduced the potential energy and risk of injury from falls (Boden et al., 2003). Examples that could be effective include rules changes, the imposition of stiffer penalties or the rigid enforcement of existing rules that prevents a wrestler from lifting his opponent off the matt or tossing his opponent through the air. In judo, banning the ability of a competitor to hyperextend the elbow (or dislocate it) until his opponent taps out (gives up) would likely reduce the risk of elbow injuries in that sport.

Targeting the environment

Targeting issues of athlete fatigue as well as ensuring safe equipment and environment would also reduce the risk of elbow problems. Athletes should be instructed to rest when fatigued. This is especially true when their partner is dependent on their elbow's strength and function (pairs figure skating, cheerleading) or when they are participating in a high energy sport such as gymnastics in which a fall could be catastrophic. Equipment and apparatus should be checked for proper function before competition begins. If competition apparatus is unstable or set at the wrong height, it may predispose the athlete to a fall. There is good literature to support that the use of elbow pads in rollerbladers reduces their risk of elbow injuries especially of contusions and abrasions (Schieber et al., 1996; Jerosch et al., 1998; Sheiker & Casell, 1999). Elbow injuries in rollerbladers are most strongly correlated with their willingness to perform advanced tricks and maneuvers. The use of elbow protection in sports at risk of direct contusion such as hockey, lacrosse, or racquetball may reduce the risk of these contact injuries. In addition better designs and fitting with improved shock absorption may assist to a diffuse the load of the more significant direct injuries (Table 10.3).

Targeting overuse

While avoiding a single catastrophic injury, particularly for the individual athlete, is important, the most effective aim for elbow injury prevention should target the most common injuries; that is, overuse injuries. The foundational knowledge of injury risk, risk factors, and mechanisms should serve as our guide to developing an injury prevention plan for the elbow that can be applied to all sports but also one that can be individualized to create a sport-specific plan. Athlete's at risk of elbow injuries due to a history of previous elbow injuries or due to their participation in at risk sports golf, baseball, softball, javelin, tennis, and wrestling should be more thoroughly evaluated on preparticipation physical examinations. The presence of elbow stiffness or pain should be addressed with appropriate therapy prior to release for unrestricted training. Extension loss of greater than 15° at the elbow or an abnormal carrying angle secondary to development or previous injury will likely lead to abnormal mechanics and future overuse injury. For all overhead and upper extremity dominant athletes, the screening program should also include a thorough assessment of shoulder function and motion. Posterior capsular tightness evidenced by a loss of internal rotation has been directly associated with both shoulder and elbow complaints. Fortunately in a large majority of cases, the shoulder tightness responds to a focused program of capsular stretches including cross-over stretches, internal rotation stretches, and "sleeper" stretches. The latter are performed as the athlete lays on his side trapping the effected scapula between his body and the bed followed by internal rotation stretches in various positions.

Table 10.4 Interval throwing program: baseball. All throws should be on an arc with a crow hop. Warm-up throws should be 10–20 tosses at 30 ft. Perform each step 2–3 times before progressing. If pain occurs go to previously level. Distances should be shortened for Little Leaguers.

Step	Throwing program
Step 1 & 2: 45-ft Phase	
	1. Warm-up, 25 tosses, 5-min rest, repeat
	2. Warm-up, 25 tosses, 5-min rest, repeat twice
Step 3 & 4: 60-ft Phase	
	3. Warm-up, 25 tosses, 5-min rest, repeat
	4. Warm-up, 25 tosses, 5-min rest, repeat twice
Step 5 & 6: 90-ft Phase	
	5. Warm-up, 25 tosses, 5-min rest, repeat
	6. Warm-up, 25 tosses, 5-min rest, repeat twice
Step 7 & 8: 120-ft Phase	
	7. Warm-up, 25 tosses, 5-min rest, repeat
	8. Warm-up, 25 tosses, 5-min rest, repeat twice
Step 9 & 10: 150-ft Phase	
	9. Warm-up, 25 tosses, 5-min rest, repeat
	10. Warm-up, 25 tosses, 5-min rest, repeat twice
Step 11 & 12: 180-ft Phase	
	11. Warm-up, 25 tosses, 5-min rest, repeat
	12. Warm-up, 25 tosses, 5-min rest, repeat twice
Step 13 & 14: progression to pitching: flat ground stage	
	13. Warm-up, 60-ft/15 tosses, 90-ft/10 tosses, 120-ft/10 tosses, 60-ft/20 tosses using pitching mechanics from flat ground
	14. Step 13, 10-min rest, repeat
Step 15: pitching: mound stage	
	15. Progression to pitching from mound

Targeting training

When athletes return to play after a significant period of rest or injury, their return should be slow and progressive. Acute and intense increases in the training regimen at the beginning of the season, prior to major competitions, or during injury recovery have been associated with recurrence or overuse injury. A slow progressive recovery program has the best opportunity for successful return to play without recurrence (Tables 10.4, 10.5 and 10.6). In addition to conditioning, coaches should also assure that athletes also have a gradual progression in skills from fundamental to more complex. This plan would avoid the risk of the immature baseball player throwing a curveball with poor mechanics or of the young cheerleader/gymnast attempting a stunt beyond her skill level and risking a catastrophic fall on her outstretched hand.

Targeting the athlete at risk

The at-risk athlete should also be screened at the time of his preparticipation examination for coordinated movement, strength and symmetry along the entire kinetic chain. Scapular dyskinesia can be assessed by inspecting the athlete from posterior and asking them to protract, retract, and elevate their shoulders with their arms at the sides, hands on their hips, and with their arms abducted 90° (Box 9.1). Any side-to-side asymmetry should be

Table 10.5 Interval rehabilitation program: tennis (Reinhold et al., 2005).

Week #	Monday	Wednesday	Friday
Week 1	12FH	15 FH	15FH
	8BH	8BH	10BH
	10-min rest	10-min rest	10-min rest
	13FH	15FH	15FH
	7BH	7BH	10BH
Week 2	25FH	30FH	30FH
	15BH	20BH	25BH
	10-min rest	10-min rest	10-min rest
	25FH	30FH	30FH
	15BH	20BH	25BH
Week 3	30FH, 25BH	30FH, 25BH	30FH, 30BH
	10 Serves	15 Serves	15 Serves
	10-min rest	10-min rest	10-min rest
	30FH, 25BH	30FH, 25BH	30FH, 25BH
	10 Serves	15 Serves	15 Serves
Week 4	30FH, 30BH	30FH, 30BH	30FH, 30BH
	10 Serves	10 Serves	10 Serves
	10-min rest	10-min rest	10-min rest
	Play 3 games	Play set	Play 1.5 sets
	10FH, 10BH	10FH, 10BH	10FH, 10BH
	5 Serves	5 Serves	5 Serves

*FH = forehand shots; BH = backhand shots.

Table 10.6 Interval rehabilitation program: golf (Reinhold et al., 2005).

Week #	Monday	Wednesday	Friday
Week 1	10 putts	15 putts	20 putts
	10 chips	15 chips	20 chips
	5-min rest	5-min rest	5-min rest
	15 chips	25 chips	20 putts/20 chips
Week 2	20 chips	20 chips	15 short irons
	10 short irons	15 short irons	20 med irons
	5-min rest	10-min rest	10-min rest
	10 short irons	15 short irons	20 short irons
	15 med irons	15 chips	15 chips
	5 iron off tee	putting ad lib	putting ad lib
		15 med irons	15 medium irons
Week 3	15 short irons	15 short irons	15 short irons
	20 med irons	15 med irons	15 med irons
	10-min rest	10 long irons	10 long irons
	15 short irons	10-min rest	10-min rest
	15 med irons	10 short irons	10 short irons
	5 long irons	10 med irons	10 med irons
	10-min rest	5 long irons	10 long irons
	20 chips	5 woods	10 woods
Week 4	15 short irons	Warm-up	Warm up
	15 med irons	Play 9 holes	Play 9 holes
	10 long irons		
	10 drives		
	15-min rest		
	Repeat		
Week 5	Play 9 holes	Play 9 holes	Play 18 holes

addressed with focused rehabilitation. Evaluation of core strength and coordination is also important. During the preseason screening evaluation, all overhead athletes should be asked to perform a single-legged squat on both a stable and an unstable surface (foam pad, balance board, mini-tramp). The observer should look for poor balance in the upper body with arm swaying or inability to maintain single leg stance, hyperflexion of the lumbar spine instead of a true knee squat, and gluteal weakness evidenced by knee internal rotation or dropping the contralateral pelvis (Figure 5.7). Any abnormalities discovered should be addressed with focused training and has been shown to reduce the incidence of elbow problems in athletes (Kibler & Sciascia, 2004).

Targeting early recognition

Educational programs may also target the reduction of injury incidence and severity. Athletes in throwing, weight-bearing and weight-lifting sports need to be educated to offer complaints of elbow pain when present. Delayed diagnosis can lead to poorer prognosis. For example, young gymnasts should never participate in the presence of undiagnosed pain for fear of making the pathology worse. Mild degrees of osteochondritis dissecans can be treated with rest and have a significantly better prognosis than advanced degrees of osteochondritis dissecans with loose bodies. Indeed gymnasts compared to all sports have the worst prognosis regarding return to sport when the osteochondritis dissecans is severe. Another example is the mature athlete with a prodrome of bicipital tendonitis or medial collateral ligament pain. Continued participation and loading can lead to complete rupture, while early treatment and rest may avoid the need of surgical intervention completely.

Focused, sport-specific injury prevention intervention plans should target the three most studied sports regarding overuse elbow injuries; golf, tennis, and baseball. These plans can easily be translated to other sports using baseball as a model for throwing sports, tennis as a model for racquet sports, and golf as model for stick sports.

Targeting golf

Golf has a surprisingly high rate of elbow injuries, particularly for the amateur athlete (see Table 10.1). The length of the golf club increases the force moment that magnifies the energy that crosses the elbow joint. As noted earlier, this mechanism has been associated with the development of golfer's elbow or a tendinopathy on the medial aspect of the elbow. Prevention centers on an increased awareness of the risk as well as improving the mechanics of the golf swing including impact. Avoid taking large divots. Optimize swing mechanics. Equipment modifications may also be helpful with more flexible shafts to absorb shock, appropriate grips for hand size, and broader head designs with peripheral weighting to maximize the sweet spot.

Targeting tennis

A majority of elbow injuries related to tennis are related to either repetitive varus forces with active wrist extension during the backhand or repetitive valgus extension overload during the serve. Reduction of the risk of tennis elbow begins with the proper equipment. The grip should not be too small placing the extensors on tension and at risk of injury. For beginners and intermediate level players, high tension racquets are unnecessary for success and may be avoided while skills are advancing. Oversized heads and other equipment designs that help to absorb the shock of impact or assure optimal contact may also be helpful. Counterforce bracing has also been popular to decrease the focal loads on the lateral aspect of the elbow. Many athletes have switched to a two-fisted backhand because it allows them increased power, more control, and reduced forces over the lateral aspect of the elbow. Athletes with a history of or at risk of tennis elbow should consider switching to a two-fisted backhand to diminish the loads.

The next most common injury pattern in tennis players are related to the repetitive valgus-extension overload that occurs with overheads and the tennis serve. This pattern mimics that seen in throwing athletes. Strains or rupture of the medial collateral ligament, compression injuries of the capitellum, and posterior impingement lesions have been identified just like those seen in baseball. Indeed the severity may be magnified by the increased fulcrum provided by the additional racquet extension to the site of impact. Prevention plans include athlete education to optimize early identification and initiation of treatment; preparticipation screening identifying risks in both the elbow and the shoulder, conditioning programs that focus on every facet of the kinetic chain (Box 10.1). To avoid overuse elbow problems in the skeletally immature, an evaluation of the number of serves, overheads, and backhands performed in a given session or week may be of benefit. This has clearly been effective in reducing the risk of injury in skeletally immature throwers (Lyman et al., 2002; Dugas, 2006; Olsen et al., 2006). Indeed, there is a good support to this plan in skeletally immature throwers in little league baseball.

Targeting baseball and overhead throwers

To begin targeting the throwing athlete, most athletes are placed on a routine program of rotator cuff strengthening, scapular stabilization exercises, core strengthening and posterior capsular stretches. Those with deficits are asked to participate in a supervised program until the deficits are corrected (Box 10.2). The second key intervention for overhead throwers is educating the athlete regarding overuse and monitoring the number of throws they perform and the amount of rest between each outing. This is especially true for the skeletally immature athlete. Controlled number of pitch counts per week and season with prescribed numbers of days or rest between outings has been directly correlated with reduced risk of elbow injuries in both the immature and the mature throwers (Table 10.7) (Lyman et al.,

Box 10.1. Injury prevention protocol for tennis

1. Low-to-high pull with resistance against weight or tubing
   - Begin reaching low across body outside of contralateral foot
   - Explosive lift the arm into full abduction and external rotation
   - Slowly return to the first position
   - Repeat 1–3 sets, 15–20 repetitions

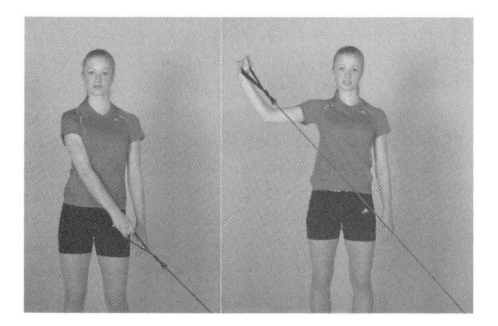

2. Straight arm rowing with resistance against weight or tubing
   - Begin with arms straight in front with in line tension
   - Pull arms into extension while squeezing shoulder blades together as if rowing a boat
   - Repeat 1–3 sets, 15 repetitions

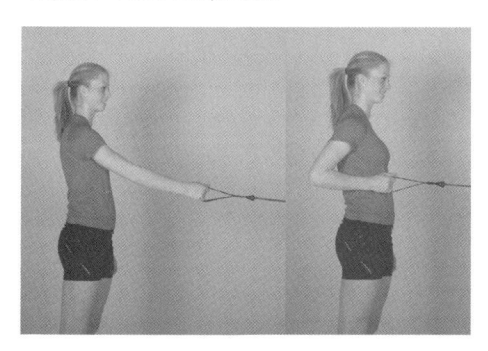

3. Standing external rotation with resistance against weight or tubing
   - With the arm at the side & 0° of abduction & neutral rotation
   - Externally rotate against resistance
   - 1–3 sets, 15–20 repetitions

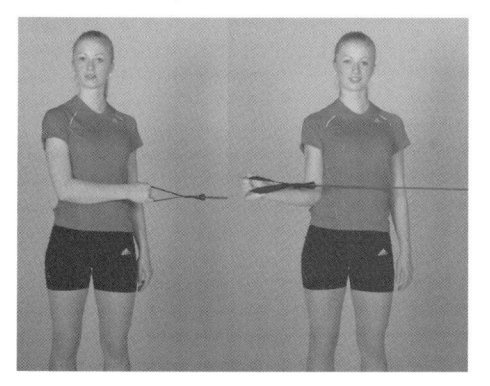

4. 90–90 external rotation with resistance against weight or tubing
   - Begin with the arm at 90° of abduction and neutral position
   - Externally rotate against resistance
   - 1–3 sets, 15–20 repetitions

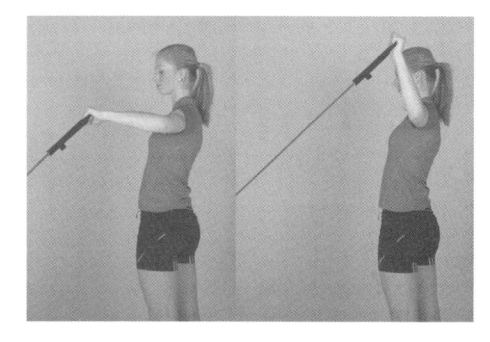

5. Wrist extension (strengthening) with resistance against weight or tubing
   - While seated and forearms resting comfortably on thigh
   - Extend wrists from a flexed, palm down position to full extension
   - 1–3 sets, 15–20 repetitions

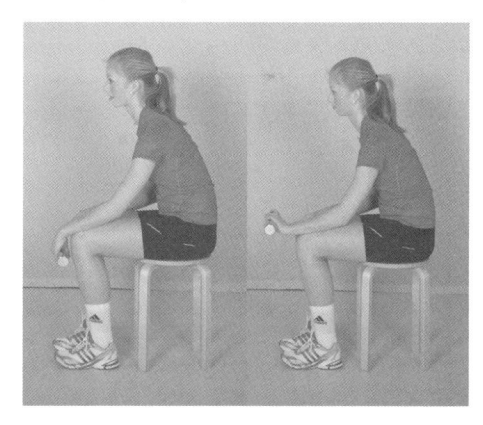

6. Wrist flexion (strengthening) with resistance against weight or tubing
   - While seated and forearms resting comfortably on thigh

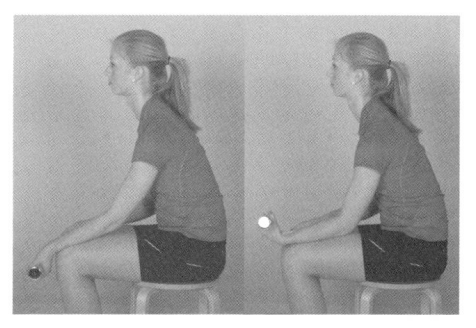

(*Continued*)

Box 10.1 (Continued)

- Flex wrists from a extended, palm up position to full flexion
- 1–3 sets, 15–20 repetitions

7. Forearm pronation with resistance against weight or tubing
   - While seated and forearms comfortably resting on thigh
   - Wrap resistance tubing around hand so that it exits on the thumb side of the hand and secure the free end
   - Hand should be positioned palm up until resistance is felt in tubing 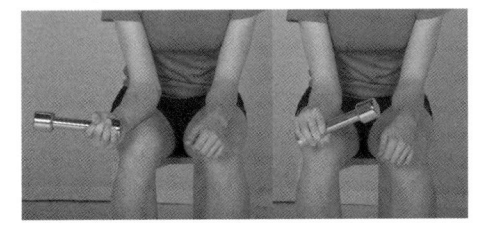
   - Twist forearm palm down against resistance
   - 1–3 sets, 15–20 repetitions

8. Forearm supination with resistance against weight or tubing
   - While seated and forearms comfortably resting on thigh
   - Wrap resistance tubing around hand so that it exits on the thumb side of the hand and secure the free end
   - Hand should be positioned palm up until resistance is felt in tubing
   - Twist forearm palm down against resistance
   - 1–3 sets, 15–20 repetitions.

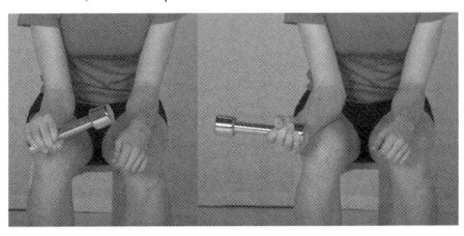

Source: Shoulder and elbow injury prevention protocol from United States Tennis Association (www.playerdevelopment.usta.com).

Box 10.2 The thrower's 10 exercise prevention program

1. Diagonal pattern D2 extension/flexion
   - Stand, using resistance tubing begin with arm in full abduction and external rotation and pull tubing down and across the body to the opposite side of the leg
   - Using resistance tubing begin with arm crossed over body bear opposite hip and pull tubing into full abduction and external rotation position

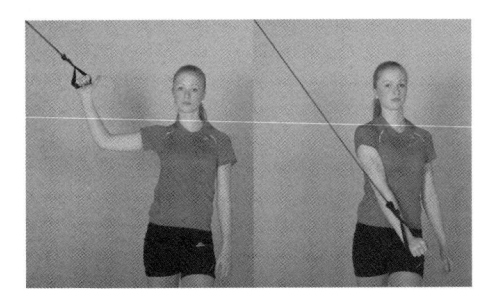

2. External/internal rotation at 0° and 90° of abduction
   - Stand, using resistance tubing begin with arm in fully internally rotated position, first with arm at 0 abduction then with arm in 90° of abduction
   - Pull on resistance while rotating into full external rotation
   - Repeat above but begin with arm in full external rotation and pull on resistance at both 0° and 90° of abduction into full internal rotation

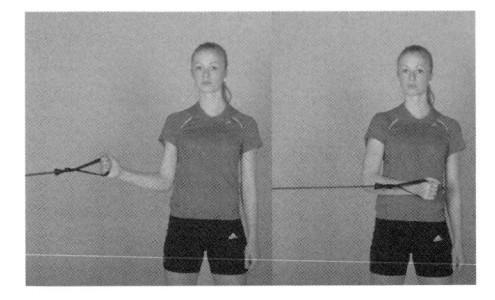

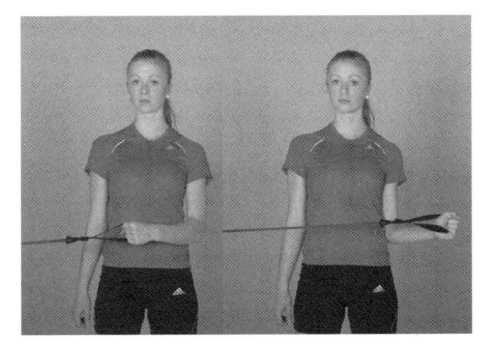

(Continued)

Box 10.2 (Continued)

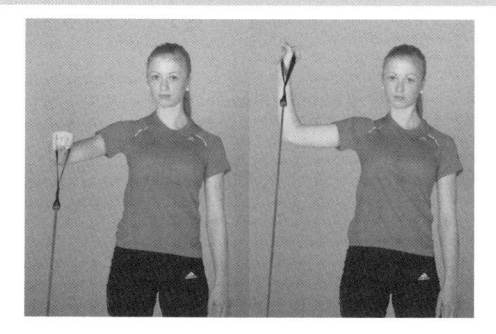

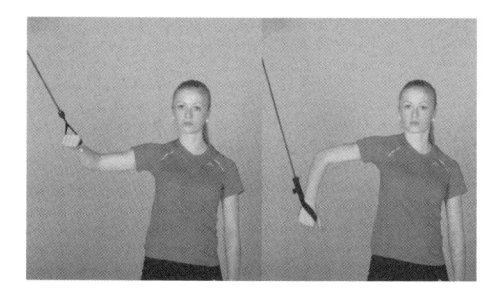

3. Shoulder abduction to 90°
   – Stand holding a 5 pound weight or against resistance tubing begin with arm at side then abduct the shoulder to 90° with elbow in full extension

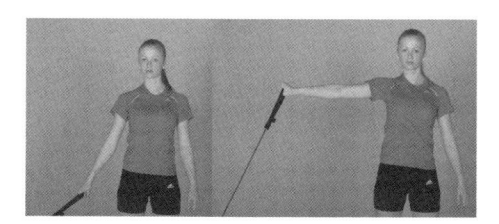

4. Scaption, internal rotation
   – Stand with arm at side and elbow straight and thumb up
   – Raise arm to shoulder level at 30° angle in front of body (in plane of scapula)
   – Hold for 2 s, lower slowly

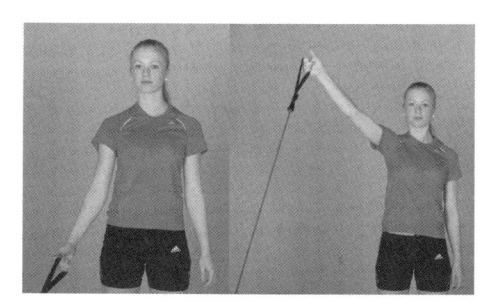

5. Press-ups
   – Seated on a chair or table, place both hands firmly with palms down
   – Slowly push downward on both hands to elevate your body
   – Hold for 2 s, lower slowly

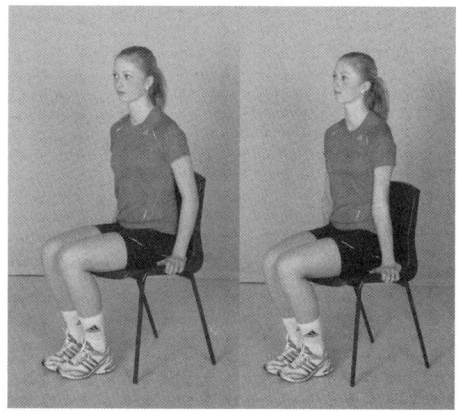

6. Prone horizontal abduction
   – Lie on table face down with arm hanging to floor, hold barbell weight or against tubing resistance, extend the arm laterally, parallel with the floor
   – Hold 2 s, lower slowly
   – Repeat both in neutral and full external rotated positions

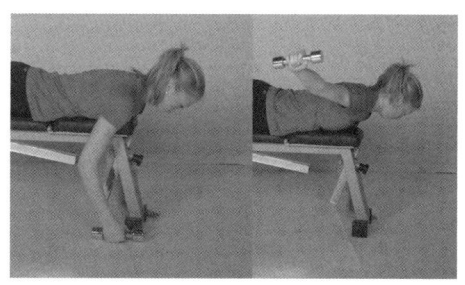

7. Prone rowing
Lie on table face down with arm hanging to floor and holding barbell weight, pull backwards, flexing the elbow as if rowing
   – Bring the dumbbell up as high as possible
   – Hold for 2 s and slowly lower

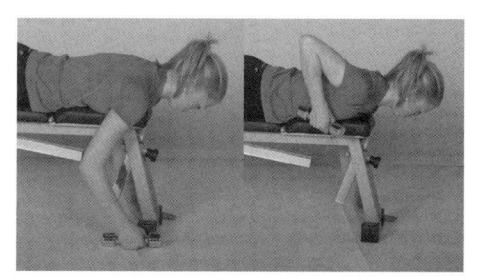

(Continued)

172 Chapter 10

> **Box 10.2 (Continued)**
>
> 8. Push-ups
> Place hands no more than shoulder width apart. Push up as high as possible rolling shoulders forward after elbow lock straight
>
> 9. Elbow flexion/extension
>   - With arm against side and in full supination, lift barbell weight or against resistance tubing, hold 2 s and lower slowly
>   - Lift arm overhead and support elbow. 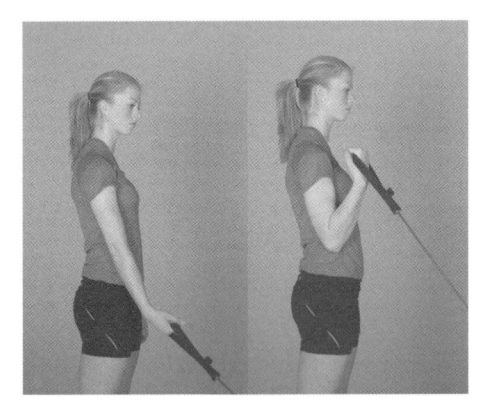 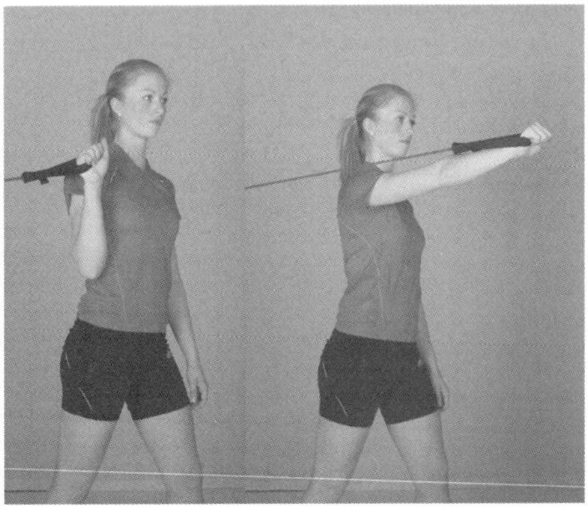
>   - Straighten elbow over head against resistance or barbell weight. Hold 2 s and slowly lower
>
> 10. Wrist extension/flexion, supination/pronation
>   - Supporting the forearm on a table with the palm faced down, extend the wrist against weight or tubing resistance
>   - With the palm faced up, flex the wrist against weight or tubing resistance
>   - With the wrist in neutral position use a hammer, off-centered weight, or tubing to resist placing the arm in to a palms-up position
>   - With the wrist in neutral position use a hammer, off-centered weight, or tubing to resist placing the arm in to a palms-down position 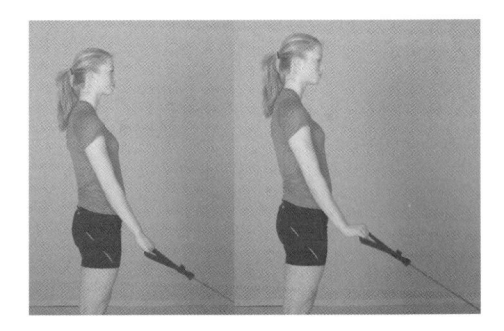 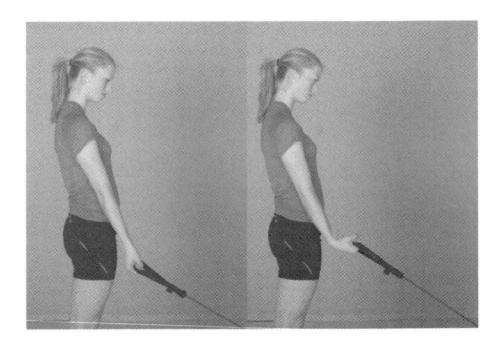
>
> Source: From James Andrews, American Sports Medicine Institute. Video illustrations available at http://www.asmi.org/sportsmed/throwing/thrower10.html.

2002; Dugas, 2006; Olsen et al., 2006). These guidelines are based on performance pitch counts and not tosses from other positions; however, the clinician should ask the athlete if they participate in more than one league, pitch at full speed between games, or perform showcase events. In any of those cases, the full speed pitch count should be applied to the pitch count guidelines. Prevention guidelines for the skeletally immature also include recommendations regarding the appropriate age to add certain types of pitches (Table 10.8). It should be emphasized to the young thrower that a proper throwing mechanic

Table 10.7 Pitch count guidelines in Youth Baseball from USA Baseball and the American Sports Medicine Institute.

Age group	Throwing program
9–10 year olds	– 50 pitches per game
	– 75 pitches per week
	– 1000 pitches per season
	– 2000 pitches per year
11–12 year olds	– 75 pitches per game
	– 100 pitches per week
	– 1000 pitches per season
	– 3000 pitches per year
13–14 year olds	– 75 pitches per game
	– 125 pitches per week
	– 1000 pitches per season
	– 3000 pitches per year

Table 10.8 Guidelines for the institution of pitch types in Little Leaguers from USA Baseball and the American Sports Medicine Institute.

Pitch type	Age (years)
Fastball	8–10
Change-up	10–13
Curveball	14–16
Knuckle ball	15–18
Slider	16–18
Fork ball	16–18
Screwball	17–19

and not some new tricky pitch will most improve their performance and outcomes.

Take-home message

The elbow serves an integral role in many sports making the importance of maintaining optimal function and avoiding injuries is an important goal for athletes. Not all elbow injuries, particularly many of the traumatic ones, are avoidable. Nonetheless, the incidence of those may be reduced by following the rules of play, optimizing equipment, and avoiding fatigue for at risk athletes. The best target for injury prevention of elbow injuries should target the repetitive overuse injuries. For children, reducing exposure by imposing pitch counts or throwing limits can reduce the incidence of injury and early identification and rest can prevent them from becoming more severe. A simple rule for coaches of skeletally immature athletes is that they should not play through pain. The return to play for all injured elbows should be gradual and progressive. In thrower's this is done via a throwing protocol which begins with light tosses and progresses in distance and speed. If the athlete returns too quickly he risks reinjuring his elbow. A universal program to reduce the risk of elbow injuries must look beyond the elbow joint itself and include training and coordination of the entire kinetic chain. Preseason screening programs to identify core weaknesses including such things as single leg squats on unstable surfaces and evaluation of scapular dynamics can help to identify the athlete at risk.

References

Boden, B.P., Tachetti, R., Mueller, F.O. (2003) Catastrophic cheerleading injuries. *American Journal of Sports Medicine* **31**, 881–888.

Dugas, J.R. (2006) Prevention of overuse in the adolescent thrower. *Sports Medicine Update, American Orthopaedic Society for Sports Medicine* **1**, 4–7.

Jerosch, J., Heidjann, J., Thorwesten, L., Lepsein, U. (1998) Injury pattern and acceptance of passive and active injury prophylaxis for inline skating. *Knee Surgery Sports Traumatology and Arthroscopy* **6**, 44–49.

Kibler, W.B., Sciascia, A. (2004) Kinetic chain contributions to elbow function and dysfunction in sports. *Clinics in Sports Medicine* **23**, 542–552.

Lyman, S., Fleisig, G.S., Andrews, J.R., Osinski, E.D. (2002) Effect of pitch type, pitch count and pitching mechanics on risk of elbow and shoulder pain in youth pitchers. *American Journal of Sports Medicine* **30**, 463–468.

Olsen, S.J., Fleisig, G.S., Dun, S., Loftice, J., Andrews, J.R. (2006) Risk factors for shoulder and elbow injuries in adolescent pitchers. *American Journal of Sports Medicine* **34**, 905–912.

Reinhold, M.M., Wilk, K.E., Reed, J., Crenshaw, K., Andrews, J.R. (2005) Interval sports programs: guidelines for baseball, tennis, and golf. *Journal of Orthopaedic and Sports Physical Therapy* **32**, 293–298.

Schieber, R.A., Branche-Dorsey, C.M., Ryan, G.W., Rutherford Jr., G.W., Stevens, J.A., O'Neil, J. (1996) Risk factors for injuries from in line skating and effectiveness of safety gear. *New England Journal of Medicine* **28**, 1680–1682.

Sheiker, S., Casell, E. (1999) Preventing in-line skating injuries: how effective are the countermeasures? *Sports Medicine* **28**, 325–335.

Further reading

Andrews, J.R., Zarins, B., Wilk, K. (1998) *Injuries in Baseball*. Lippincott-Raven Publishers, Philadelphia, PA.

Cain, E.L., Dugas, J.R., Wolf, R.S., Andrews, J.R. (2003) Elbow injuries in athletes: a current concepts review. *American Journal of Sports Medicine* **31**, 621–635.

Caine, D.J., Nassar, L. (2005) Gymnastics injuries. *Medicine and Science in Sports and Exercise* **48**, 18–58.

Field, L.D., Altchek, D.W. (1995) Elbow injuries. *Clinics in Sports Medicine* **14**, 59–78.

Fleisig, G.S., Barrentine, S.W., Escamilla, R.F., Andrews, J.R. (1996) Biomechanics of overhand throwing with implications for injuries. *Sports Medicine* **21**, 421–437.

Hutchinson, M.R., Laprade, R.F., Burnett, Q.A., Moss, R., Terpstra, J. (1995) The incidence and prevalence of injuries at the United States Tennis Association's national boys championships. *Medicine and Science in Sports and Exercise* **27**, 826–830.

Hutchinson, M.R., Wynn, S. (2004) Biomechanics and development of the elbow in the young throwing athlete. *Clinics in Sports Medicine* **23**, 531–544.

McCarroll, J.R. (2001) Overuse injuries of the upper extremity in golf. *Clinics in Sports Medicine* **20**, 469–479.

NCAA (2006) *NCAA Injury Surveillance System*. National Collegiate Athletic Association, Indianapolis, IN.

Stockard, A.R. (2001) Elbow injuries in golf. *Journal of the American Osteopathic Association* **101**, 509–516.

Chapter 11
Preventing injuries to the head and cervical spine

Paul McCrory[1], Michael Turner[2] and Andrew McIntosh[3]

[1]Centre for Health, Exercise and Sports Medicine, University of Melbourne Parkville, Australia
[2]Chief Medical Adviser, British Horseracing Authority and Lawn Tennis Association; formerly CMA to British Olympic Association and Snowsport, UK
[3]School of Risk and Safety Sciences, The University of New South Wales, Sydney Australia

Epidemiology of head and cervical spine injuries in sports

Sports involving collision, body contact, projectiles, and/or high speeds are associated with a risk of head and neck injury. The range of potential head and neck injuries—from facial lacerations to intracranial hemorrhage, from mild neck strains to spinal cord lesions makes this area of injury management particularly difficult.

Fortunately, most sports-related head and neck injuries are mild. However, severe and sometimes fatal injuries do occur which makes the need to prevention of such injuries critical. It is worth also observing that head and neck injuries do not always occur on the sports field; a child spectator died in 2002 after being struck in the head by an ice hockey puck in the United States and in 2001, a track marshal was killed during a Formula 1 championship race.

These tragic examples indicate that injury prevention must be multi-faceted, addressing, in these cases, the "built" environment, training, and supervision.

Sports Injury Prevention, 1st edition. Edited by R. Bahr and L. Engebretsen Published 2009 by Blackwell Publishing
ISBN: 9781405162449

Pathophysiology of head and neck injury

Non-penetrating brain injury (or closed head injury) may be divided into primary and secondary injuries. Primary injury is the result of mechanical forces producing tissue deformation at the moment of injury. These deformations may result in either functional disturbance or structural disruption of cell membranes. The injury may also set in train a complex cascade of biochemical, immunological, or coagulopathic changes that may cause further damage.

Secondary damage occurs as a complication of primary injury and includes hypoxic and ischemic damage, brain swelling, hydrocephalus, and infection. Sports concussion by definition has no macroscopic neuropathological damage and it is speculated that the critical physiological change occurs at the cell membrane level. There has also been recent evidence to suggest a significant genetic basis to head injury outcomes (Aubry et al., 2002; McCrory et al., 2005).

Concussion and mild traumatic brain injury

Sports concussion has been defined as a complex pathophysiological process affecting the brain, induced by traumatic biomechanical forces (Aubry et al., 2002; McCrory et al., 2005). Several common features that incorporate clinical, pathological, and biomechanical injury constructs that may be utilized in defining the nature of a concussive head injury include:

1. Concussion may be caused either by a direct blow to the head, face, neck, or elsewhere on the body with an "impulsive" force transmitted to the head.

2. Concussion typically results in the rapid onset of short-lived impairment of neurological function that resolves spontaneously.

3. Concussion may result in neuropathological changes, but the acute clinical symptoms largely reflect a functional disturbance rather than structural injury.

4. Concussion results in a graded set of clinical syndromes that may or may not involve loss of consciousness. Resolution of the clinical and cognitive symptoms typically follows a sequential course.

5. Concussion is typically associated with grossly normal structural neuroimaging studies.

In Table 11.1, the incidence of concussion is presented using common exposure risk. It can be seen that sports where high velocity impacts (e.g., equestrian sports) occur, the risk of head injury is the greatest.

Catastrophic head and spinal cord injury

Catastrophic head and spinal cord injury occur in virtually all sports. In total 497 persons have died while playing American football in the United States since 1945; of these 69% died from fatal brain injuries and 16% from spinal cord injury (Levy et al., 2004). Data from the US Catastrophic Injury Registry suggests that the incidence of catastrophic head and spinal cord injury has been dropping since the late 1960s and the effect of the introduction of rule changes (e.g., mandatory helmet use, banning spear tackles) in the 1970s led to no appreciable change in the downward trend of injury rates.

Even though the overall rate of spinal cord injury in rugby is low, there is a likely risk in rugby associated primarily with the tackle and scrum.

Table 11.1 Risk of concussion in elite sports.

Sport	Incidence per 1000h of exposure[1]
Horse racing	25.0
Kickboxing	4.8
Australian football	4.2
Professional boxing	3.9
Rugby union football	3.9
Cricket	2.0
Ice hockey	1.5
Football/Soccer	0.4
American football	0.2
Skiing/snowboarding	0.05
Baseball	0.0043

The numbers reported are average estimates based on the studies available.
[1] Incidence is reported for adult, competitive athletes as the number of injuries per 1000h of competition.

Although this is suggested by retrospective studies and theoretical modeling, no prospective study of rugby spinal cord injury has been performed before and after the introduction of rule changes to reduce scrum-related injury. Studies of "spinal" injury in rugby union demonstrate that the scrum and tackling constitute high risk injury mechanisms for non-catastrophic neck injury. However, the number of spinal cord injuries is too low in the study to provide a meaningful statement as to spinal cord injury risk due to these mechanisms (Fuller et al., 2007). Interestingly there is some data to suggest that the spinal cord injury rate differs significantly with age, with schoolboy rugby players having spinal cord injury rates approximately one-third that of adult players.

With regard to fatal head injury, the only comparative data between sports and/or recreational activities was performed in the United Kingdom a number of years ago (Lyens et al., 1984). The findings are somewhat surprising insofar as sports that have a perception of high injury risk (e.g., boxing) have surprisingly few fatalities, whereas aquatic sports have relatively high fatality rates (Table 11.2).

Most commonly played sports (with the exception of equestrian sports) have relatively low fatality rates and although a fatal event may expose an underlying anatomical or physiological abnormality in the individual concerned there is no conclusive evidence that pre-event screening (e.g., MR or CT brain scans in boxers) will prevent fatalities.

Table 11.2 Sport-related fatalities in England and Wales.

Sport	Fatality rate[1]
Climbing/mountaineering (excl. hiking and fell walking)	>793
Air sports	>640
Motor sports	146
Water sports/windsurfing (excl. sailing and fishing)	67.5
Sailing/yachting	44.5
Fishing	37.4
Horse riding (excl. hunting and polo)	34.3
Rugby (union and league)	15.7
Boxing/wrestling	5.2
Football (Soccer)	3.8
Cricket	3.1

[1]Fatality rates per 100,000,000 occasions (days) of participation.

Key risk factors: how to identify athletes at risk

In general, risk factors for injury can be classified into either intrinsic or extrinsic (Meeuwisse, 1991; Milburn, 1993). Intrinsic or internal factors relate to innate qualities of the individual such as their age or genetic make-up. Conversely, extrinsic factors are those related to the environment. Analysis of the epidemiological literature reveals a number of risk factors, which may be associated with increased risk of sports concussion (Table 11.3). Other than for sports concussion, there is surprisingly little published prospective risk factor analysis for catastrophic head and neck injury.

Injury mechanisms

General

Head and cervical spine injuries in sport arise mainly due to impacts either with opposing players, the ground or equipment. Participants are exposed to impacts in many sports, for example, football (of all types), projectile sports (cricket, baseball, and hockey), high-speed winter sports, aerial sports (gymnastics), martial arts, and wrestling.

Table 11.3 Summary of intrinsic and extrinsic risk factors in sports concussion.

Proposed risk factors	Comments
Intrinsic factors	
Age	Confounding factors include (a) increased exposure with increasing age and (b) potential mismatch of ability players in junior competitions.
Genetic predisposition	The current literature is based largely on studies involving case series and retrospective designs in patients with moderate to severe head trauma.
	In studies where potential confounding factors are controlled (e.g., age, GCS score on admission, neurosurgical management), no association is found between apolipoprotein E4 genotype and outcome (Nathoo et al., 2003).
Behavior ("risk compensation")	Use of protective equipment such as helmets, may result in higher risk taking behavior.
Extrinsic factors	
Characteristics of the playing surface	The main confounding factor is ground hardness, which may impact on speed of the game and subsequent forces of collisions and risk of contact injuries.
Playing position	The common trend is that positions of highest risk tend to reflect those in which collision rates and velocity of impact are highest.
Level of play	Confounding factors include (a) increased potential for mismatch of player size and ability at some lower levels and (b) modified rules, which may limit player contact.
Biomechanics of head impact (site, closing velocity, and duration of impact)	Significant limitations include (a) not all concussions are clearly seen on video footage and (b) mathematical assumptions are made in estimates of acceleration.
Previous injury	Most studies rely on retrospective recall of concussion, which is known to be inaccurate. Furthermore, important confounding factors such as style of play (e.g., tackling technique) are often overlooked.

The mechanics of head and cervical spine injuries have been studied extensively using mathematical, experimental, and observational methods. These studies arose initially out of the need to prevent blunt trauma amongst road users and to assess the effects of pilots operating in environments with high "g forces." Due to the recognition that sports participants experience many similar injuries to road users and that the loading patterns can be similar, there has been a transfer of knowledge and theoretical approaches into sport.

In simple terms, the head and neck are injured due to exposure to forces that exceed the "strength" of the brain, skull, blood vessels, and vertebrae. The magnitudes of the force and/or other relevant characteristics, moment, and acceleration, are determined largely by the energy transfer in the impact. Other factors are important such as, anatomical point of impact, the shape and stiffness of the impacted/impacting object, the direction of loading; amount of translational and/or angular motion of the head, and, for the neck, the presence of axial loading. The strain that results from these forms of loading is the primary cause of injury. However, strain is difficult to measure in these situations.

The tackle in rugby, Australian and American football, and body checking in ice hockey are associated with risks of minor to severe impact injury, including spinal cord injury. In rugby, approximately half of all injuries arise in the tackle.

Factors that may give rise to injury risks in the tackle include: high tackles; high velocity tackles; tackles in which the tackler may have been in the peripheral vision of the ball carrier; "big hits" in which the ball carrier is tackled by more than one player ("grapple" tackle is an example of a controversial multiplayer tackle in rugby league) (Figure 11.1); and, a general lack of skill for the tackler. Apart from high tackles and spear tackles, where the ball carrier is speared head first into the ground, the other types of tackle are legal.

Biomechanics of head injury

How do head impacts in motor vehicle accidents compared with those in football? It is very difficult to measure or simulate the complex dynamics of these real-life impact events because of energy attenuation by muscle, joint, or connective tissue forces applied through the neck to the head, and soft tissue deformation.

A number of studies using video analysis, finite element analysis and injury modeling have attempted this in both Australian and American football. The basic biomechanical injury mechanisms however, are the same, namely; forces applied directly to the

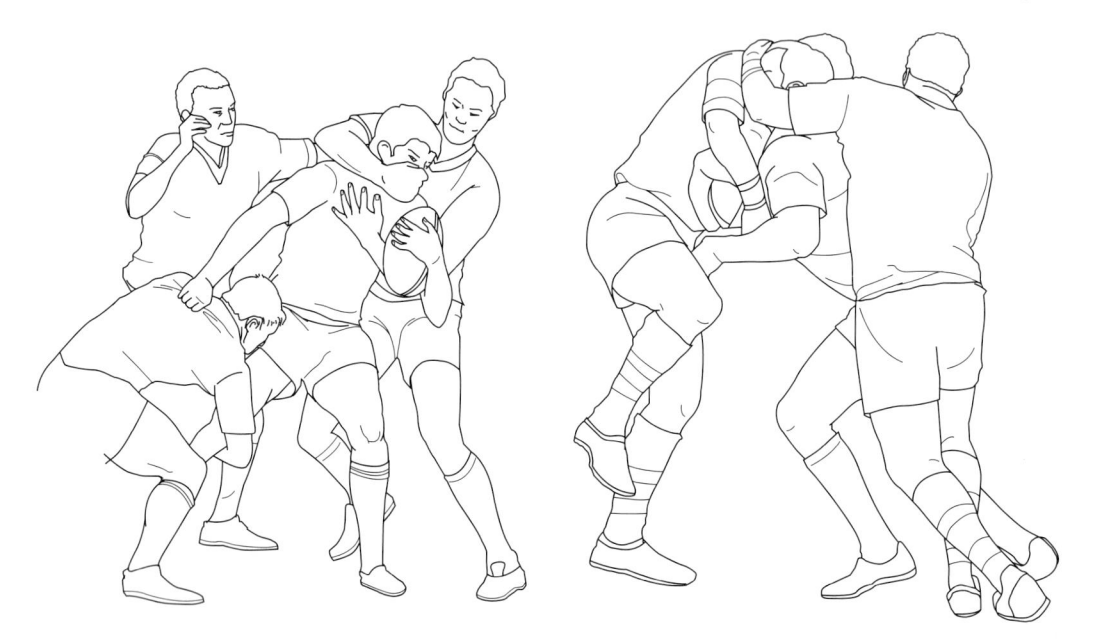

Figure 11.1. Examples of "grapple tackles" in rugby league where multiple opponents tackle the ball carrier and attempt to get their arms around the neck while flexing the head forward

head or via the trunk and neck accelerate the head producing internal stresses within the brain, which in turn may result in anatomical or physiological injury. The resultant brain injury is related to the magnitude of the impact force, the location of impact and the resultant head and brain acceleration. Loading of the skull can deform it leading to fractures, brain contusions, pressure effects, and/or intracranial hemorrhages.

Interestingly, biomechanical data from sports head injury studies show that in the majority of impacts the resulting head accelerations are not trivial but they are lower than those observed in motor vehicle accidents. Linear head accelerations in the order of 100g are associated with concussion in sport, whereas the probability of skull fracture or intracranial haemorrhage becomes very high with accelerations greater than 200g. Angular acceleration has been associated with axonal injury and bridging vein rupture that leads to subdural hemorrhages. Strain rate and intracranial pressure effects during impacts have also been identified as possible causes of brain injury. These are difficult to measure directly, but can be approximated using computer simulations.

Biomechanics of spinal cord injury

Sport-related spinal cord injury is often due to a combination of axial compression of the cervical spine and either flexion or extension (Figure 11.2). The resultant

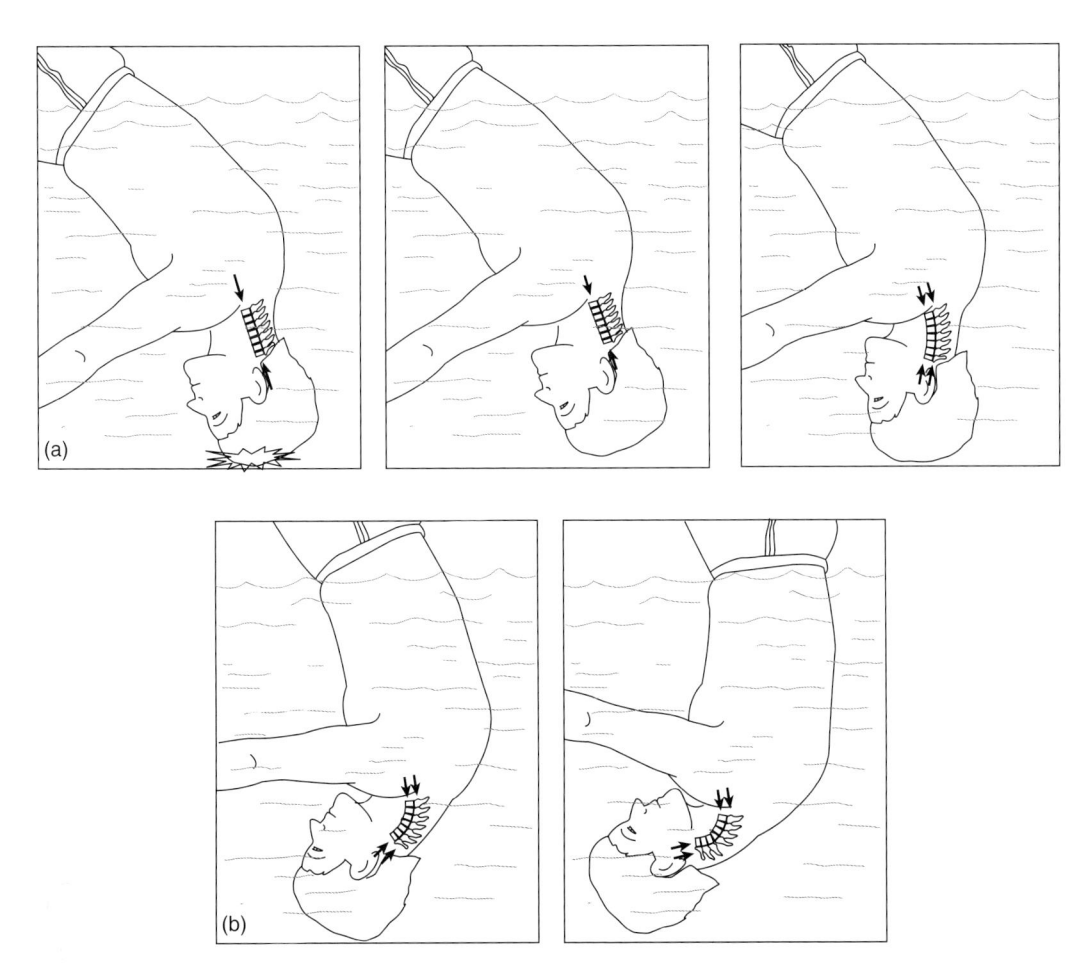

Figure 11.2. Spinal injury mechanisms: (a) the key mechanism in sport-related cervical spine injuries is axial load and forward flexion of the neck as illustrated in a diver; (b) Axial load and forward flexion of the neck results in vertebral compression and anterior wedging of the vertebral bodies

force compresses the vertebral segments and if the tolerance of the vertebrae is exceeded, a "burst fracture" and/or uni-/bi-facet dislocation occurs which then damages the cervical spinal cord through direct compression.

Examples of sport-specific mechanisms are given later.

The rugby scrum

The rugby scrum has received substantial attention over the years with regard to spinal cord injury. A rugby scrum consists of two opposing packs of eight players divided into the three front row, two back row, and three "loose" forward. The front rows of each team's scrum pack engage through their heads and shoulders in a forceful driving motion. This can result in high axial compressive neck forces combined with a bending moment and/or shear forces. During the 2003 Rugby World Cup there was one case of cervical dislocation during a scrum engagement that was a career-ending injury.

Milburn et al. measured the forces applied to an instrumented scrum machine, and found that the total horizontal forward force on engagement ranged between 4.4 kN for high school players and 8 kN for the Australian national team (Andersen et al., 2004). After the initial engagement, the sustained force reduced by approximately 20%. The forces on engagement have the potential to exceed axial neck load and bending moment tolerance limits. As a result, scrum laws for under 19 year olds are now designed to eliminate an impact on engagement and permit each front row to orient itself well, thus reducing neck loads. No study has reported on the effectiveness of the "under 19 law," although it is widely viewed as being successful and these principles are influencing future developments in the scrum.

Head and neck injury prevention

Injury prevention methods have been categorized under headings drawn from Haddon's Matrix (Table 11.4). Examples from the literature have been used to demonstrate the effectiveness of each method. For these methods to be successful, they must either be able to minimize the energy involved in impacts and collisions or reduce the forces applied to the body to levels that can be tolerated without injury. In the context of formal sports it is possible to eliminate some injury risks by pre-crash measures; elimination or substitution of hazards, or engineering methods. Sensible removal of structures from the playing field, and the provision of barriers between the playing field and spectators are obvious engineering methods for preventing injuries.

Administrative controls (Laws and Rules)

Rules are one of the most common methods used to prevent injury, however there have been few structured intervention studies that have identified the benefits associated with specific rules. If the rules are not followed, for example, spear tackling, illegal scrum engagement, or high tackles, the enforcement of the rule occurs after the potential injurious event. Post-injury penalization of players might serve to prevent the illegal play in conjunction with a pre-injury explanation of the rules, their rationale, and development of a safe culture.

Body checking in ice hockey, especially involving the head, has led to a concern that this form of contact should be eliminated through rule changes due to its association with head injury. As with spear tackling in American football, which was made illegal, there is a view that the use of helmets has increased hazardous play due to players' perceptions that they are at a lower risk of injury, often referred to as risk compensation. In American football, the intentional use of the helmet or faceguard as the primary point of contact has also been made illegal. Apart from reducing tackle-related injuries through rules, no study has reported on the effects of tackle training as a method for preventing injury.

Head injury in football (soccer) has been investigated recently. While heading the ball does not appear to cause concussion per se, the contest for the ball in the air does. During the contest, players can be struck in the head by the opponent's elbow, shoulder, or head, causing injury (Figure 11.3). Approximately 50% of all concussions were attributable to this mechanism (Cantu, 2000). As a direct

Table 11.4 Injury prevention matrix applied to sporting head and neck injury prevention: potential measures to prevent injuries.

	Pre-impact	Impact	Post-impact
Athlete	Tackling technique Neck strengthening Preparticipation screening	Technique: Good head position in tackle, good body posture in scrum engagement	Provide appropriate medical care Education Correct rehabilitation
Surroundings	Preparation and inspection of playing area and surface	Improve padding of goalposts Develop low impact sideboards	Access for emergency medical coverage
Equipment/other athletes	Training Availability of personal protective equipment	Improve energy attenuation of helmets/head protectors and mouthguards Improve impact characteristics of ball Teach opponents to disengage if spinal injury is called	First-aid equipment Spinal stretcher Ambulance
Administrative	Medical review Player exclusion rules and return to play guidelines Team culture, competitiveness, risk awareness and compensation Rules of the game	Enforcement of rules	Removal of player from field Post-match penalization of dangerous player Injury management guidelines

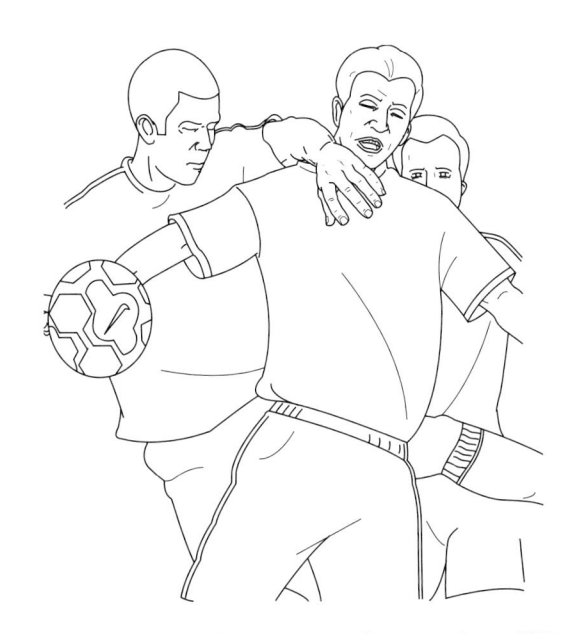

Figure 11.3. Arm to head contact is the cause of over 50% of all concussions in football (soccer)

result of this research, FIFA modified the playing rules before the 2007 World Cup to make contact to an opponent's head with the elbow/upper arm during such heading contests a "red card" offence.

Preparticipation screening for head and neck injury

Unlike most sporting injuries, head and neck injuries do not have clear-cut risk factors that have been conclusively shown to influence either incidence or the outcome of injury (Table 11.3). Because of this most "risk factors" are theoretical in their application. Preparticipation screening while commonly advocated relies more on clinical common sense than the weight of scientific evidence.

One such method for preventing head and neck injury requires participants to undergo medical screening programs to identify players at risk of injury due to anatomical abnormalities (e.g., MR or CT brain scan), pre-existing brain injury (e.g., neuropsychological testing), or genetic markers (e.g., ApoE). Although intuitively sensible, it is important to realize that excluding player participation based on this approach may not be scientifically or medicolegally defensible.

In some situations, congenital spinal canal stenosis has been postulated as a risk factor for cervical cord injuries. Although the risk of future cord injury may be increased when canal stenosis is present and the athlete has previously sustained a cord injury, this increased risk cannot be quantitated with any certainty (Ackery et al., 2007). Furthermore, the risk of future cord injury in an asymptomatic athlete with canal stenosis is unknown at present. Advice regarding the risk of injury in this latter situation is at best anecdotal and no intervention studies are reported in the literature.

Training

Training to improve strength, fitness, individual and team skills is an accepted part of sport. While training programs have been shown to reduce lower limb injury, for example, the benefits of neck strengthening, skills or fitness on reducing head and neck injury have not been formally addressed. Considering the high associations between body contact and injury in American football, rugby, and ice hockey, it is possible that skills may theoretically reduce injury. Improving tackling skills in rugby, for example, head placement, may eliminate some accidental head impacts. Skills to track a ball, avoid ball contact, and mishits may also help to reduce neck and head injury, however they have not been formally assessed.

Environment: ground hardness and surface

Australian Rules Football is a fast, kicking and running game played at professional and amateur levels across Australia and associated with a high rate of concussion (Table 11.1). Recent studies have debated whether ground hardness is a direct factor in the etiology of injury or whether it indirectly contributes to higher injury rates as it enables higher running speeds and higher energy impacts. With regard to direct head impacts and concussion, various studies have noted significant differences in the impact energy attenuation properties of grass compared to artificial surfaces.

Personal protective equipment: helmets

Helmets and padded headgear are used in many projectile and contact sports to prevent head injury.

Recent published meta-analysis studies of pedal cycle helmets in transport and recreation have confirmed the fact that light weight helmets are effective in preventing head and facial injuries in cyclists.

In some sporting competitions it has become mandatory to wear a helmet and/or faceguard, for example, baseball, softball, American football, ice hockey, as well as competitive alpine skiing and snowboarding. Helmets in American football and ice hockey have evolved from padded headgear to helmets comprising a hard shell, a liner, and a faceguard. Canadian and NOCSAE standards for ice hockey and football helmets, respectively, were established in the early 1970s. Recently, there has been much debate over the use of padded headgear in soccer.

Helmets are designed to attenuate the impact energy and distribute the impact force applied to the head. If a helmet can reduce the head impact force and head's acceleration to below relevant tolerance levels and under sport-specific impact scenarios, then a helmet can function to reduce the risk of brain injury.

The results of published studies show that all of the currently available commercial padded headgear for rugby and Australian football has a very limited ability to reduce concussive impact forces based on existing head injury models. Even if the more generous injury thresholds are applied to the data, all headgear tested lose any protective capacity once the impact energy is greater than 20J. This is reflected in randomized controlled trials of headgear in rugby and Australian football showing a lack of efficacy in concussion prevention with soft-shell helmets.

Studies of the effectiveness of helmets in sports where the use (other than in alpine racing) is not mandatory are emerging (Table 11.5).

While alpine sport injuries appear to be increasing over time, the use of helmets to prevent head injuries is associated with a 22–60% reduction in head injury rates (McCrory & Turner, 2005). The greatest limitations to the widespread application of protective helmets in these sports are the lack of an internationally accepted helmet standard, the availability of helmets and the variable fitting of helmets, especially with children.

Protective equestrian helmets are also widely recommended. Such helmets need to be certified to an appropriate materials testing standard. At

Table 11.5 Levels of evidence regarding helmet effectiveness.

Sport	Effect of helmet use on concussion incidence	Level of evidence	Comments
American football	Inconclusive	III	
Pedal cycling	Reduction	I	Ecologic or observational only
Ice hockey	No change	II	
Cricket	Unknown	IIII	Lab evidence only
Rugby	No change	I	High-quality RCT
Skiing	Reduction	II	Several high quality case control studies
Australian football	Unknown	II	One underpowered study only
Soccer	No change	III	Observational only
Equestrian	Unknown	III	Indirect evidence only

present, regulatory authorities mandate the use of helmets and body protectors in professional competition. It is recommended that an approved safety helmet be worn at all times when mounted. The British Standard (EN 1384.1996) is designed for competitive riding and is compulsory for professional jockeys and similar standards for horse riding helmets exist in other countries. Interestingly, since helmets were made compulsory for professional jockeys in 1993–1994, no significant changes in concussion rates have been observed. The numbers of fatal brain injuries over the same time period are too small to be adequately analyzed in this regard.

Indirect evidence exists that head protectors may play a role in injury reduction at least in non-professional equestrian riders. Both United States and United Kingdom data showed a fivefold drop in horse-related injury presentations between 1971 and 1992, due largely to a reduction in head injury presentation. Although not a causal relationship, this change was associated with an increase in helmet use over the same time period. Strategies to increase helmet use in riders have been studied extensively (Marshall et al., 2003).

Research to date, both field and laboratory, indicates that padded headgear (soft-shell helmets) does not reduce the incidence of concussion or serious head injury in Rugby Union football however it seems to reduce superficial injuries. Similarly the data from football (soccer) and Australian football suggests that the currently available helmets are unlikely to reduce concussion incidence.

Studies of the effectiveness of cricket helmets have been confined to the laboratory and indicate that the level of protection is greatly reduced with high-speed ball impacts.

Personal protective equipment: mouthguards and face shields

The use of correctly fitting mouthguards and face masks can reduce the rate of dental, facial, and mandibular injuries. In the case of face shields, there is evidence that they also reduce the rate of concussion whereas randomized controlled trials have demonstrated that mouthguards have little or no effect on reducing concussions and any suggested benefit for the prevention of brain injury is largely anecdotal.

Equipment: baseball

In baseball, softer balls have been used to reduce the risk of head injury in comparison to standard balls. Marshall et al. observed a 28% reduction in the risk of injury in baseball for games using the reduced impact ball compared to the standard ball (Nathoo et al., 2003). The softest impact ball was observed to be associated with the lowest risk of injury (48% reduction in risk) and the authors reported on a study noting that adult and child players found it difficult to identify the differences between standard and safety balls in pitching, throwing, and batting.

Neck muscle strengthening

It is often suggested that neck muscle conditioning may be of value in reducing impact forces transmitted to the brain. Biomechanical concepts dictate that the energy from an impacting object is dispersed over the greater mass of an athlete if the head is held rigidly. Although attractive from a theoretical standpoint, there is little scientific support for this viewpoint and no prospective published studies to support this approach. Video analysis of concussive injury seen in Australian football, rugby and soccer demonstrates that approximately 95% of concussive impacts are an accidental part of play and the players concerned were unaware of impending impact and hence unable to tense their neck muscles in an attempt to withstand the impact. This same issue may apply to protecting the spine.

Secondary injury prevention: post-impact measures

The role of injury prevention in the post-impact phase has not been adequately addressed in the published literature. It is intuitively likely that correct first-aid or paramedical management will reduce the risk of head or spinal cord injury complications. The management of the concussion or mild traumatic brain injury itself at best follows expert consensus guidelines (Level III evidence) in the absence of scientifically tested management strategies.

As the ability to treat or reduce the effects of concussive injury after the event is minimal, education of athletes, colleagues, and those working with them as well as the general public is a mainstay of progress in this field.

When head and cervical spine injuries are expected, the medical staff must have appropriate qualifications (e.g., AMST, EMST) and training to deal with them. They must have all the appropriate equipment to hand (hard collars, sandbags, lifting frame, and/or a spinal board) and have a method of rapid disposal on site (paramedic ambulance or helicopter) to an appropriate hospital (i.e., with neurosurgical trauma expertise). Administrative bodies supervising sideline doctors need to ensure that all medical staff have the appropriate and up-to-date qualifications.

Athletes and their health care providers must be educated regarding the detection of concussion, its clinical features, assessment techniques and principles of safe return to play. Methods to improve education including various web-based resources (e.g., www.concussionsafety.com), educational videos, outreach programs, concussion working groups, and the support and endorsement of peak sport groups such as FIFA, IOC, and IIHF.

The promotion of fair play and respect for opponents are ethical values that should be encouraged in all sports and sporting associations. Similarly coaches, parents, and managers play an important part in ensuring these values are implemented on the field of play and hopefully these may play a role in injury prevention.

Take-home message

Head and neck injury is common across all sports. Some sports (such as equestrian sports) have relatively high risks for participants. By contrast catastrophic injury is rare. Despite the significance and cost of head and neck injury, there have been few formal evaluations of injury prevention methods. Approaches that are considered successful or have been proven to be successful in preventing injury include: modifying the baseball; implementing helmet standards and increasing wearing rates in cycling, ice hockey, equestrian sports, and skiing and snowboarding; use of full face guards in ice hockey; changing rules associated with body contact; and, implementing rules to reduce the impact forces in rugby scrums. Soft-shell helmets and padded headgear appear in current designs to make little difference to rates of concussion. Neck injury has been addressed through laws and skill development, with little formal evaluation. Epidemiological, medical, and human factors research methods are required in combination with biomechanical and technological approaches to reduce further injury risks in sport.

References

Ackery, A., Hagel, B.E., Provvidenza, C., Tator, C.H. (2007) An international review of head and spinal cord injuries in alpine skiing and snowboarding. *Injury Prevention* **13**, 368–375.

Andersen, T., Arnason, A., Engebretsen, L., Bahr, R. (2004) Mechanism of head injuries in elite football. *British Journal of Sports Medicine* **38**, 690–696.

Aubry, M., Cantu, R., Dvorak, J., Graf-Baumann, T., Johnston, K., Kelly, J., Lovell, M., McCrory, P., Meeuwisse, W., Schamasch, P. (2002) Summary and agreement statement of the First International Conference on Concussion in Sport, Vienna 2001. Recommendations for the improvement of safety and health of athletes who may suffer concussive injuries. *British Journal of Sports Medicine* **36**, 6–10.

Cantu, R. (2000). Cervical spine injuries in the athlete. *Seminars in Neurology* **20**, 173–178.

Fuller, C.W., Brooks, J., Kemp, S. (2007) Spinal injuries in professional rugby union: a prospective cohort study. *Clinical Journal of Sport Medicine* **17**, 10–16.

Levy, M., Ozgur, B., Berry C. (2004) Analysis and evolution of head injury in football. *Neurosurgery* **34**, 649–655.

Lyens, R., Lefevre, J., Renson, L., Ostyn, M. (1984) The predictability of sports injuries: a preliminary report. *International Journal of Sports Medicine* **5**, 153–155.

Marshall, S., Mueller, F., Kirby, D., Yang, J. (2003) Evaluation of safety balls and faceguards for prevention of injuries in baseball. *Journal of the American Medical Association* **289**, 568–574.

McCrory, P., Turner, M. (2005) Equestrian injuries. *Medicine and Sport Science* **48**, 8–17.

McCrory, P., Johnston, K., Meeuwisse, W., Aubry, M., Cantu, R., Dvorak, J., Graf-Baumann, T., Kelly, J., Lovell, M., Schamasch, P. (2005) Summary and agreement statement of the 2nd International Conference on Concussion in Sport, Prague 2004. *British Journal of Sports Medicine* **39**, 196–204.

Meeuwisse, W.H. (1991) Predictability of sports injuries. What is the epidemiological evidence? *Sports Medicine* **12**, 8–15.

Milburn, P.D. (1993) Biomechanics of rugby union scrummaging. Technical and safety issues. *Sports Medicine* **16**, 168–179.

Nathoo, N., Chetry, R., van Dellen, J.R., Connolly, C., Naidoo, R. (2003) Apolipoprotein E polymorphism and outcome after closed traumatic brain injury: influence of ethnic and regional differences. *Journal of Neurosurgery* **98**, 302–306.

Further reading

Cantu, R. (Ed) (2000) *Neurologic Athletic Head and Spine Injuries*. Philadelphia, WB Saunders & Co.

Cantu, R.C., Aubry, M., Dvorak, J., Graf-Baumann, T., Johnston, K., Kelly, J., Lovell, M., McCrory, P., Meeuwisse, W., Schamasch, P., Kevin, M., Bruce, S.L., Ferrara, M.S., Kelly, J.P., McCrea, M., Putukian, M., McLeod, T.C. (2006) Overview of concussion consensus statements since 2000. *Neurosurgical Focus* **21**, E3.

Cantu, R.C., Herring S.A., Putukian, M.; The American College of Sports Medicine. (2007) Concussion. *New England Journal of Medicine* **356**, 1787.

Dvorak, J., McCrory, P., Kirkendall, D.T. (2007) Head injuries in the female football player: incidence, mechanisms, risk factors and management. *British Journal of Sports Medicine* **41**, i44–i46.

Grindel, S., Lovell, M., Collins, M.W. (2001) The assessment of sport-related concussion: the evidence behind neuropsychological testing and management. *Clinical Journal of Sport Medicine* **11**, 134–144.

Guskiewicz, K.M., Bruce, S.L., Cantu, R.C., Ferrara, M.S., Kelly, J.P., McCrea, M., Putukian, M., McLeod, T.C.; National Athletic Trainers' Association (2006) Research based recommendations on management of sport related concussion: summary of the National Athletic Trainers' Association position statement. *British Journal of Sports Medicine* **40**, 6–10.

Guskiewicz, K.M., Marshall, S.W., Bailes, J., McCrea, M., Harding Jr., H.P., Matthews, A., Mihalik, J.R., Cantu, R.C. (2007) Recurrent concussion and risk of depression in retired professional football players. *Medicine and Science in Sports and Exercise* **39**, 903–909.

Iverson, G. (2007) Predicting slow recovery from sport-related concussion: the new simple-complex distinction. *Clinical Journal of Sport Medicine* **17**, 31–37.

Johnston, K.M., McCrory, P., Mohtadi, N.G., Meeuwisse, W. (2001) Evidence-based review of sport-related concussion: clinical science. *Clinical Journal of Sport Medicine* **11**, 150–159.

McCrory, P., Collie, A., Anderson, V., Davis, G. (2004) Can we manage sport related concussion in children the same as in adults? *British Journal of Sports Medicine* **38**, 516–519.

McCrory, P., Johnston, K. M., Mohtadi, N.G., Meeuwisse, W. (2001). Evidence-based review of sport-related concussion: basic science. *Clinical Journal of Sport Medicine* **11**, 160–165.

Chapter 12
Preventing tendon overuse injuries

Jill Cook[1], Mads Kongsgaard[2], Karim Khan[3] and Michael Kjær[4]

[1]Centre for Physical Activity and Nutrition Research School of Exercise and Nutrition Sciences, Deakin University, Melbourne, Australia
[2]Institute of Sports Medicine, Bispebjerg Hospital, Copenhagen, Denmark
[3]Professor, Center for Hip Health and Mobility, University of British Columbia, Vancouver, Canada
[4]Department of Rheumatology, Institute of Sports Medicine, Bispebjerg Hospital, University of Copenhagen, Copenhagen, Denmark

Introduction

Tendons, force transducers interposed between muscles and bones, transmit the force of muscle contraction to bones to allow movement. Optimal tendon function is required for optimal performance. Tendons are subjected to large mechanical forces during movement but healthy tendons are well adapted to this peak demand.

Despite this peak load tolerance, tendon overuse injury (tendinopathy) is one of the most frequent injuries among elite and recreational athletes. Such overuse injuries most often affect tendons such as the Achilles, patellar, or supraspinatus tendon (Table 12.1). In sports characterized by forceful and explosive muscle contractions, the prevalence of patellar tendinopathy can reach 45–55% in populations of jumping athletes such as elite volleyball and basketball players. The prevalence of Achilles tendinopathy is also considerable in a variety of different sports such as running (about 10% of all athletes) and different ball games (e.g., football). Overuse injuries in the upper limb occur in athletes (throwing and racquet sports), but are also prevalent in an older population, particularly manual workers.

Overuse tendon injury presents as tendon pain, but tendon pathology and tendon pain can develop independently; pathology appears to precede

Sports Injury Prevention, 1st edition. Edited by R. Bahr and L. Engebretsen Published 2009 by Blackwell Publishing ISBN: 9781405162449

Table 12.1 Prevalance of tendinopathy at various anatomical sites according to sport.

Sport	Anatomical region of tendon	Prevalence
Running	Achilles/iliotibial band/fascia plantaris	10% of runners
Football	Achilles	5–10% of all elite players
Volleyball	Patella	55% of elite-players
Basketball	Patella	45% of elite players
Track and fields	Patella/Achilles	10% of elite athletes
Badminton	Achilles/patella	5% of all players
Handball	Supraspinatus/other rotator cuff	5% of elite players
Baseball	Supraspinatus/other rotator cuff	20% of all players

The numbers reported are estimates based on the studies available.

pain in most cases. Tendons that rupture are often painfree, but have an extensive pathology and the force imposed on them is greater than the tendon integrity (Kannus & Jozsa, 1991). The mechanisms of tendon injury have not been identified and this greatly limits the ability of coaches and clinicians to prevent and treat tendon injuries.

In tendinopathy, where so little is known about the basics of the condition, prevention strategies are limited and not supported by evidence. To fully comprehend tendon injury mechanisms and the prevention of tendon injuries, it is important to understand tendon structure and function. Thus, we briefly introduce the structure, function and mechanics of normal tendon. Then we review the etiology of tendinopathy and propose opportunities for injury prevention.

Basic tendon structure

All muscles basically have two tendons, a short one at their proximal end (origin of muscle) and a somewhat longer one at their distal end (insertion of muscle) underlining that the mechanical properties of the tendons will have a great impact upon the function of the entire muscle–tendon–bone complex. Tendons and muscles join, and integrate, at the myotendinous junction—the site where the tendon infiltrates or interdigitates the muscle body to provide a large contact surface between the two structures. Distally, the tendon joins bone in the osteotendinous junction, a complex transition from soft to hard tissue. Because the muscle–tendon junction is primarily affected in a muscle strain injury, we will not consider the structure and function of the myotendinous junction in this chapter.

The structural design of different tendons varies substantially; some are short and thick, and others long and thin. Structure depends on the specific function of each tendon. Long tendons, such as the Achilles tendon, provide the body with energy-returning springs so that movement is energy efficient. Short, broad tendons, such as the quadriceps tendon, serve as pure force-transducers for their attached muscles.

Tendon matrix proteins: the building blocks of the tendon

The basic load-bearing element of tendon is collagen which exists as fibrils (Figure 12.1) that are embedded in a hydrated viscous proteoglycan-rich substance called the ground substance. Together, the collagen and the ground substance are called the extracellular matrix. The various components of the extracellular matrix are produced by the tendon cells (tenocytes, specialized fibroblasts) that are elongated spindle-shaped cells and are located between the collagen fibrils (Figure 12.1). If you were to digest tendon collagen fibrils down to their core component you would come across

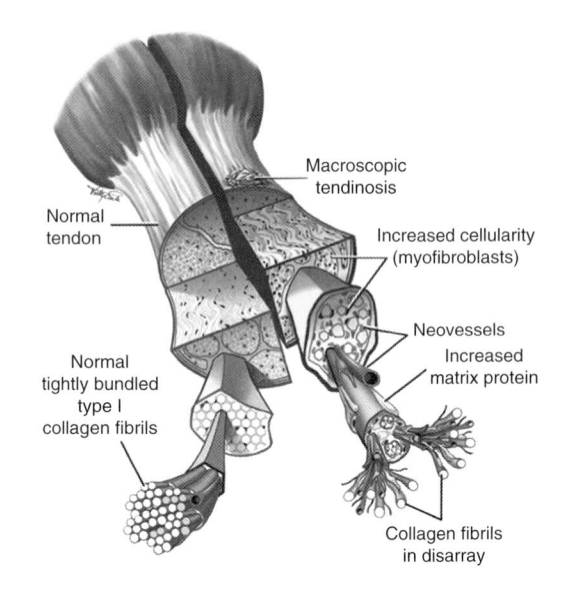

Figure 12.1. Bundles of type I collagen fibrils provide the load-bearing element of tendon (left side of the illustration). These fibrils are embedded in a hydrated viscous proteoglycan-rich substance called the ground substance. In pathological tendon, the fibrils lose their organized structure and disarray is obvious (right side of the illustration). Reproduced with permission from Clinical Sports Medicine (3/e) page 22, McGraw-Hill Publishing, Sydney, 2007.

triple helical collagen molecules. The individual collagen molecules inside the fibrils are interconnected and stabilized by cross-links thereby securing the force transduction along the fibril from one end of tendon to the other. Although there are more than 20 different collagen proteins, tendons predominantly consist of fibrillar type I collagen as well as smaller amounts of other collagen types including type II, III, and V. The various collagen molecules exhibit different mechanical properties and the general mechanical properties and function of the whole tendon is therefore highly influenced by the distribution of collagen types.

The matrix between the collagen fibrils is comprised of proteoglycans that are important for the alignment of collagen fibers. Proteoglycans are hydrophilic (attract water, hence the "swelling" in injured tendons, see later) and composed of polysaccharide chains of glycosaminoglycans that are bound to protein cores. Proteoglycans act as glue between the various collagen networks binding all the extracellular matrix molecules together. Proteoglycans also regulate matrix assembly and stabilize the extracellular matrix architecture. Further, proteoglycans control the hydration of the extracellular matrix and spacing between collagen fibrils and they bind various growth factors to regulate the tendon milieu. Together with other glycoproteins such as elastin, fibronectin, and laminin, the collagen and ground substance create a meshwork that does not rely on single molecules but rather on the polymers and networks that the molecules create.

The architecture of the tendon

The structural properties of the collagen fibril determine the mechanical properties of the tendon. This means that small fibrils increase the elastic properties and larger fibrils increase the strength via greater cross-sectional area and increased numbers of intramolecular cross-links. Approximately 95% of the fibers run longitudinally with the tendon orientation. Tendon fibrils can span the entire tendon length which implies that the tendon mechanical properties including strength and stiffness are highly dependent upon the dimensions and composition of the single fibrils. However, other factors such as collagen-type distribution, inter- and intra-fibrillar interactions as well as total tendon cross-section are important for the overall function and strength of tendons.

The intrafibrillar cross-linking of collagen molecules is an important mechanism for integrity between collagen molecules that contribute to the strength and force-transducing capability of the tendon fibril. Increased cross-linking increases tendon stiffness and elastic modulus, reduces the failure strain but does not appear to significantly affect rupture stress. Tendons in older individuals have an increase in non-enzymatic cross-linking in the form of glycation (incorporation of sugar) and this increases tendon stiffness.

Several collagen fibrils combine to make up a tendon fiber (Figure 12.1). Bundles of fibers surrounded by connective tissue (endotenon) comprise a fascicle bundle. The endotenon surrounding the collagen fibers and fascicles carries blood vessels, nerve fibers, and lymphatics into the tendon. Loose connective tissue (epitenon)

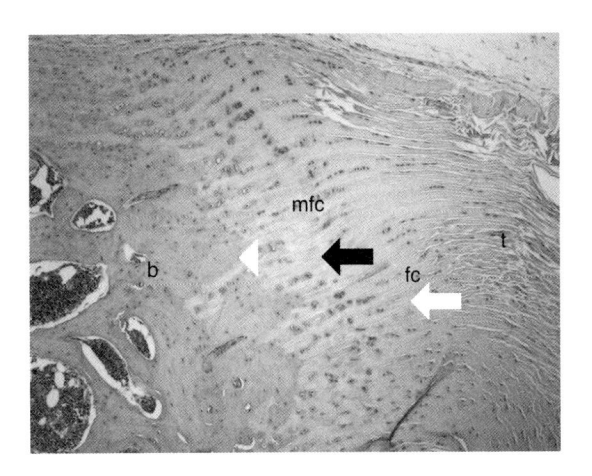

Figure 12.2. The area where the tendon inserts into bone the highly specialized "osteotendinous junction." There is a transition through four consecutive structural zones: the tendon zone (t), fibrocartilage (fc), mineralized fibrocartilage (mfc), and bone (b). Note the gradual transition from the tendon tissue to fibrocartilage; more rounded chrondocyte-like cells (white arrow) and type II collagen (black arrow) increase in prominence to make the tissue appear more "cartilage like." The fibrocartilage zone is terminated by a distinct border with the mineralized fibrocartilage zone (white arrowhead), this then intercalates with bone

surrounds the whole tendon. In areas where tendons slide relative to adjacent tissues the tendon may also be enveloped by another loose connective tissue sheet called the paratenon. Together, the epitenon and paratenon is called the peritendon and these structures allow the tendon to glide with minimal resistance during movement.

The area where the tendon inserts into bone is the highly specialized "osteotendinous junction." Here, the viscoelastic tendinous tissue transfers force to the rigid bone, and there is a gradual change in the mechanical properties that is achieved by transition through four consecutive structural zones; the tendon zone, fibrocartilage, mineralized fibrocartilage, and bone. The transition from the tendon tissue to fibrocartilage is gradual; more rounded chrondocyte-like cells and type II collagen increase in prominence to make the tissue appear more "cartilage like." Moving even further toward bone, the fibrocartilage zone is terminated by a distinct border beyond which the mineralized fibrocartilage zone begins, this then intercalates with bone (Figure 12.2).

Tendon mechanics and strength

Normal tendons can sustain strain levels up to 20% before suffering initial failure (Figure 12.3). When testing human tendons in vivo, strain levels at maximal isometric muscle contractions have ranged 7–18% depending on the tendon investigated. However, the "single strain" condition is not the only way that tendons can be injured. In sportspeople, tendons are mostly subjected to repeated or prolonged loading. This can cause fatigue damage, even though each single loading is well below the maximal strength of the tendon—this is defined as fatigue damage.

Although a completely stiff structure would provide the most efficient force transduction from muscle to bone, tendons are quite elastic. Thus, when a tendon is loaded and elongated, tendon force is built up, and energy is stored within the tendon. This stored energy can be released from the tendon and utilized to create or prevent joint movement. This process conserves energy and improves efficiency of locomotion. It is estimated that the elastic energy contributes as much as 60% of the energy demand during locomotion. Although a thin and long tendon will assist energy storage and release, it may be more vulnerable to injury. A thicker tendon, which would yield less strain energy, would reduce the stress across the tendon and thereby provides the tendon with a greater safety margin. Thus, from an injury prevention standpoint a presumably healthy (physiological) hypertrophic tendon adaptation to exercise would be advantageous since it will reduce the amount of stress on the tendon.

Unquestionably, tendons are remarkably strong, a tendon with a cross-sectional area of $1\,cm^2$ (approximately corresponding to a normal adult patellar tendon) will be able to withstand a tensile load of $10,000\,N$ or $1000\,kg$—perhaps 10–15 times body weight. The strength of tendons is related to the cross-sectional area (number and thickness of parallel fibrils) of the tendon and the tensile quality of the tendinous tissue (related to factors such as intrafibrillar cross-links and collagen type distribution). In other words, the greater the cross-sectional area, number of cross-links and type I collagen content of a given tendon, the greater loads can be withstood by the tendon before failure occurs if all other factors are equal. The tensile strength of a non-injured tendon is normally several times higher than the strength of its attached muscle leaving most tendons with a substantial tensile safety margin. However this may not be the case for all tendons during all circumstances. Patellar tendon forces have been estimated to be as high as $8000\,N$ during landing and $9000\,N$ during sprinting and tendon loads in the human Achilles tendon reach $9000\,N$ during running. Thus, some tendons, including the patellar and especially the Achilles, may operate close to their maximal strength tolerance.

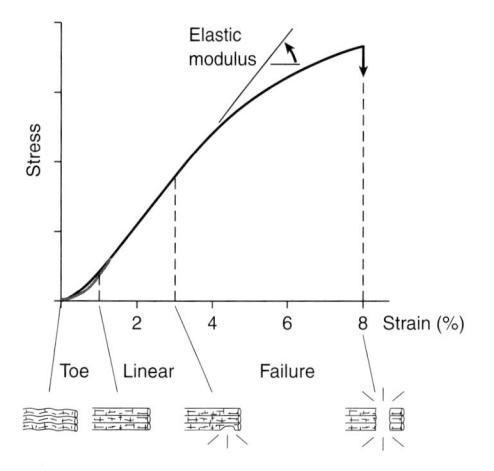

Figure 12.3. Stress strain curve. There is a "toe" region where strain can increase with little increase in stress. Then there is a "plastic" region where increased strain causes a linear increase in stress. The term "plastic" means the change is reversible. Beyond the plastic region is tendon failure—frank rupture of tendon tissue. The elastic modulus is a measure of how "stiff" a tendon is; the stiffer the tendon, the steeper the slope of the curve

Tendon adaptation to loading

Mechanical loading stimulates collagen production dramatically—a single bout of exercise doubles the synthesis rate of collagen, and maintains this elevated level for 2–3 days. This increased synthesis is dose- or intensity-dependent. In short-term exercise, collagen degradation is also elevated, resulting in little overall gain in collagen production.

After several weeks of exercise stimulus, degradation returns to normal levels so that overall collagen synthesis is increased (Kjær, 2004).

These new findings indicate that tendon tissue responds much more dynamically to loading than previously thought and that intermittent loading could cause a negative balance between new collagen formation and collagen degradation. Also, the fact that matrix protein formation is already elevated after one acute bout of exercise and remains elevated for around 48 h after exercise indicates that from "a matrix point of view," it would be sufficient to train every other day to optimally stimulate matrix tissue of the tendon. Thus, the apparent mismatch between how quickly tissues such as skeletal and heart muscle adapt to loading, and how frequently such tissues tolerate the training stimulus, and the fact that connective tissue such as the tendon has a more "delayed" and slower adaptation pattern, may explain why tendon can be the weak link in situations of intense training or overloading.

Although physical training is associated with a chronic elevation of collagen turnover, it is not clear to what extent this leads to net collagen synthesis and tendon growth. Although trained men (but not trained women) have greater Achilles tendon cross-sectional area than their untrained counterparts, 9 months of running training did not increase the cross-sectional area of the Achilles tendon. As training strengthens tendon mechanically, it is likely that several factors other than just the amount of collagen in the tendon are important in the training-induced adaptation of healthy tendon in humans.

Some investigators have suggested that endurance training results in qualitative changes (improved tissue mechanics) but not quantitative (increased tendon size) changes, whereas other investigators have concluded that tendons react to endurance training by both quantitative and qualitative augmentations.

Tendon pathology

Tendon pathology induces dramatic changes in tendon structure, with changes in both the cells and the extracellular matrix that results in poorer mechanical properties and capacity to sustain load. The matrix changes are extensive and responsible for the fundamental decrease in load-bearing capacity of the tendon. Ground substance is increased and becomes more cartilage-like in composition, primarily seen in a change from small to large proteoglycans with more glycosaminoglycan chains. Collagen is disrupted, and altered in type from type I to smaller diameter fibers of type II, and III, and there is an increase in vascularity and neural ingrowth to the tendon (Figure 12.4). Overall, it seems that extracellular matrix homeostasis is important to maintain normal tendon function and that disruptions of the matrix balance is an early sign or mechanism in tendon injury development.

We still lack a biomarker in human tendon that can provide an early warning sign of emerging overloading of the tendon. Clinically, tendon pathology can be detected by abnormal imaging (ultrasound or MR) (Figure 12.5). However, the correlation between pain and abnormal imaging is poor; tendons with abnormal imaging are not always painful, likewise tendons that appear normal to imaging can be painful.

Mechanism of tendon overuse injury

Despite the high incidence and prevalence of tendinopathies the exact etiology remains elusive. It is, however, generally accepted that overuse injuries are related to repetitive tensile loading and strain of the tendon. Thus, a tendon overuse injury implies an injury in response to repeated strains above a certain threshold. The response is driven by cell detection of load that causes increased protein production in the cell. Eventually the injury will manifest itself by increased ground substance, fibril disorganization, neovascularization and potentially pain and swelling.

As mentioned earlier, sporting activities that utilize energy storage capacities of the tendon or forceful eccentric components may maximally challenge the tendon's fatigue resistance and reparative capacity especially if there is little recovery time between exercise sessions. With enough

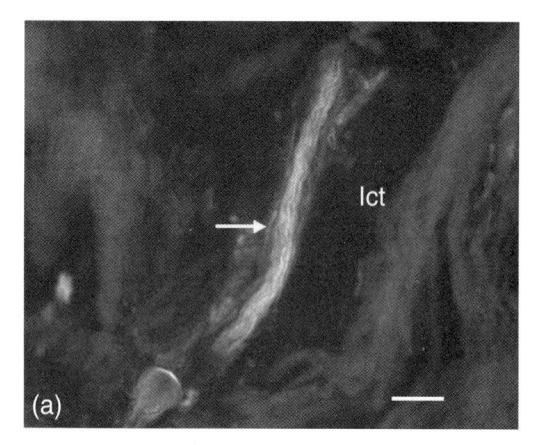

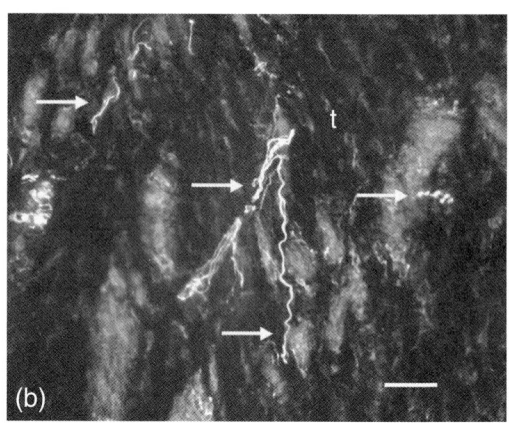

Figure 12.4. This photomicrograph compares neural tissue in (a) normal patellar tendon and (b) injured patellar tendon. In the side affected by chronic tendinopathy, there is increased spread and sprouting of nerve fibers (arrows) and they are not restricted to the loose connective tissue (lct) around the tendon. They invade the tendon itself (labeled a "t" in the image). Reproduced with permission from Øystein Lian, Johan Dahl, Paul W. Ackermann, Frede Frihagen, Lars Engebretsen, Roald Bahr. Pronociceptive and Antinociceptive Neuromediators in Patellar Tendinopathy. *American Journal of Medicine* 34, 1801–1808 (2006). Published by Sage Publications.

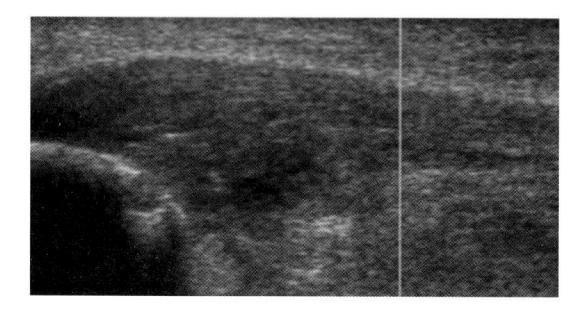

Figure 12.5. Tendon pathology can be detected as a hypoechoic appearance when the tendon is scanned using gray scale ultrasound

time between bouts of acute loading, tendons recover, but stress reapplied without sufficient recovery may lead to injury. This reminds us of the fine line between optimal loading for adaptation and loading that puts the tissue under too much reparative stress. It could be suggested that the tendon fibroblast increases protein synthesis in response to mechanical loading, but that this cannot increase further with higher-intensity exercise. This might explain why too much exercise (e.g., excessive jumping) can result in a suboptimal adaptation of the tendon and subsequent tendinopathy.

The development of tendinopathy may also be related to the structural properties of the tendons. Both the Achilles tendon and the patellar tendon have a non-uniform cross-sectional area distribution along their length and that the regions where tendinopathy most often occur in these tendons have the narrowest cross-sectional area. Thus, tendon overload injuries may arise at sites of stress concentrations (high force per area) in the tendons at these specific regions. However, it is unlikely that tendon stress is the sole factor in the etiology of tendinopathies. The majority of tendinopathies occur in the tendon closer to the attachment to bone. The tissue at the osteotendinous junction display inferior modulus and maximum stress compared to mid-tendon tissue.

Risk factors for tendon overuse injuries

Age

The prevalence of tendon pain and rupture increases with age, and this may be due to changes in tendon structure and mechanics. As tendons age they decrease protein content and increase cross-links, consequently the tendon is stiffer.

Tendons also thicken with age, and an increase in cross-sectional area may compensate for decreased "quality" of the tendon.

Younger tendons are also vulnerable to tendon pathology and in the adolescent population the prevalence of patellar tendon pathology in jumping athletes is similar to adults. At all ages, overload can produce pain in an already pathological tendon.

Sex

The prevalence of lower limb tendinopathy appears to be less in sporting women than among men with comparable training history, men have twice the risk of developing tendon pathology and pain compared to women (Lian et al., 2005). Possible reasons for this difference require investigation. Candidate hypotheses include that (i) men with larger muscles may be able to impose greater loads on their tendons, or subject them to more loading cycles, (ii) women's and men's tendons have different capacities to adapt to an increased or decreased loading, or, (iii) sex hormones may play a key role in tendon pathogenesis.

Genes

Researchers have unraveled the relationship between Achilles tendinopathy and genes for two proteins: tenascin-C and type V collagen. Certain types of genes (polymorphisms) in both the tenascin-C and collagen V genes were associated with Achilles tendinopathy and this association has been confirmed in a second population. Further research is ongoing, and if the link is clearly demonstrated, this may be the first demonstrated (non-modifiable) risk factor for tendinopathy. It is noteworthy that patients with a previous Achilles tendon rupture have a 200-fold risk of sustaining a contralateral rupture (Arøen et al., 2004). This strongly indicates either a genetic predisposition or other unknown predisposing factors in these individuals. Further evidence to support a strong genetic link is that the incidence of tendon ruptures in western countries far exceeds that in Africa and East Asia but at the same time it has convincingly been shown that Afro-American individuals have a substantially higher prevalence of tendon ruptures than matched Caucasian Americans (Owens et al., 2007).

Body composition

A recent cohort study has demonstrated that waist measurement was associated with patellar tendinopathy. This study reported that waist circumference in males of greater than 83 cm resulted in a 74% probability of morphological tendon abnormalities (via ultrasound), whereas males with waist of less than 83 cm had a 15% probability of tendon changes (Malliaras et al., 2007).

Body mass index has been associated with onset of tendinopathy. Nineteen out of 41 studies in a systematic review showed a significant association with adiposity and tendon health. In those having rotator cuff surgery there was a strong relationship between body mass index and risk of rotator cuff tendinopathy. A longitudinal study showed that the strongest predictor for developing upper limb tendinopathy was a body mass index of greater than 30. Further research is needed to identify the mechanisms for such associations, but like other musculoskeletal conditions it is likely that the mechanisms are more complex than just an increase in load on the tendon (Pottie et al., 2006).

Range of joint movement

A decreased range of ankle dorsiflexion range of movement is associated with both Achilles and patellar tendon pathology, and is likely to relate to increased tendon forces with landing. Interestingly, plantar fasciitis and Achilles tendinopathy have been also associated with an increased range of dorsiflexion.

Chronic disease

Glycation cross-links are increased in subjects with diabetes, making tendons stiffer and more prone to overload. Cross-linking is crucial in order to secure normal tendon function and tensile strength but increased cross-links and therefore stiffness, may be detrimental by reducing the strain to tissue failure. Spondyloarthropathy manifests as bone–tendon junction disease similar to athletic tendinopathy. These diseases have systemic and familial links, as does diabetes (especially type 1). In addition, type 2 diabetes is associated with increased abdominal adiposity, and interactions between risk factors for tendinopathy have not been clarified.

Muscle strength and flexibility

Muscle strength of the attached muscle has not been clearly shown to be a factor in the onset of tendon pathology. Athletes who can jump higher have more patellar tendon pathology in some studies (Lian et al., 2003), other studies do not support this (Malliaras & Cook, 2006). Reduced muscle flexibility has been shown to be associated with patellar tendinopathy, both the hamstrings and quadriceps have been implicated (Witvrouw et al., 2001).

Other factors

The amount of loading has been shown to be associated with patellar tendon pain and pathology. The type of flooring has also been implicated, a harder floor will increase tendon load (Ferretti et al., 1984).

Take-home message

Athletes who load heavily with training in sports and have a big energy storage and release component are vulnerable to tendon pathology. Each sport has its own collection of vulnerable tendons: the patellar tendon in jumping athletes, Achilles in running and court sports, and the adductor tendons in football players. This vulnerability is ameliorated or enhanced in individuals by intrinsic risk factors and a range of other unknown factors. Coaches are well aware that two athletes can train identically yet one will develop tendon pathology and pain and the other will remain symptom-free.

Although we can identify tendon pathology clinically with imaging, this does not allow us to predict which athletes will develop pain, and of these, which will develop pain sufficient to stop participation. At best, imaging might allow the coach or medical practitioner to be aware of which athletes are at risk (Fredberg et al., 2007), plan training so overload is minimal, and monitor and modify tendon load as necessary. Although this is far from satisfactory, tendon pain and pathology remain outside the injuries that can be easily controlled.

Preventing tendon overuse injuries

Because tendon pathology appears to result from an interaction between several individual and environmental risk factors, prevention is not merely a matter of following a single recipe for all athletes. A tendon that is not overloaded will not develop tendinopathy—it appears that repeated stretch-shortening cycles with body weight over time are required to generate tendon pathology and pain. However, as individuals appear to have a wide variation in load tolerance, it is not currently possible to provide "research evidence" for a narrow, defined load that minimizes risk of tendon overuse injury.

Adaptation to loading

The ability of tendinous tissue to respond to mechanical loading of the muscle–tendon unit is of great interest as inadequate adaptations may promote the development of injury and an adequate adaptation may reduce the risk of tendinopathy despite substantial tendon loading.

Tendinous tissue has traditionally been regarded as rather sluggish and static with a limited ability to react and adapt to exercise and training. However research has shown that tendinous tissue is highly capable of adjusting its metabolism to match an increase in loading and that the tissue can adapt to training. Interestingly, also in tendinopathic tendons, regular exercise does result in an upregulation of collagen synthesis, indicating that even in a diseased state, tendons benefit from a certain degree of controlled loading (Langberg et al., 2007).

Specific types of exercise: high intensity and strength training

There has been very little investigation of tendon responses and adaptations to intermittent high loads as those seen in jumping, sprinting and heavy strength training. Patellar tendon hypertrophy occurs in response to 12 weeks of heavy resistance training the increase in cross-sectional area occurred at the proximal and distal ends but not at the mid-tendon (Kongsgaard et al., 2007). This is supported by a study that showed high-resistance training reduced tendon pain (Frohm et al., 2007).

Specific types of exercise: eccentric training

Eccentric exercise places high load on tendon and it has been used extensively to rehabilitate painful tendons (Kingma et al., 2007). Its use as a prevention has been investigated only recently and a study of soccer players has shown that it did not reduce the risk of injury. In fact those with patellar tendon pathology at the beginning of the season were more likely to be injured if they did the preventative eccentric exercise (Fredberg et al., 2007). In a similar study in volleyball players, eccentric training in season did not improve tendon pain (Visnes et al., 2005).

Stretching

Stretching is used to prevent injury, in tendons the type of stretching may be critical. Dynamic stretching may be superior to static stretching as it alters the mechanical properties of the tendons (Witvrouw et al., 2007), whereas static stretching in many tendinopathies will increase the compressive load, known to cause pathological alterations in tendons. In athletes although static stretching may be relevant for the muscle, the best tendon response is to dynamic stretching.

Adjusting training load

Although overload has been clearly linked to tendon pain and pathology, athletes have widely ranging load tolerance. Thus, we are unable to prescribe simple protocols for adjusting load. However, energy storage and release causes tendon pathology, hence it is easy to say if you cycle or swim you are unlikely to get a tensional tendon overload (swimmers may get compressive overload of the rotator cuff). Outside of this recommendation, load management becomes more difficult, frequency of load appears important; training more than once in every 2 days does not allow the tendon to respond fully to each load stimulus. Nothing is known about modifying volume and intensity of load. A recent study that investigated gradual introduction of running compared to a standard running training program did not find any difference in injury between groups, because of individual variations in injury susceptibility very large numbers in such studies may be needed to clearly show if a difference exists (Buist et al., 2008).

Take-home message

Because tendon's response to different kinds of exercise and loading varies, coaches cannot follow "one-size fits all" approach. Tendons possess adaptational capabilities and in most circumstances will adapt adequately to different levels of exercise if they are given enough time. However, as tendinous tissue is somewhat slower to adapt than muscle tissue it is suggested that sudden increases or changes in exercise loads and modes should be avoided wherever possible. It would appear prudent for training changes to be prescribed cautiously to allow the tendon enough time to adapt and recover and prevent the development of injury. Abdominal fat, lack of fitness, and certain biomechanical factors are risk factors for overuse tendinopathy so these should be addressed in active individuals. Imaging (including ultrasound and MR imaging) does not appear to contribute to the clinical approach to tendinopathy prevention at this stage.

References

Arøen, A., Helgø, D., Granlund, O.G., Bahr, R. (2004) Contralateral tendon rupture risk is increased in individuals with a previous Achilles tendon rupture.

Scandinavian Journal of Medicine and Science in Sports **14**, 30–33.

Buist, I., Bredeweg, S.W., van Mechelen, W., Lemmink, K.A., Pepping, G.J., Diercks, R.L. (2008) No effect of a graded training program on the number of running-related injuries in novice runners: a randomized controlled trial. *American Journal of Sports Medicine* **36**, 33–39.

Ferretti, A., Puddu, G., Mariani, P.P., Neri, M. (1984) Jumper's knee: an epidemiological study of volleyball players. *Physician and Sports Medicine* **12**, 97–103.

Fredberg, U., Bolvig, L., Andersen, N.T. (2007) Prophylactic training in asymptomatic soccer players with ultrasonographic abnormalities in Achilles and patellar tendons: the Danish Super League Study. *American Journal of Sports Medicine* December 13 [Epub ahead of print].

Frohm, A., Saartok, T., Halvorsen, K., Renström, P. (2007) Eccentric treatment for patellar tendinopathy: a prospective randomised short-term pilot study of two rehabilitation protocols. *British Journal of Sports Medicine* **41**, e7.

Kannus, P., Jozsa, L. (1991) Histopathological changes preceding spontaneous rupture of a tendon. A controlled study of 891 patients. *Journal of Bone and Joint Surgery (American)* **73**, 1507–1525.

Kingma, J.J., de Knikker, R., Wittink, H.M., Takken, T. (2007) Eccentric overload training in patients with chronic Achilles tendinopathy: a systematic review. *British Journal of Sports Medicine* **41**, e3.

Kjær, M. (2004) Role of extracellular matrix in adaptation of tendon and skeletal muscle to mechanical loading. *Physiology Review* **84**, 649–698.

Kongsgaard, M., Reitelseder, S., Pedersen, T.G., Holm, L., Aagaard, P., Kjær, M., Magnusson, S.P. (2007) Region specific patellar tendon hypertrophy in humans following resistance training. *Acta Physiologica Scandinavia* **191**, 111–121.

Langberg, H., Ellingsgaard, H., Madsen, T., Jansson, J., Magnusson, S.P., Aagaard, P., Kjær, M. (2007) Eccentric rehabilitation exercise increases peritendinous type I collagen synthesis in humans with Achilles tendinosis. *Scandinavian Journal of Medicine & Science in Sports* **17**, 61–66.

Lian, Ø.B., Engebretsen, L., Bahr, R. (2005) Prevalence of jumper's knee among elite athletes from different sports: a cross-sectional study. *American Journal of Sports Medicine* **33**, 561–567.

Lian, Ø., Refsnes, P.E., Engebretsen, L., Bahr, R. (2003) Performance characteristics of volleyball players with patellar tendinopathy. *American Journal of Sports Medicine* **31**, 408–413.

Malliaras, P., Cook, J. (2006) Reduced ankle dorsiflexion range may increase the risk of patellar tendon injury among volleyball players. *Journal of Science and Medicine in Sport* **9**, 304–309.

Malliaras, P., Cook, J., Kent, P. (2007) Anthropometric risk factors for patellar tendon injury among volleyball players. *British Journal of Sports Medicine* **41**, 259–263.

Owens, B., Mountcastle, S., White, D. (2007) Racial differences in tendon rupture incidence. *International Journal of Sports Medicine* **28**, 617–620.

Pottie, P., Presle, N., Terlain, B., Netter, P., Mainard, D., Berenbaum, F. (2006) Obesity and osteoarthritis: more complex than predicted! *Annals of Rheumatic Disease* **65**, 1403–1405.

Visnes, H., Hoksrud, A., Cook, J., Bahr, R. (2005) No effect of eccentric training on jumper's knee in volleyball players during the competitive season: a randomized clinical trial. *Clinical Journal of Sports Medicine* **15**, 227–234.

Witvrouw, E., Bellemans, J., Lysens, R., Danneels, L., Cambier, D. (2001) Intrinsic risk factors for the development of patellar tendinitis in an athletic population. A two-year prospective study. *American Journal of Sports Medicine* **29**, 190–195.

Witvrouw, E., Mahieu, N., Roosen, P., McNair, P. (2007) The role of stretching in tendon injuries. *British Journal of Sports Medicine* **41**, 224–226.

Further reading

Bahr, R. (2003) Preventing sports injuries. In R. Bahr & S. Mæhlum (eds.) *Clinical Guide to Sports Injuries*, pp. 41–53. Human Kinetics, Champaign, IL.

Bahr, R. (2007) Principles of sports injury prevention. In P. Brukner & K. Khan (eds.) *Clinical Sports Medicine*, pp. 78–101. McGraw-Hill, Sydney.

Cook, J.L., Purdam, C.R. (2003) Rehabilitation of lower limb tendinopathies. *Clinics in Sports Medicine* **22**, 777–789.

Ljungqvist, A., Schwellnus, M.P., Bachl, N., Collins, M., Cook, J., Khan, K.M., Maffulli, N., Pitsiladis, Y., Riley, G., Golspink, G., Venter, D., Derman, E.W., Engebretsen, L., Volpi, P. (2008) International Olympic Committee consensus statement: molecular basis of connective tissue and muscle injuries in sport. *Clinics in Sports Medicine* **27**, 231–239.

Maffulli, N., Renström, P.A.F.H., Leadbetter, W.B. (2005) *Tendon Injuries: Basic Science and Clinical Medicine*. Springer-Verlag, London.

Woo, S.L.-Y., Renström, P.A.F.H., Arnoczky, S.P. (eds) (2007) *Tendinopathy in Athletes*. Blackwell Publishing, Massachusetts.

Chapter 13
Implementing large-scale injury prevention programs

Randall W. Dick[1], Claude Goulet[2] and Simon Gianotti[3]

[1]Research/Injury Surveillance System National Collegiate Athletic Association, Indianapolis, Indiana, USA
[2]Department of Physical Education, Laval University, Québec, Canada
[3]Sport and Road Injury Prevention, Accident Compensation Corporation, Institute of Sport and Recreation Research New Zealand, Faculty of Health and Environmental Science, Auckland University of Technology, New Zealand

Introduction

It is well documented that regular sport participation or physical activity can improve health and quality of life. Moreover, in combination with a proper diet and a healthy lifestyle, physical activity is an influential factor in the control of body weight. From a public health perspective, the benefits of physical activity are clear.

There is, however, a cost of physical activity—namely the burden of injuries. Injuries resulting from sports and recreational activities are a significant health problem in many countries. There is now irrefutable evidence that the sports injury problem is not restricted to professional sports. For more than two decades, about every fifth unintentional injury treated in a health care setting in industrialized countries has been associated with sports or physical activity. This makes sport and recreational activity injuries probably the most ironic injury type. On one side, public health authorities are actively promoting regular sport and physical activity participation. On the other hand, it is known that if not practiced in safe environments, sport and recreational activity injuries could significantly reduce the public health benefits of regular sport and physical activity participation. In a public health perspective, it supports the importance of implementing large-scale injury prevention programs.

Implementing large-scale injury prevention programs poses many challenges. Drawing mainly from our experience and from published literature in the fields of sport and recreational activity injury prevention (see Chapter 2), we have produced a list of five key elements to consider in the development and implementation of large-scale prevention programs. These key elements are as follows.

Approach the injury problem at hand with a multi-dimensional view

It is essential to analyze any injury problem through a systematic approach and a multi-dimensional view (see Chapter 2). It maximizes the probability that all possible solutions to the problem will be addressed. Based on some of the latest conceptual advances made in the field of injury prevention, we also suggest that the following guiding principles be considered in the analysis process: (1) Consider the cost/benefit ratio when selecting an intervention strategy; (2) consider the impact an intervention might have on the nature of the sport; (3) choose interventions adapted to the problem at hand: either inform, convince, or contrive (see Section "Active versus passive measures" in Chapter 2); and (4) Encourage partnership.

Sports Injury Prevention, 1st edition. Edited by R. Bahr and L. Engebretsen Published 2009 by Blackwell Publishing ISBN: 9781405162449

Beliefs confuse the issue; get the facts

Sport is an area where changes occur slowly because of deep-rooted beliefs. You need well-documented facts on the injury problem as well as the effects of the proposed measures before trying to convince the targeted group—whether it be elite athletes, recreational participants or owners of sport facilities.

Work toward a consensus; develop coalitions

Even if you are in a position to impose mandatory safety measures, make sure you develop strong grass-roots support for your intervention. As a sport injury prevention specialist, identify the key stakeholders and work with them on solutions that they are willing to apply. Be prepared to support these partners with information and training.

Recognize the limits of information campaigns; develop back-up technological systems

Public awareness campaigns are important, but they are not enough. Well-informed people are still human beings; which means that knowledge does not necessarily result in behavior change. One of the most efficient ways to improve sports safety is through the modification of the environment (see Section "Active versus passive measures" in Chapter 2).

Try to change the perception that more safety brings less fun

Safety is often perceived as something that will take fun away from sport and recreational activities. In fact, safety measures can allow participants more enjoyment from their activity by giving them "peace of mind." In general, outdoor specialists understand this positive side of safety. Safety is often what makes their activity possible. We can all learn from their attitude toward safety skip line after end of PP.

The aim of this chapter is to present five practical examples of large-scale programs that have been implemented by the National Collegiate Athletic Association (NCAA) in the United States of America, by the Accident Compensation Corporation (ACC) in New Zealand, and by the provincial government in the Canadian province of Québec. Each example will incorporate the five key elements previously discussed within the context of the four step injury prevention model (IPM): (1) describing the magnitude of the injury problem, (2) understanding the causes, (3) introducing measures likely to reduce the future risk and/or severity of injuries, and (4) evaluating their effect (Figure 2.1). These examples and approaches should help key stakeholders in sports injury prevention to implement efficient large-scale injury prevention programs to improve the social and health benefits of sport participation.

The American National Collegiate Athletic Association model

The NCAA is an organization of approximately 1100 colleges and universities established in 1906 to govern athletics competition in a fair, safe, equitable, and sportsmanlike manner and to integrate intercollegiate athletics into higher education. The association conducts its business through a committee structure made up of diverse representatives from member institutions. Nationally, more than 380,000 student–athletes participate in NCAA sports that offer national championships.

Recognizing its organizational health and safety roots, the NCAA has maintained an Injury Surveillance System (ISS) for intercollegiate athletics since 1982. The primary goal of the system is to collect injury and exposure data from a representative sample of NCAA institutions in a variety of sports. Relevant data are then shared with appropriate NCAA sport and policy committees to provide a foundation for evidence-based decision-making on health and safety issues. The NCAA model of a sport organization with (1) a committee structure with the authority to develop enforce policy, (2) data collections systems such as the ISS to provide an information foundation for decision-making, and (3) a review process to assess policy effectiveness has been beneficial in a variety of injury prevention initiatives.

Example 1: Wrestling with weight loss—The NCAA Wrestling Weight Management Program

The problem (IPM Steps 1 and 2)

In a span of 33 days in late 1997, three collegiate wrestlers died while engaging in a program of rapid weight loss. All were in the presence of coaches.

According to the Centers for Disease Control and Prevention's (CDC, 1998) review of the cases, the wrestlers were attempting to lose an average of 8 pounds over a 3- to 12-h period by wearing rubber suits and exercising vigorously in hot environments. The wrestlers were attempting to lose this weight AFTER dropping an average 21 pounds over the previous 2–3 months.

There were no previous recorded deaths in NCAA wrestling associated with making weight but the sport in general had a reputation for rapid and severe weight fluctuations similar to those reported in these three cases.

Understanding the facts and the belief structure (IPM Steps 1 and 2)

The sport of wrestling had a variety of issues to consider before addressing the problem.

1. Established guidelines: Position statements associated with weight loss in wrestling from organizations such as the American College of Sports Medicine (ACSM, 1996) had existed for many years. The three deaths brought attention to weight loss behaviors that, in some cases, had been contrary to medical guidelines for many years.

2. Safety: The NCAA ISS had shown wrestling as a sport at very high risk for injury relative to other sports monitored by the system (Agel et al., 2007). Many of the injuries may have been directly or indirectly associated with improper weight loss practices or their after-effects.

3. Competitive equity: Weight was acknowledged to be the competitive equity variable in the sport of wrestling. Weight classes were established to assure that opponents were paired against athletes of similar weight. Prior to these fatalities, collegiate wrestlers were able to make weight at least 24 h prior to competition, When the actual competition took place, both opponents generally weighed significantly more than the designated weight class they had qualified for the previous day (mean 3.3 kg in one study; Horswill et al., 1994). There also could be a significant weight differential between the two individuals (mean 1.5 kg in one study; Scott et al., 1994) nullifying any competitive equity associated with weight class.

4. Wrestler mindset: Wrestlers believed that self-discipline, commitment and sacrifice they learned from making weight would help make them better wrestlers. Cutting 3–7% body weight and then regaining it the next day was perceived to allow one to gain a strength and size advantage over a "smaller/weaker" opponent.

Working toward consensus: identifying the stakeholders

In the aftermath of the wrestling deaths, the NCAA joined with other organizations to create a joint resolution which said, in part: "Eliminate from wrestling any and all weight control practices which could potentially risk the health of the participants."

Two NCAA committees, the National Wrestling Coaches Association, USA Wrestling, the national governing body for wrestling and various medical organizations were involved in the discussions. Coaches, student-athletes, exercise physiologists, athletic trainers, physicians, athletic administrators, sport governing body officials, and lawyers were all represented. Since weight cutting mostly occurred in the practice environment, and could not be regulated effectively by competition rules, the wrestling coach was identified as a key stakeholder. While certain policies could be implemented and enforced, the wrestling coach, and his or her attitude toward weight cutting leading up to competitions, ultimately would determine the success of the program.

NCAA weight management program components (IPM Step 3)

The NCAA weight management program (Figure 13.1) was based on four guiding principles:
- Enhance safety and competitive equity
- Minimize incentives for rapid weight loss

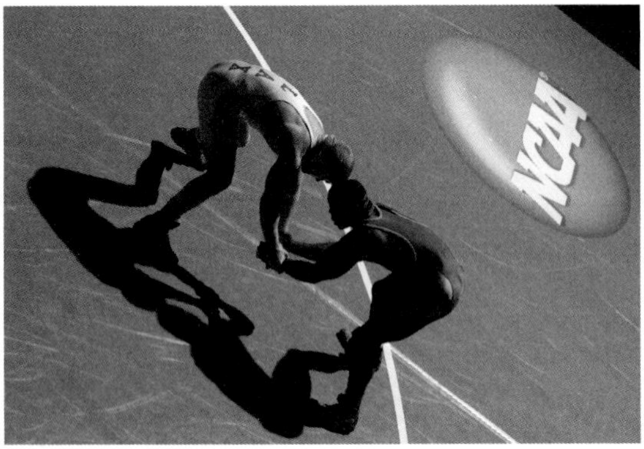

Figure 13.1. The NCAA Wrestling Weight Management Program shows promise for increased safety and competitive equity for wrestling participants of all ages

- Emphasize competition, not weight control
- Implement practical, effective, and enforceable guidelines.

Specific components included: establishing weight classes that better reflect the collegiate wrestling population, establishing a permanent healthy weight class (lean body weight plus at least 5% body fat) early in the season with time to achieve it safely, establishing weigh-ins as close to the match as possible, eliminating the tools used to accomplish rapid dehydration, and requiring CPR certification of all wrestling coaches.

Evaluation of the weight management program (IPM Step 4)

To evaluate effectiveness, research investigating the changes in weight and body composition relative to performance over the course of the season was initiated. Research conducted over the entire wrestling season showed that the most successful wrestlers chose to participate at a body composition well above the minimum allowable value of 5% and that reducing the time between weigh-ins and competition was effective in reducing rapid weight loss. A weight management program coupled with reducing time between weigh-ins and competition was even more effective.

Discussion

The successful NCAA model includes injury surveillance (facts), input from diverse constituents (consensus), a committee structure with the capability to enact and enforce formal policy, and specific research to determine policy effectiveness. The NCAA wrestling weight management program has become a model program for the sport and has been accepted by collegiate wrestlers and coaches. The sport has become more fun for participants as the emphasis has switched from weight loss to skill development. In the 2004–2005 academic year, this program involved 224 intercollegiate wrestling programs, touching almost 6000 student-athletes. In 2006 the National Federation of State High School Associations (NFHS) implemented a similar weight management program at the United States high school level impacting over 250,000 student-athletes. These programs show promise for increased safety and competitive equity for wrestling participants of all ages. A similar weight management program may be beneficial at higher levels of wrestling and in other Olympic weight category sports such as rowing and boxing.

The New Zealand model

In New Zealand, determining the size and scope of a particular sport injury problem is relatively simple. This is largely due to the existence of a mandatory no-fault 24-h injury scheme providing coverage for injury treatment and rehabilitation costs. The scheme is administered by the Accident Compensation Corporation (ACC). In the last ACC financial year (1 July 2006 to 20 June 2007—2006/2007), the 4.1 million New Zealanders made 422,000 sport and recreation claims, costing the Corporation $NZ 329 million. There is no disincentive for making a claim; people are not discriminated, risk rated or penalized for the number of claims they make. The cost of claims and the legislation governing the ACC provides incentive for investing in large-scale injury prevention programs. ACC has a cost-outcome model to determine investment levels and programs are expected to provide a return on the investment. ACC currently targets moderate to serious injury claims for its sport cost-outcome model. Although moderate to serious injury claims may make up only a small proportion of all sport claims, 7.4% in 2006/2007, they represent around 75% of the cost.

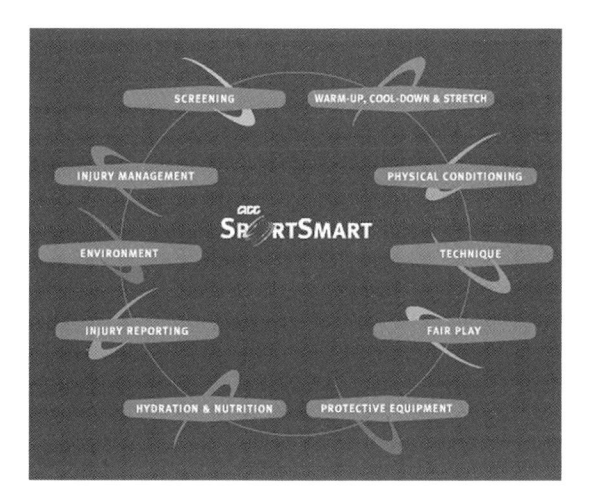

Figure 13.2. The New Zealand Accident Compensation Corporation SportSmart model is a 10-point action plan for sports injury prevention

In 1999, ACC developed the SportSmart model, a 10-point action plan (screening, warm up/cool down, physical conditioning, technique, fair play, protective equipment, hydration/nutrition, injury reporting, environment, injury management) (Figure 13.2) for sports injury prevention and has since developed a range of sport-specific injury prevention programs based on this model. This initiative relies on a coalition between ACC and the respective national sporting body. Two specific applications of the SportSmart model are discussed in the following section.

Example 2: The RugbySmart Program—preventing injuries in rugby union

The injury problem (Steps 1 and 2)

Rugby Union (rugby) represents the largest percentage (15%) of sport moderate to serious injury claims to ACC. It is also a sport that has been associated with serious spinal injuries. Due to their severity and life changing impact, these injuries draw media attention and focus on to rugby.

In 1996, the New Zealand Rugby Union (NZRU) implemented a compulsory safety course for coaches and referees, with the focus on preventing serious spinal injuries. Analysis of the compulsory safety course showed that it was not achieving the desired effect, despite early reported results. In 2000, ACC and NZRU formed a coalition to tackle the injuries. ACC data identified neck/back/spine, shoulder, knee, ankle, and leg (excluding knee and ankle) injuries to target in addition to serious spinal injuries. These body parts were predominantly injured in contact situations of the scrum, tackle, ruck, and maul phases of the game. Improving technique in these phases lowers the risk of injury and moderate to serious injury claims. The program targeted community-level (non-professional) 15–44-year-old rugby players due to their impact on the ACC scheme; they represented 34% of the players, but 92% of the rugby moderate to serious injury claim costs.

Understanding the facts and belief structure

While there was acknowledgment that the incidence of serious spinal injuries needed attention, the NZRU compulsory safety course was widely viewed as undesirable and was not well received by the rugby community. Common reasons included:
1. Coaches/referees were volunteers and were difficult to recruit; having to undertake a compulsory safety course was yet another commitment on the coaches time.
2. The focus was on the consequences of a serious injury. Highlighting the problem had the potential to turn people away from coaching/refereeing.
3. Coaches perceived that they knew most of the information imparted in the compulsory course and that it was the same every year.

In summary, a system to deliver compulsory safety education was in place but it needed to be made more suitable to the audience to achieve buy-in and acceptance.

Working toward consensus: identifying the stakeholders

By developing a coalition, both groups could achieve appropriate outcomes. ACC desired a reduction in the number of injuries, as it provided for the cost of rehabilitation and replacement of earnings, whereas the NZRU wanted to make the game a competitive, safe, and popular sport.

The new program, RugbySmart, was developed based on SportSmart and implemented in the 2001 rugby season with ACC investment. The NZRU compulsory safety course evolved to RugbySmart and was repackaged to focus more on causes of injury rather than consequences. In addition to NZRU and Rugby Development Officers, coaches and referees also were identified as stakeholders. RugbySmart targeted coaches and referees as (i) reaching 137,000 players via coaches/referees was more effective than targeting each player directly and more effective than relying on clubs and schools and (ii) coaches were identified by both players (and coaches) as having an important role in injury prevention.

The RugbySmart program (Step 3)

RugbySmart involves the screening of a DVD at a compulsory workshop, as originally put in place by NZRU. The DVD contained aspects of the 10-point action plan, with an emphasis on areas where injury issues have been identified, such as the scrum, tackle, and ruck (Figure 13.3). The workshop was conducted by Rugby Development Officers (for coaches) and Referee Education Officers (for referees), and these positions were funded by NZRU.

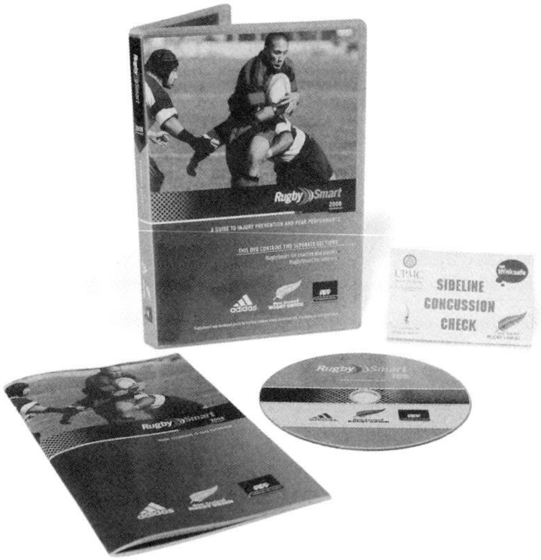

Figure 13.3. The RugbySmart DVD used in the workshops is a key factor in implementing injury prevention in rugby that has resulted in decreases in serious spinal injuries and injury claims in targeted injury areas

Having a DVD ensured consistency of delivery and supported the facilitator. RugbySmart, like its NZRU predecessor was compulsory for coaches and referees to attend. Team were withdrawn from competition and referees were not assigned games if they did not attend. While the compulsory education aspect was appealing to ACC and ensured a captive audience, it also created resistance to the program. This was largely overcome by developing a product that appealed to the coaches and referees. For example, promoting correct or winning technique as safe and then demonstrating skills that focused on the improved technique was a successful strategy. The skills demonstrated were in a straightforward manner, allowing coaches to master them and easily incorporate into trainings.

Evaluation of the RugbySmart program (Step 4)

RugbySmart was evaluated in several ways and the results were used to develop the program further, keeping it fresh and relevant. NZRU is one of the few sports in NZ to have an accurate and reliable player registration system, providing a moderate to serious injury claims rate per 100,000 players to determine the effectiveness of RugbySmart. Evaluation justified continued investment in the existing program as well as in further areas that warrant investigation. The return on the investment was $7:78 for every ACC $1 invested (Gianotti & Hume, 2007). The results of the RugbySmart program showed a decrease in serious spinal injuries in the scrum (Quarrie et al., 2007), decreases per 100,000 players in moderate to serious injury claims in targeted injury areas (Gianotti et al., 2008), and increases in desired training behaviors in safe scrum, ruck, and tackle at practices/trainings (Gianotti et al., 2008).

Example 3: The SoccerSmart Program—preventing injuries in football (soccer)

The injury problem (Steps 1 and 2)

Based on the initial success of RugbySmart, ACC was keen to implement SportSmart into other sports. Football was targeted as it represented the second largest percentage of sport claims (7.2%) to ACC. While ACC and New Zealand Football (NZF) had previously developed some injury prevention initiatives, they were small and involved using the generic SportSmart model rather than a football-specific one. Attention was also focussed on secondary/tertiary prevention (e.g., training for the treatment of soft-tissue injuries).

The ACC system could, like in rugby, pinpoint the type and nature of football injuries. Initially the focus was all moderate to serious soccer injury claims. However, in 2005 the system targeted players aged 15–44 years who represent the greatest percentage of football moderate to serious injury claims (85%) with knees (38%) and ankles (19%) being the most predominate injury sites. To address these injuries, the SportSmart model was adapted for football to provide relevance to the target group. Feedback from initial projects with NZF had highlighted the need for this specificity. In addition, the world governing body for football FIFA's Medical and Research Committee (F-MARC) had developed a program called "The 11" which ACC were keen to see implemented.

Understanding the facts and belief structure

While there was success with the RugbySmart concept, football required a completely different approach to build a coalition due to the following:
1. Financial considerations: Rugby has an annual budget 10–50 times that of other sports with the same playing numbers. Investing in the community aspect of the game on this scale was difficult to repeat in other sports. NZF has fewer staff and could not afford to devote the time necessary to develop and implement an injury prevention program.
2. Non-governed participation: There are different forms of football that NZF does not control. ACC data collection did not distinguish between forms of football (e.g., indoor soccer, 6-a-side, 11-a-side), as it is a no-fault system. This impacted on the ability to undertake evaluations.
3. Inaccurate playing numbers: NZF does not keep accurate playing numbers and relies on estimates.

This is a further hindrance to evaluation and also limits the development of a cost-outcome model to help secure ACC investment.
4. Public perceptions. Football is considered a safer sport than rugby. It does not produce serious spinal injuries and parents have been known to remove their children from rugby in favor of football due to injury risk perception.

Working toward consensus: identifying the stakeholders

To encourage an increased emphasis on injury prevention and to engage NZF, ACC increased its investment in the sport. This provided for NZF to employ a person whose primary responsibility would be injury prevention, but who would also be available for other NZF duties. Having a person essentially inside NZF devoted to injury prevention gave this topic credibility and emphasis in the sport. This was essential in developing a coalition with NZF. The remaining ACC investment was for injury prevention resources, ensuring the injury prevention person had an established and targeted budget rather than bidding and competing for existing NZF funds. While ACC was prepared to make this investment, it still took NZF 18 months to formally agree to a coalition. This was more reflective of a busy sport rather than a reluctance to be involved in injury prevention. Key discussion points included compulsory training of coaches and rule changes. NZF was not in the same position as NZRU to make injury prevention training compulsory for coaches and the sport also was concerned about the expectation to implement rule changes and the subsequent implications.

The SoccerSmart program (Step 3)

In 2004, NZF (formally New Zealand Soccer) and ACC adapted SportSmart to create SoccerSmart. Despite the governing bodies name change, from soccer to football, the SoccerSmart brand was retained because of its market recognition. Football coaches were identified as a suitable initial target and SoccerSmart was included in all existing NZF coach education courses, as well as a stand-alone workshop. Resources were created to be included in each course pack. These included booklets, wallet

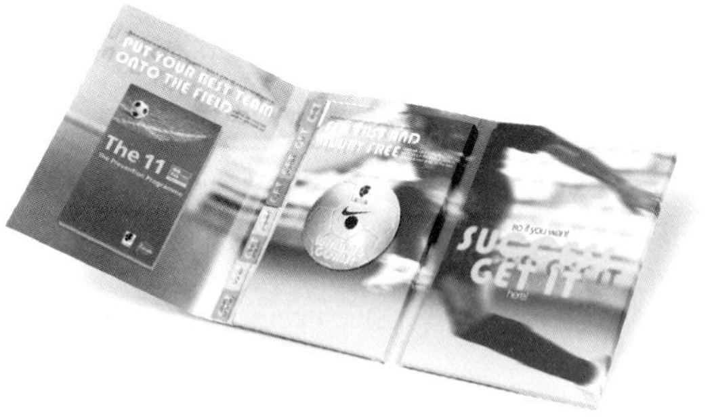

Figure 13.4. The SoccerSmart resources targeting has shown a claims reduction against forecast for knee and ankle injuries in 15–44-year-old soccer players

cards (pocket-sized folded information sheets), and posters that addressed all 10 SoccerSmart action points. Resources were designed to be used by coaches and passed on to players. FIFA's "The 11" resources were also included in the SoccerSmart course packs (Figure 13.4). SoccerSmart (similar to RugbySmart) focused on injuries or injury-related issues that were more prevalent in the sport of football, as determined from the ACC claims database. These included tackling, physical fitness, and prematch issues. Special care was also taken with the language and phrases used in SoccerSmart, to ensure suitability for the audience.

Evaluation of SoccerSmart program (Step 4)

As with all injury prevention ACC invests in, moderate to serious injury claims are used for evaluation. Unlike Rugby, NZF could not provide accurate playing numbers, nor an accurate estimate of the prevalence of indoor soccer. As such, moderate to serious injury claims were assessed against a forecast, made by ACC, as part of its cost-outcome approach (see Further reading). In 2006/2007, the return on the investment for all soccer moderate to serious injury claims was $2.41 (Gianotti & Hume, 2007) and there was 2.5% fewer claims against forecast for 15–44 year olds in knees and ankles. This resulted in ongoing investment in the SoccerSmart program. However, the actual number of football moderate to serious injury claims is increasing, which is purported to be due to the anecdotal reports of marked growth of the game.

Hence a forecast is used on the absolute number of moderate to serious injury claims.

Discussion

The NZ examples show a passive model that can be adapted to other sports and is effective in achieving injury prevention outcomes. In these examples, education plays more of a role than enforcement and engineering of the injury prevention matrix (see chapter 2) since there is no ability to enforce rules or make a sport undertake injury prevention by withholding injury coverage. A strong coalition with the national body (NZRU, NZF) is crucial for the implementation of an effective sports injury prevention program. While investment and funding is also important, this investment would not have been as effective if the national bodies were not supportive. This is particularly important for large-scale implementation of injury prevention programs.

The Canadian Province of Québec model

Injuries resulting from sports and recreational activities are a significant health problem in Québec. The Canadian Community Health Survey of Statistics Canada revealed that in 2003 in Québec, injuries which occurred in a sport and leisure venue represented 21% of all injuries resulting in limitation of normal activities or medical consultation, compared with 35% of injuries at home, and 8% on the road. Moreover, participation in sport and recreational activities was the leading cause of non-intentional injuries in Québec in 2003 (25%), before occupational injuries (23%). Of course, sport and recreational activity injuries are not all severe: there are more deaths on Québec roads than on sports fields and, generally, road injuries are more severe. However, the public health burden of sport and recreational activity injuries is manifest in their morbidity. A population-based survey done for the Québec Ministry of Education, Leisure, and Sport estimates that during the year 2004, 514,000

Québec residents aged between 6 and 74 years consulted a health professional to treat a sport and recreational activity injury (88/1000 participants). These data clearly show the scale of the sport and recreational activity injuries problem and the importance of establishing safe environments.

In 1979, to significantly contribute to the establishment of safe environments, the government of Québec adopted the *Act Respecting Safety in Sports* which created the Québec Sports Safety Board (Régnier & Goulet, 1995; Government of Québec, 1988). Since 1998, through its mission to "foster the development of recreation and sport in a safe and healthy environment and promote an active lifestyle for all Québecers," the Safety Promotion Unit of the Québec Ministry of Education, Leisure, and Sport supervised the execution of the *Act Respecting Safety in Sports*. In accordance with this act, one of the Safety Promotion Unit's orientations is to "ensure that the safety and physical security and well-being of participants are provided for during sports and recreation activities."

With respect to the *Act*, the Safety Promotion Unit is empowered to

1. Gather, analyze, and disseminate information on sports safety.
2. Conduct, or cause others to conduct, research on sports safety.
3. Educate the public on safety in relation to the practice of sports.
4. Prepare safety training methods for persons who work in the sports field.
5. Give technical assistance to sports federations or unaffiliated sports bodies in preparing safety regulations.
6. Assist any person requesting advice on means to ensure sports safety.

Two examples of the application of the Québec Model are presented in the following example.

Example 4: Bodychecking injuries in minor ice hockey

The injury problem (Steps 1 and 2)

Ice hockey is one of Canada's most popular winter sports, with more than 500,000 registered players in the Canadian Hockey Association. In 2004–2005, it was estimated that 9%–31% of all Canadian boys participated in organized leagues.

In the 1970s, faced with an increase in ice hockey violence and poor performances at the international level, Canadian administrators and other individuals involved with North American hockey began to question their basic philosophies of the game. This awareness sparked increased research in ice hockey which was followed, in some cases, by changes in the rules, particularly at the minor level. One of the major changes was the abolition of bodychecking for players 12 years old and under. Bodychecking is defined as an individual defensive tactic designed to legally separate the puck carrier from the puck by use of physical contact.

In 1985, to allow Midget age players (15–16 years old) who wanted to play junior hockey to finish high school in their home towns, the Canadian Hockey Association decided to raise all age groups by 1 year, thus making the Pee Wee category 12–13 years old. With those age changes, the "no bodychecking" rule was reconsidered. After a brief discussion during their general meeting of 1985, the Canadian Hockey Association adopted a new rule allowing bodychecking for Pee Wee category.

In the province of Québec, faced with a controversy on the risk of injuries associated with the new rule, Hockey Québec (the Québec Ice Hockey Federation) asked the Québec Sports Safety Board for its opinion on the matter.

Understanding the facts and belief structure

Realizing that no hard scientific data were available on the effect of bodychecking on the safety of Pee Wee players, the Québec Sports Safety Board sponsored an appropriate research study (Régnier et al., 1989). Consistent with the first key element mentioned earlier, the multidisciplinary nature of the research group allowed its members to study the following topics:

1. The attitudes and beliefs of coaches, parents, and players toward bodychecking.
2. The morphological and biomedical differences among Pee Wee players.

3. The number and types of penalties within leagues playing with and without bodychecking.
4. The injury rate among Pee Wee leagues playing with and without bodychecking.
5. The modeling effect of professional hockey.
6. The training of coaches in the teaching of bodychecking.
7. The effects on participation.

The most influential study result relative to public awareness was that Pee Wee players were 12 times more likely to suffer a fracture in leagues that allowed players to bodycheck. The rate of fracture was 1 per 22 games in leagues where bodychecking was allowed compared to 1 per 263 games in leagues where bodychecking was not allowed. The weight and height difference between players was shown to be one of the most important risk factors of injury. Morphologic and strength differences between the smallest and the largest players competing at the Pee Wee level revealed an average weight and height difference of 37.2 kg and 31.5 cm, respectively. Furthermore, a 70% difference in the force of impact during bodychecking between a group of small players and larger players was observed.

Working toward consensus: identifying the stakeholders

With those results, the next step was to convince the minor ice hockey administrators to ban bodychecking at Pee Wee level. Some factors had major influence. The involvement of a well-respected team of university researchers in the study was important, bringing credibility to the process. Moreover, the public health network of the province highly supported the actions to ban bodychecking at Pee Wee level and information campaigns in the media were launched to influence public awareness. Finally, the Minister responsible for the administration of the *Act Respecting Safety in Sports* was lobbied for his support of the proposal.

The preventive measure (Step 3)

Based on those results, Hockey Québec decided to ban bodychecking for all Pee Wee leagues in Québec (Robidoux & Trudel, 2006). Today, Québec is the only province or territory where bodychecking is still banned for this age group. In the other provinces, there is still controversy about the issue. Government reports and academic studies have identified some problems related to bodychecking and further educational initiatives have been launched. For example, the Canadian Hockey Association has been actively providing courses on the appropriate bodychecking techniques for coaches, players, managers, referees, trainers, and parents. Only a few training initiatives have been evaluated and the overall effectiveness of these courses on injury prevention has not been established.

Evaluation (Step 4)

It is estimated that in 20 years, this large-scale measure prevented 4000 young growing players to suffer from a fracture. Moreover, there is no evidence that the ban of bodychecking at Pee Wee level reduced the level of competitiveness of Québec players at national or international levels of competition.

Example 5: Full–face protection to prevent facial injuries for adult ice hockey players

The injury problem (Steps 1 and 2)

Even if ice hockey is one of the leading contributors to sports-related injuries in Québec, it provides the sport and public health communities with an impressive success story of injury prevention: the quasi-elimination of eye and facial injuries through the use of face protectors.

In the mid-1970s, Canadian and US ophthalmologists documented a significant incidence of serious eye injuries in ice hockey players. This public awareness brought together safety specialists, amateur ice hockey governing bodies, and sport equipment manufacturers in an attempt to improve available eye and face protective equipment and to increase its routine use in the sport.

These efforts led to the adoption of a Canadian and a US standard on face protectors for ice hockey players. The standards led in turn to the adoption of regulations imposing the use of a certified full-face protector for all minor league players (18 years or under) in the United States starting with the 1976 season, and in Canada starting with the 1978 season. However, the large population of adult hockey players remained at risk because full face protection was not required beyond age 18.

Understanding the facts and belief structure

The effect of the use of certified full-face protectors by minor league players have been well documented in Canada and in the United States of America. For instance, no eye injuries have been recorded for a player wearing a full-face protector certified by the Canadian Standard Association. But the most eloquent demonstration of the effectiveness of full-face protectors was based on reports from Canadian ophthalmologists. In 1974–1975 the average age of hockey players suffering from an eye injury in Canada was 14 years. In 1983–1984, 5 years after full-face protectors were imposed on all minor league players by the Canadian Hockey Association, the average age of the victims rose to 24 years (Pashby, 1985). From these results, it was determined that the main population at risk of eye injury in hockey had become the thousands of adult recreational hockey players participating in organized leagues not subject to the Canadian Hockey Association regulation.

Many studies conducted in Québec between 1982 and 1987 confirmed these conclusions as to the vulnerability of 90,000 adult recreational players not wearing full facial protection. Observations in a representative sample of arenas in Québec revealed that only 25% of these players wore facial protection in 1987 in spite of previous social marketing campaigns promoting the voluntary use of full-face protectors. A major challenge was introducing a new piece of equipment to a generation that had not grown up with it.

It was clear that the use of full-face protectors by adult ice hockey players needed to increase by enacting regulation requiring their use. But, before the implementation of such regulation it was important to convince the players to comply with the regulation.

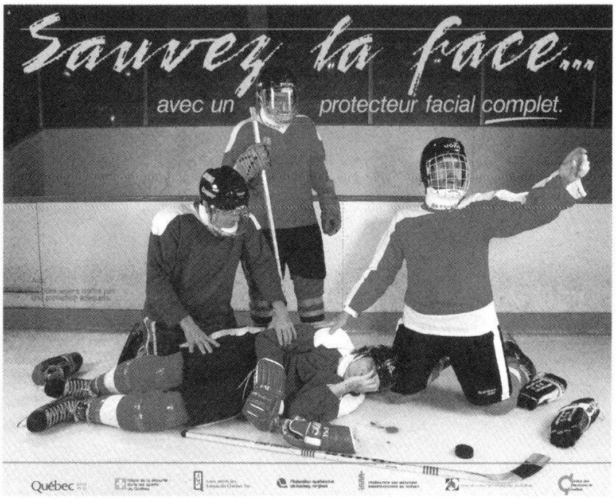

Figure 13.5. Mandating full-face protection in adult league Québec ice hockey players has shown a dramatic decrease in eye injuries and a positive promotional cost/health care savings ratio

Working toward consensus: identifying the stakeholders

As was the case for the ban of bodychecking at Pee Wee level (Example 4), the regulation imposing the use of full-face protectors by adult ice hockey players was supported by the public health network of the province, and by groups of ophthalmologists in Canada and in the United States of America. This support significantly enhanced the credibility of the regulation. Social marketing campaigns promoting the use of full-face protectors were also undertaken (Figure 13.5). The Minister responsible for the administration of the *Act Respecting Safety in Sports* also had to be convinced.

The preventive measure (Step 3)

To significantly reduce the incidence of eye injuries to adult ice hockey players, the Québec Sports Safety Board enacted a regulation imposing full-face protectors on all adult ice hockey players participating in an organized league.

The evaluation (Step 4)

The regulation imposing full-face protector had an immediate and long-lasting effect on the use rate of full-face protectors among adult recreational hockey players in Québec. One year after the adoption of the regulation, the use of full face protectors rose from 25% to 88% (it was 75% in 2005) with a corresponding reduction in eye injuries. The relatively few eye injuries still reported involve adult players who choose not to comply with the regulation and young participants in non-organized situations. Moreover, there is no evidence that the introduction of the full-face protector induced more neck injuries or aggressive behaviors from the players.

An update of a previous study (Régnier et al., 1995) evaluating the economic impact of this second regulation from 1988 to 2000 showed a cost/savings ratio of 1/13.7; every dollar invested by the government in the development, promotion, and enforcement of the regulation generated 13.70 of savings in health care costs.

Discussion

From the Québec experience, what would be the answer to the question "Is legislation the answer for safety in sport?" We would certainly like to answer "no," if for no other reason that it is not easy to constrain. In an ideal world, every stakeholder group (participants, manufacturers of equipment, owners of facilities, coaches, instructors, teachers, and others) would adopt safe, or safer practices on their own. But our past experience shows that this is not always the case. In fact, the presence of a governmental body such as the Québec Sports Safety Board is often essential to serve as a catalyst and a unifying force to channel and co-ordinate interventions. On the other hand, legislation alone is not the answer. In the Québec context, the powers defined in the *Act Respecting Safety in Sports* should be viewed as only one of a number of possible intervention strategies that range from education to coercion. The injury problems were approached with a multi-dimensional view, well documented facts were gathered to assess the problem, and coalitions were developed.

Summary

Implementing large-scale injury prevention programs poses many challenges. However as the examples in this chapter have shown, they can be successful and positively impact thousands of recreational to elite sport participants. In summary, we revisit the five key elements of a large-scale injury prevention program and consider specific lessons learned from our examples that are consistent with these criteria.

Approach the injury problem at hand with a multidimensional view

Both the New Zealand and Québec models had a cost/benefit ratios that were a specific part of the evaluation process. This information justifies existing efforts and creates momentum for future work (e.g., the success of the RugbySmart program helped with the development of the SoccerSmart initiative.) Without this information, sport injuries could be considered insignificant. Regarding the impact on sport, ice hockey equipment rules changes could have other effects on the game (e.g., one could argue that more aggressive play occurs because equipment makes one feel invincible). These impacts, both positive and negative, need to be identified before implementation and followed in the evaluation phase. All examples involved partnerships; a broad group of constituents to agree upon the issue and to have ownership in the solution. Pee Wee ice hockey fractures, rugby head and spinal injuries, or wrestling weight loss practices are examples of targeting a specific population and a set of injuries that has the greatest possibility of safety success in terms of both injury reduction and rehabilitation cost minimization. Focus specifically on these key issues, generate success and acceptance, and then expand as needed.

Beliefs confuse the issue: get the facts

Understanding the existing incentive to cut weight allowed for specific effective wrestling rules modification to be developed. Injury surveillance was essential in developing the scope of the problem in wrestling and in monitoring effectiveness in the RugbySmart intervention. Existing high-profile injury prevention efforts (FIFA "11"), position stands (ACSM Wrestling Weight Loss Guidelines), established models (RugbySmart, mandatory full face protection in youth hockey), and surveillance systems (NCAA ISS, ACC) were important in educating affected parties of existing medical consensus and provided a credible template. Targeted research identified the issues in the Québec bodychecking issue. Build an evaluation process into implementation and celebrate success. Follow-up research documented success in the wrestling weight loss, RugbySmart and Québec eye injury examples. These publicized successes led to further initiatives, funding and application. Success breeds success. However, understand that successes in large-scale initiative may not match results from more controlled environments due to the inherent complexities associated with educating and evaluating a much larger, less-controlled population.

Work toward a consensus: develop coalitions

Even if you are in a position to impose mandatory safety measures, make sure you develop strong grass-roots support for your intervention and identify the key stakeholders (often coaches). While the NCAA model has the capability to mandate rules, the weight management model was developed with input from a broad base to achieve ownership in the solution. In the New Zealand and Québec models, a governmental entity, national governing body, or designated position clearly responsible for the safety of sports and recreational participants with appropriate funding carried two strong messages: (1) injuries resulting from sports and recreational activities are a significant public health problem and (2) something can be done to prevent them from happening. Yet the ability for these entities to gather diverse viewpoints and ultimate consensus enhanced the success of the prevention initiatives. Having high-profile champions (coaches or athletes) promoting the cause also helps the development and acceptance process.

Recognize the limits of information campaigns: develop back-up technological systems

Public awareness campaigns are important, but they are not enough. Well-informed people are still human beings; which means that knowledge does not necessarily result in behavior change. To maximize effectiveness in educational efforts, injury prevention programs need to be engaging, current, and sport-specific, using the right language (less scientific, more plain speak) to reach the target audience. Associated resources must be stimulating and promote the enhanced performance and enjoyment benefits of programs along with injury prevention. These resources need to be designed to make it easier for the coach, referee or sporting participant to take positive action, thus increasing acceptance of injury prevention. However, backup plans are important. In the wrestling example, a long-standing position statement did not alter people's behavior as much as restricting the use of dehydration devices such as saunas and rubber suits. Field sports can minimize injury risk by well-maintained surfaces, a passive environmental modification. In ice hockey, the mandate of full-face protection and the ban of bodychecking provided socio-legislative environmental changes that had a positive impact on reducing injuries.

Try to change the perception that more safety brings less fun

One of the strong motivations drawing people to recreational activities, in particular to those practiced outdoors such as skiing, is the sense of liberty they provide. Safety is often perceived as something that will take fun away from these activities. Initiatives should promote value and fun as well as safety. For example, safety allows participation, an important selling point for coaches, players, and the national governing bodies that oversee them. Coaches, players, and referees should be alerted to injury prevention successes as soon as possible to maximize acceptance, increase participation, and further reinforce the critical role they play. Once the heavy burden of constant weight management was removed, wrestlers could spend more time on becoming better technical wrestlers. Emphasizing topics like nutrition that resonated beyond the athletic field (New Zealand model), also can have a positive impact on injury prevention on the field.

Conclusion

Conceptual advances made in the field of injury prevention in recent years show that solutions to sport and recreational injury problems have to be developed and implemented from an intersectorial perspective. The examples cited in this chapter emphasize this concept as well as the value of working from an established model or framework. We conclude this chapter with an example of a Summit on Sport Safety, organized and conducted by the province of Québec, Canada in the mid-1990s. The resulting framework established the roadmap and the initial collaboration opportunities to drive various injury prevention initiatives in the Province for the next decade. It is a model that can serve as a starting point for future initiatives in any country.

The Québec Sports Safety Board Summit on Sports Safety

In order to serve as a catalyst and a unifying force to channel and co-ordinate interventions from disparate groups, each holding part of the solution to this problem, the Québec Sports Safety Board sponsored the first summit on sport and recreation safety. The summit brought together over 80 associations and governmental agencies from education, health, and sports and recreation, both from the private and public sectors. The following stages leading to the summit were.

1. Consultation meetings: Close to 100 experts and representatives of organizations participated in five meetings. They were asked to precisely define their field of intervention and their expectations regarding the summit. It was clear that participants wanted an "action" oriented event rather than an abstract process.
2. Sports safety survey: In order to complete the consultation meetings, a questionnaire was posted to 7000 contributors from diverse sectors of intervention. Among other topics, the participants had to give their opinion on priorities for action over the years to come.
3. The program: From the consultation activities, the summit's management committee selected 13 areas of intervention resulting in the creation of 13 working groups.
4. Participant preparation: Each working group held at least one meeting before the summit. The aim of these meetings was to begin developing goals with a view to the actions required to reach those goals.
5. The Summit: The aim of the summit was to solidify each working group's action plan.

The result was 13 three-year action plans. One hundred and ten specific actions were identified, ranging from regulation modifications to social marketing campaigns. Most of the participating agencies committed themselves to carry out the actions falling within their responsibility. A flexible, easy to use follow-up system has been established to track progress and maintain the momentum of each group toward honoring their commitment.

Beyond the action plans, the most important outcome of the summit was the consolidation of a real network of organizations coming from different fields and the public and private sectors. For the first time these stakeholders were exchanging information and expertise on the common problem of safety in sport and recreational activities in Québec.

In 1990, Québec was the province with the lowest rate of sport and recreational injuries in Canada: 67/1000 participants compared with 100/1000 for the rest of the country. In 2003, Québec was still the province with the lowest rate of sport and recreational injuries in Canada. Although it is impossible to directly link these observations to the interventions identified in the Sport Summit, they strongly suggest trends in the right direction. Our evaluation is that, at the very least, the work of the government of Québec and its partners over the last 29 years has contributed to the creation of a much safer climate for sports in the province.

References

Agel, J., Ransome, J., Dick, R.W., Oppliger, R., Marshall, S.W. (2007) Descriptive epidemiology of collegiate men's wrestling injuries: National Collegiate

Athletic Association Injury Surveillance System, 1988–1989 through 2003–2004. *Journal of Athletic Training* **42**, 303–310.

American College of Sports Medicine (1996) ACSM position stand on weight loss in wrestlers. *Medicine and Science in Sports and Exercise* **28**, 9–12.

Centers for Disease Control (1998) Hypothermia and dehydration-related deaths associated with intentional rapid weight loss in three collegiate wrestlers—North Carolina, Wisconsin and Michigan, November–December 1997. *Morbidity and Mortality Weekly Report* **47**(6), 105–108.

Gianotti, S.M., Hume, P.A., Quarrie, K.L. (2008) Evaluation of RugbySmart: a rugby union community injury prevention programme. *Journal of Science and Medicine in Sport*. In press. Government of Québec (1988) *An act respecting safety in sports*. Éditeur officiel du Québec, Québec.

Horswill, C.A., Scott, J.R., Dick, R.W., Hayes, J. (1994) Influence of rapid weight gain after the weigh-in on success in collegiate wrestlers. *Medicine and Science in Sports and Exercise* **26**, 1290–1294.

Pashby, T.J. (1985) Eye injuries in Canadian amateur hockey. *Canadian Journal of Ophthalmology* **20**, 2–4.

Quarrie, K.L., Gianotti, S.M., Hopkins, W.G., Hume, P.A. (2007) Effect of nationwide injury prevention programme on serious spinal injuries in New Zealand rugby union: ecological study. *British Medical Journal* **334**, 1150.

Régnier, G., Goulet, C. (1995). The Québec Sports Safety Board: a governmental agency dedicated to the prevention of sports and recreational injuries. *Injury Prevention* **1**, 141–145.

Régnier, G., Boileau, R., Marcotte, G., Desharnais, R., Larouche, R., Bernard, D., Roy, M.A., Trudel, P., D. Boulanger (1989) Effects of body-checking in the pee-wee (12 and 13 years old) division in the province of Québec. In C. Castaldi, & E.F. Hoerner (eds.) *Safety in Ice Hockey,* pp. 84–103. American Society for Testing and Materials, Philadelphia, PA.

Régnier, G., Sicard, C., Goulet, C. (1995) Economic impact of a regulation imposing full-face protectors on adult recreational hockey players. *International Journal for Consumer Safety* **2**, 191–207.

Robidoux, M., Trudel, P. (2006). Hockey Canada and the bodychecking debate in minor hockey. In D. Whitson & R. Gruneau (eds.) *Artificial Ice: Hockey, Culture, and Commerce,* pp. 101–122. Broadview Press, Peterborough, Ontario.

Scott, J.R., Horswill, C.A., Dick, R.W. (1994) Acute weight gain in collegiate wrestlers following a tournament weigh-in. *Medicine and Science in Sports and Exercise* **26**, 1181–1185.

Further reading

For information on the NCAA, see www.ncaa.org.
For information on the NCAA ISS, see www.ncaa.org/ISS.
For information on the New Zealand Accident Compensation Corporation (ACC), see www.acc.co.nz.
For information on SportSmart, please see www.sportsmart.org.nz.
For information on ACC RugbySmart, please see www.rugbysmart.co.nz.
For information on ACC SoccerSmart, please see www.soccersmart.co.nz.
For information on the Act Respecting Safety in Sports, see "Laws and Regulations" in www.publicationsduQuébec.gouv.qc.ca/accueil.en.html

Chapter 14
Planning for major events

Michael Turner[1] and Jiri Dvorak[2]

[1]Lawn Tennis Association and British Horseracing Authority; British Olympic Association and Chief Medical Adviser to Snowsport, UK
[2]FIFA Medical Assessment and Research Center (F-MARC), Schulthess Clinic, Zurich, Switzerland

Introduction

Major events are held all over the world on a regular basis and providing appropriate medical cover for the athletes, support staff, and spectators, as well as initiating injury prevention strategies, should be a priority for every organizer.

A major event may involve only two teams competing in front of 17,000 spectators for less than 2 h on a single day but the variation is infinite. When planning a major event it is customary to appoint a Chief Medical Adviser for the event and it is essential that this individual is familiar with the hazards and risks involved in such an undertaking. In many instances this will be the same individual, or team of professionals, and it should be a priority that medical staff with experience of all the particular challenges are recruited to advise and cover the event. This is especially so in high-risk sports where medical staff unfamiliar with the sport may well find that they are ignorant of the environment and equipment in use (motor sport, equestrian sports, water sport, winter sports).

Depending on how far in advance the Chief Medical Adviser is appointed, there should be opportunities to implement emergency and injury prevention strategies and to introduce effective risk management procedures. However, these opportunities might not allow for the implementation of the standard injury prevention strategies outlined in previous chapters because these are primarily aimed at sports governing bodies, coaches, equipment manufacturers, and athletes themselves.

For example, all major events involving professional football (soccer) and American Football take place in purpose built stadia. Teams travel with their own medical support staff and there is no possibility of an event Chief Medical Adviser having any impact on the quality of the pitch, the protective equipment worn by athletes, the training technique of players, the falling technique of players, or the rules of the sport. The medical staff providing support at these events will normally have done so on numerous previous occasions and the opportunity to implement injury prevention strategies at this stage is non-existent.

What is a "major event"?

Global events are often deemed to be "major" as a result of the huge television audiences that they attract (the 2006 FIFA World Cup was watched by 26.3 billion people in 214 countries) but this chapter will focus on those events with a large number of spectators in attendance or a large number of participants.

The largest number of spectators

For the purpose of this review, we have utilized the figures of spectators in attendance only and have

Sports Injury Prevention, 1st edition. Edited by R. Bahr and L. Engebretsen Published 2009 by Blackwell Publishing ISBN: 9781405162449

identified a selection of global events that attracted an average of 17,000 or more spectators per day. The largest daily crowds are seen at the New York Marathon (2.5 million spectators) and the London Marathon (500,000) and the other major events in this category include the Tour de France cycling (434,000/day), Sydney 2000 Olympics (418,000/day), NASCAR (186,100/day), Kentucky Derby horse racing (156,400/day), Melbourne Cup horse racing (106,500/day), and Salt Lake 2002 Winter Games (95,300/day).

By comparison, the US professional sports attracted a large number of spectators over the whole season but only modest numbers attended the individual events. The figures for 2006 are as follows:

Major League Baseball—94.9 million spectators over 2419 games (30,970/event)

College Football—32.6 million spectators over 709 games (46,039/event)

NBA Basketball—21.6 million spectators over 1230 games (17,558/event)

NHL Ice hockey—20.8 million spectators over 1230 games (16,955/event)

The other sports that attract over 10 million spectators include NPB baseball (Japan—19.9 million), NFL football (USA—17.3 million), Premier League soccer (GB—12.8 million), Bundersliga 1 soccer (Germany—12.5 million), La Liga soccer (Spain—11.0 million), and the Tour de France cycling (10 million). The sports attracting 1–9 million spectators are national soccer leagues (Italy, France, Japan), the multi-sport, multi-national events (Olympic and Paralympic Games), NASCAR, and the Rugby Union World Cup.

The largest number of participants

Marathons and the multi-sport, multi-national events dominate this group—London marathon (35,500 participants), New York marathon (17,000), Sydney marathon (13,000), Sydney 2000 Olympics (10,651—16 days), US College football (6,095—709 games), Melbourne Commonwealth Games 2006 (4,500—11 days), Athens Paralympic Games 2004 (3,969—12 days), Salt Lake 2002 Winter Games (2,399—16 days), and NFL American football (1,692—256 games).

Factors to consider

The recommendations that follow are the result of a detailed review of selected major international and national sporting events that occur around the world. This "basket" of over 40 events involved 102,432 amateur and professional competitors taking part in 9,313 days of competition watched on site by over 292 million spectators (this does not include the TV audiences).

Given the vast variety of these events, the first duty of all medical staff at any sport event is to retrieve and analyze the following basic information:
- Number of sports—single or multiple
- Number of participants—individuals and/or teams
- Number of support staff—coaches, physical therapists, medics, sports scientists
- Number of spectators and VIPs
- Number of countries involved—national only, international
- Number of venues—single or multiple
- Accessibility of venues—static stadium, mobile, global
- Frequency of event—once only, repeated annually, monthly, weekly
- Number of days medical cover is required (including training and preparation days)—1 day only, weeks, months
- Special needs of the athletes—wheelchair event, blind competitors
- Special challenges of the sport—high speed, motor vehicles, horses, water, ice, snow
- Medical services traveling with the individuals or teams—team doctors, physical trainers to national squads
- Medical cover at locations other than the competition venue—hotels, athletes' village, training areas, on-call cover
- Need for specific medical subspecialties
- Governing body requirements for medical cover at events
- National legislation or guidelines in force regarding the medical cover at major events
- National legislation guidelines in force regarding temporary licenses of accompanying physicians

- Major Incident Medical Management and Support procedures (for dealing with a catastrophe on site and access to local hospital facilities)
- Accreditation of medical staff—access to venues and restricted areas
- Payments to medical staff—volunteers, travel and accommodation expenses, honorarium, uniforms, reimbursement of supplies provided by the individual.

This chapter provides an opportunity to explore some of the "best practice" issues for medical staff who have never had the opportunity to supervise or regulate an event of this size and complexity. Although many of the topics under consideration will not be seen as strictly "injury prevention measures," the underlining principle is that managing any injury in an effective and rapid fashion may well prevent further damage to the individual concerned. This will in turn lead to a reduction in the rehabilitation time and can be considered as part of the injury prevention—injury mitigation spectrum.

It is generally accepted that, following a spinal cord injury, 50% of the resulting disability is caused by the inept handling of the injured person (lack of immobilization strategy, spinal board, etc.). It can therefore be seen that having the appropriate equipment and trained personnel can significantly impact the outcome of injury and this could reasonably be included in a review of injury prevention. In addition, anything that increases the anxiety or stress levels in an athlete may well lead to a decrease in performance and event planning should be aimed at eliminating any concerns that relate to medical issues.

It is not only the competitors who are at risk in this context but also avoidable fatalities can occur amongst spectators at big sporting events. At the Winter Games in Lillehammer (Norway 1994) over 20,000 people were camped out in tents along the route of the 50 km cross-country track (overnight temperatures of −30°C). One spectator, having left the tent to find the communal washroom in the middle of the night, was apparently unable to find his way back to his tent and was discovered dead in the snow the following morning (Ekeland, 1995). At the Horseracing Derby (Great Britain 1995) a spectator who had arrived in a coach felt unwell during the afternoon and returned to the coach to rest. The coach was locked, and the sun was very hot, so he sheltered under the coach and fell asleep. The coach driver returned at the end of the afternoon and reversed the vehicle out of its parking place to prepare for departure. In the process, he ran over and killed the sleeping spectator. In both instances, the consumption of alcohol was thought to have played a significant part in the tragic outcome.

Further, some events representing special challenges are explicitly addressed and the specific points to be considered are outlined.

Major event planning tools

Basic planning

For basic planning purposes, the checklist shown in Table 14.1 provides a summary of all the pre-, during and post-event requirements.

Venue medical cover

Venue cover is relatively simple, as long as the venue is not spread out too much (Tour de France) and the event is not too large (Olympics). Cover for the participants is often provided by the teams themselves (team doctor and/or physical therapist) but facilities will need to be provided for them to treat the team members throughout the day (see checklist in Table 14.2):
- Squad treatment room at the competition venue
- Squad treatment room at the training area
- Squad treatment room at the accommodation area

These treatment rooms may be communal areas in events involving multiple sports (track and field).

Competition venues need additional attention because of the large number of spectators (and VIPs) who are in attendance (see checklist in Table 14.3).

Provisions for competitors

Competitors may never have visited the venue or country prior to the event and when planning a big event, the organizers must keep the needs of this group at the forefront of all health, welfare,

Table 14.1 Checklist basic planning.

Basic planning	Pre-event	During event
Climate—weather conditions	Review statistics for the last 10 years	Monitor and publish daily
Venues	Numbers Obtain detailed ground plans and carry out an on-site assessment Establish opening and closing times for each venue	Monitor daily and adapt medical support provision as required
Equipment	Review the equipment needed at every location where medical support will be provided	Monitor daily and adapt medical support provision as required
Athletes	Numbers and nationalities Date of arrival Time and dates of competitions and training	Monitor injuries daily
Support staff (incl. medical staff traveling with the teams or athletes)	Numbers Date of arrival Number of medical staff traveling with each team	Monitor injuries daily
Spectators	Numbers Time of access to and departure from each venue	Monitor injuries daily
VIPs	Numbers Program of VIP social events Accommodation arrangements	Monitor injuries daily
The Medical Team	Numbers needed Appoint core members and establish recruiting strategy for additional staff	Daily meetings
Training	Ensure that all members of the medical staff have appropriate training (e.g., Major Incident Medical Management and Support training—see later)	Monitor during event and arrange additional training if required
Specialist services	Access to outpatient consultations Availability of X-ray, MRI, blood pathology, etc.	Monitor access and speed of reporting
Hospital access	Identify nearest A+E unit and open a dialog with senior staff	Monitor access and speed of access
Central Medical Service—Polyclinic	Location and staffing (if required) Specialist services on offer to athletes—e.g., dental surgery	Provide medical service to all competitors, support staff, and VIPs
Communications	Establish a method of secure communication between all members of the medical staff that will protect confidentiality	Monitor daily and adapt provision as required
Record keeping	Establish a unified system for recording and analysis of all injuries and incidents	Monitor daily and adapt provision as required
Education	Prepare briefing information for visiting teams Prepare written Standing Orders for every event and every venue	Update daily by e-mail, text, or website
Insurance	Ensure that all medical staff are covered by appropriate insurance in case of accident or injury (not malpractice insurance)	Inform Insurers immediately if any accident or injury takes place that involves medical staff
Legal issues	Ensure that organizers are aware of all Government Legislation concerning the medical cover at the event and that these are complied with promptly (reporting of accidents, fatal incidents, etc.)	Review daily and notify organizing committee or relevant authority if required

Table 14.2 Checklist training venue.

Venues for training	Pre-event	During event
Planning	Establish layout and whereabouts of medical rooms and athletes area Ensure that the accreditation issued to medical staff will allow access to all areas	Monitor daily and adapt as required
Outdoor venue	Inclement weather options	Monitor daily and adapt as required
Open–closed	Hours that venue will be open daily	Publish daily hours that medical facilities will be open and list staff on site
Athletes	Numbers expected	Record and monitor all injuries or incidents daily
Support staff (incl. medical staff traveling with teams or athletes)	Number expected Provision of medical room for team medical staff	Monitor daily and adapt as required
Spectators	Number expected Provision of First Aid room	Monitor daily and adapt as required
Medical provision	Appoint venue specific medical team to deal with athletes and spectators	Monitor daily and adapt as required
Equipment	Review the medical equipment needed at each location	Monitor daily and adapt as required
Communication	Establish a method of secure communication between all members of the medical staff that will protect confidentiality of the patients	Monitor daily and adapt as required
Record keeping	Ensure access to the unified system for recording and analysis of injuries and incidents	Monitor daily and adapt as required
Access for emergency services	Identify and demark areas that must be kept clear for ambulance access	Monitor daily and adapt as required
Major Incident Medical Management and Support	Identify staff who will be responsible for co-ordinating a major incident Identify the medical assembly point for major incident (triage area, transport area, etc.) Ensure that all staff get appropriate training	Monitor daily and adapt as required
Meetings and education	Prepare Standing Orders for each venue Distribute Standing Orders to all staff in attendance	Daily debrief for venue medical staff when venue closed

and safety decisions. They will also need to take into account the accommodation and transport needs of the athletes (Table 14.4).

Teams traveling with their own medical support staff

For teams traveling without medical staff, event organizers should provide adequate numbers of doctors and physical therapists to enable all participants to be treated in a rapid and professional fashion (Table 14.4).
- General access medical facility at every competition venue (will normally include a doctor and physical therapist on site)
- General access medical facility at every training venue (may only include a single physical therapist on site and a doctor on call)

Table 14.3 Checklist competition venue.

Venues for competition	Pre-event	During event
Planning	Establish layout and whereabouts of medical rooms, athletes area, VIP areas Ensure that the accreditation issued to medical staff will allow access to all areas (especially VIP areas)	Monitor daily and adapt as required
Outdoor venue	Inclement weather options	Monitor daily and adapt as required
Open—closed	Hours that venue will be open daily	Publish daily hours that medical facilities will be open and list staff on site
Athletes	Numbers expected	Record and monitor injuries and incidents daily
Support staff (incl. medical staff)	Number expected Provision of medical room for team medical staff	Monitor daily and adapt as required
Spectators and VIPs	Number expected Provision of First Aid room and mobile staff required	Monitor daily and adapt as required
Medical provision	Appoint venue specific medical team to deal with athletes and spectators	Monitor daily and adapt as required
Equipment	Review the medical equipment needed at each location	Monitor daily and adapt as required
Communication	Establish a method of secure communication between all members of the medical staff that will protect confidentiality	Monitor daily and adapt as required
Record keeping	Establish a unified system for recording and analysis of all injuries and incidents that occur during the event	Monitor daily and adapt as required
Meetings and education	Invitation for team medical staff to visit venue prior to start of competition Prepare Standing Orders for each venue	Daily debrief for venue medical staff when venue closed

Table 14.4 Checklist competitors.

Competitors	Pre-event	During event
Arrival	Numbers Date of arrival	
Accommodation—hotel or village	Location and access details Identify all security-related issues	
Training facilities—gym	Location Nearest access to medical staff and facilities	
Training venue	Location of changing and training areas Access to medical room, van, or tent Medical staff on site	Publish Opening times of team medical rooms and how to access the medical support provided by host (24 hr emergency numbers etc.)
Competition venue	Location of changing and training areas Access to medical room, van, or tent Medical staff on site	
Central Medical Service—Polyclinic	Hours of opening Rota of medical staff	
Education	Briefing literature with details of all medical services, emergency numbers, and maps (city and venues)	Update daily by e-mail, text, or website

- General access medical facility at the athlete village (will normally include a doctor and physical therapist on site)
- On call arrangements to cover "out of hours" periods when other facilities are closed.

Medical indemnity and international competition

Medical staff traveling abroad provides a particular challenge for organizers because of the medical–legal issues surrounding their national qualifications. Within the European Union, medical staff are free to practice in an unrestricted fashion but this does not apply when traveling to North America or Australia. Doctors and therapists may not be insured to practice abroad and will certainly not be entitled to obtain medicine on prescription in a foreign country. The organizers need to communicate the need for a temporary licensing procedure to all visiting physicians in advance. The organizers must therefore make arrangements for visiting medical staff to have access to:

- A pharmacy (or access to a doctor employed by the organizing committee to write the necessary prescriptions)
- A pathology laboratory—blood testing, swabs, urinalysis
- X-ray and imaging facilities
- Specialist opinion
- Dental care
- Ophthalmology, facio-maxillary surgery, orthopedic surgery, etc.

One way of ensuring that this runs smoothly is to appoint locally established doctors who can serve as mediators for the visiting medical staff and facilitate access to all services.

Medical cover for the spectators

This often poses the biggest challenge to the organizers and their Chief Medical Adviser. In many cases, nation law is in place that mandates the minimum standards of medical cover at large events and individual venues may have safety certificates that control capacity and the support services required on site. Table 14.5 provides a checklist covering spectator issues.

At any venue where large numbers of people congregate, the opportunity for the medical resources to be totally overwhelmed by a major incident must be addressed. In an era where terrorist activities occur on an annual basis, we also have instances where accidental explosions (cooking gas) or stand collapse have occurred at sporting events.

These events require close co-operation between all the emergency services (police, fire service, and ambulance service) and the medical team on site. Indeed the emergency services may not be deployed on site for 30 min or more (particularly in rural locations) and the only medical support available will be the event team.

Major Incident Medical Management and Support requires particular training and all medical staff providing cover at a big event should ensure that they have completed an appropriate training course. In the United Kingdom, the standard course takes place over 4 days.

As a result of a number of high-profile disasters at football events in the United Kingdom, the Health and Safety Executive published the *Guide to Safety at Sports Grounds* (ISBN 978 0 11 702074 0) which covers all aspects of spectator cover (Figure 14.1). These guidelines indicate the minimum level of medical cover expected for sporting events and a summary is included in Table 14.6 to help those practitioners who have no national guidelines to follow.

Very Important People

Organizers should be aware that although a few VIPs are actually former world class athletes, the vast majority are not in perfect physical shape. Despite this, they all expect to be treated as if they were potential medalists and when illness or injury occurs, all other medical resources may need to be diverted. At a single international event (UEFA Cup Final) VIPs may include Heads of State, Royalty, Prime Ministers, and Presidents of International Governing Bodies as well as their partners, children, and guests. A call to attend a collapsed VIP can severely compromise the normal spectator medical support provided and diverting the athlete medical cover is not an option. It may therefore be necessary to recruit additional

Table 14.5 Checklist spectators.

Spectators	Pre-event	During event
Arrival	Numbers expected Time of access to facility	Monitor and update daily
Duration	Days of medical cover needed Hours of access to medical staff	Monitor and update daily
Venue	Indoor stadium Outdoor stadium Outdoor urban Outdoor rural	Monitor and update daily Provision for inclement weather
Medical support	Medical room, van, or tent Triage points Number and type of medical support needed Equipment required	Monitor and update daily
Equipment	Review the medical equipment needed at each location	Monitor daily and adapt as required
Record keeping	Ensure access to the unified stem for recording and analysis of all injuries and incidents	Monitor daily and adapt as required
First Aid support	First Aid room, van, or tent Number and qualification of First Aid staff needed Equipment required	Monitor and update daily
Communication	Independent communication network for all medical staff with responsibilities for spectators	Monitor and update daily
Medical equipment for use by non-medics	Access to automated defibrillators on site	Monitor and update daily
Pharmacy	On site Nearest to venue Opening times	Monitor and update daily
Catering	Adequate for the numbers and duration	Monitor and update daily
Sanitary facilities	Adequate for the numbers and duration	Monitor and update daily
Major incident	Ensure that a details major incident plan has been agreed with the local police, fire brigade, and ambulance services Identify staff who will be responsible for co-ordinating a major incident Identify the medical assembly point for major incident (triage area, transport area, etc.)	Monitor and update daily
Education and training	Clear signage to medical facilities Standing Orders covering all aspects of spectator medical cover	Daily medical staff meeting after venue closed Update daily by e-mail, text, or website

medical resources solely to cover these individuals for the period that they are in attendance at a major event. It should also be noted that the security for these individuals is usually managed by the Military or Secret Service and access to the immediate area is impossible to achieve without the necessary accreditation and vetting. This cannot be achieved at the last minute. Table 14.7 provides a checklist for VIP medical coverage.

Selection and training of medical staff: the multi-disciplined approach

Medical support at a major event will not be restricted to doctors and physical therapists alone and consideration should be given at an early stage to the mix of staff required for any particular event or venue. These individuals may not be required to be present on site during competition or training

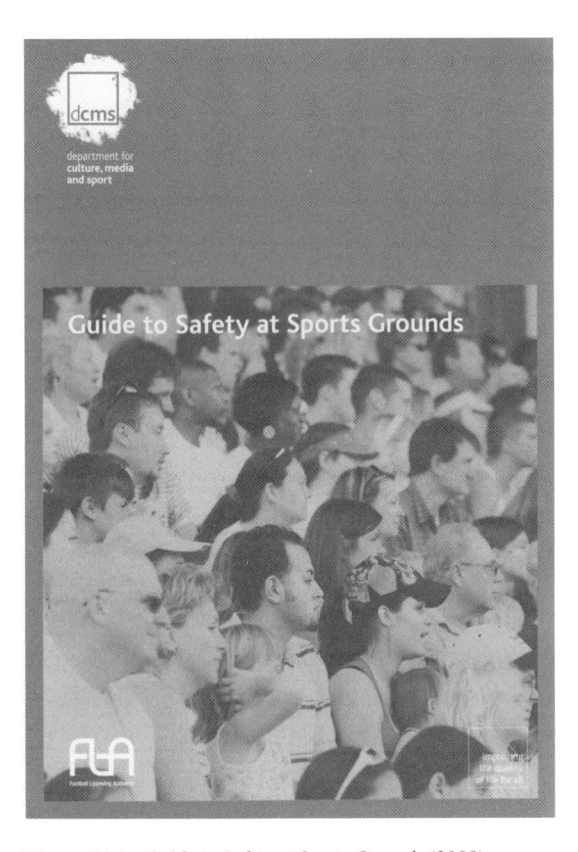

Figure 14.1. *Guide to Safety at Sports Grounds* (2008)

but will normally include a mix of doctors, paramedics, nurses, physical therapists (physiotherapists, osteopaths, chiropractors, sports therapists, massage therapists), dentists, podiatrists, sports scientists (nutritionists, sports psychologists), and First Aid trained staff. Table 14.8 provides an overview of factors to be considered related to selection and training of medical staff.

Events requiring special attention

High-risk events (including those taking place at extremes of climate or high altitude)

A number of events involve additional risk to the competitors because of the nature of the event or the location in which it takes place. These events provide a much greater challenge to medical support staff and include the outdoor winter sports and water sports, equestrian sports, and high speed sports (motor racing and motor cycle racing). These are invariably associated with a much higher incidence of significant injury and fatality.

Medical support staff at these events must be familiar with the sport concerned, the environment in which it takes place and the type of injury that can be expected. These events require all the basic cover outlined earlier but additional consideration will need to be given (see Table 14.9).

Disability sport and spectators in wheelchairs

Medical support for disability sport is essentially identical to that already outlined apart from the following areas—support staff, transport, and access. However, the support staff/athlete ratio is normally higher for events involving disabled players. Suitable accommodation and transport needs to be available for these individuals to avoid additional stress for the athletes concerned. Wheelchair competitors use one type of chair for competition and another for normal activity. When organizing transport for wheelchair events, it must be possible for competitors to travel with a spare wheelchair to the training or competition site. For events involving wheelchairs, access into and out of transport vehicles, accommodation, competition and training venues, changing rooms, medical facilities, and spectator areas must be reviewed and may need to be adapted (Table 14.10).

Marathon

The two sporting events with the largest number of competitors in this analysis are both marathons and they provide an excellent model for exploring injury prevention strategies.

The London Marathon has been run continuously since 1981. Of the 131,000 applicants in the London Marathon only 48,000 (36.6%) are accepted as participants. The age range 18–88 years with a gender bias (69% male/31% female). Of these, 35,557 will actually start the race (74.1% of the accepted application) but over 99% of these will now expect to finish the race. This figure has climbed from 88.7% in 1981 as a direct result of the management strategies

Table 14.6 Minimum level of medical cover at sport events.

Minimum of two First Aid trained staff at every event
- At least one First Aid trained person for every 1000 spectators (up to 20,000 spectators)
- Over 20,000 spectators—additional one First Aid trained person for every 2000 spectators

Each First Aid trained person must be
- Over 16 years of age
- Have no other duties or responsibilities
- Be in post before the first spectator enters the ground
- Remain in post until all the spectators have left

A designated First Aid room with specified
- Size
- Fittings and facilities
- Design and location
- Storage, equipment, and materials
- Upkeep and inspection schedule

One crowd doctor should be employed when it is anticipated that the crowd will exceed 2000 spectators
- The crowd doctor must have suitable training and experience
- The whereabouts of the crowd doctor must be known to all First Aid and ambulance staff at all times (communications)
- The crowd doctor must be on site before the first spectator enters the ground and remain on site until all the spectators have left
- The crowd doctor must have no other duties or responsibilities during this period (e.g., be a team doctor as well)

At least one fully equipped accident and emergency ambulance to be on site for all events with an anticipated attendance of over 5000 spectators

Crowds 5000 to 25,000
- One fully equipped accident and emergency ambulance (with a paramedic crew)
- An ambulance officer

Crowds of 25,000 to 45,000
- One fully equipped accident and emergency ambulance (with a paramedic crew)
- An ambulance officer
- One major incident equipped vehicle with a paramedic crew
- One control unit

Crowds of over 45,000
- Two fully equipped accident and emergency ambulance (with a paramedic crews)
- An ambulance officer
- One major incident equipped vehicle with a paramedic crew
- One control unit

introduced by the organizers of this highly successful event.

Health questionnaire and medical clearance

All applicants are required to complete a health questionnaire and to provide a statement from their own medical practitioner that they are "fit to run." The Chief Medical Adviser of the event must be prepared to monitor and manage the information provided on the health questionnaires to assist in providing the necessary medical support for participants. It should also be noted that because marathons are now used as fund raising opportunities by many charities, the majority of the participants will have no special sporting skills and a significant number may be disabled.

Education

Once accepted, each competitor should be provided with a detailed education leaflet outlining a simple training program and providing advice about nutrition, fluid intake, sleep, and rest.

Climate

This should include a review of the different strategies that might be needed under different climatic conditions. In London, experience has shown

Table 14.7 Checklist VIPs.

VIPs	Pre-event	During event
Arrival	Dates of arrival Numbers expected Requirement for interpreting service	Monitor daily and adapt as required
Accommodation	Location and numbers in hotels, staying with friends	Provision of medical services at accommodation (house call) throughout the event
Attendance at training venues	Establish impact on venue medical services	Provision of dedicated medical cover if required (see later)
Attendance at competition	Establish impact on venue medical services	Provision of dedicated medical cover if required (see later)
Security	Establish impact on venue medical services Ensure correct accreditation for medical staff (see later)	Ensure correct accreditation for medical staff (see later)
Education	Briefing literature with details of all medical services, emergency numbers and maps (city and venues)	
Health record	Submit health record pass to all participating organizations and ask them to have it completed by VIP physicians	Safely store sealed records to have them at hand in case of emergency

that an ideal temperature for a fast event is 10–12°C but the actual temperature range has been 5.9–21.0°C over 25 years. Humidity has ranged 28–96% and this will have an effect on clothing and fluid intake.

The media

Education can be greatly enhanced by utilizing media programs (particularly TV) to follow groups of novice runners as they prepare for the event. This has proven particularly effective in Australia and in Great Britain; children's TV programs are regularly used to educate children taking part in mini-marathon and "fun run" events.

Venue preparation

A typical marathon will have water stations every 1.6 km (from the 4.8 km mark) with access to sports drinks every 8 km (starting at the 8 km mark). Special drinking stations are also set up for the elite runner group where they can place their own prepared drinks—a total of eight along the 42.2 km course (approximately every 5 km). Adequate barriers will be erected to separate the competitors from the spectators and regulatory arrangements need to be coordinated with event marshals and police. In London 2006, there were 1100 marshals at the start, 3050 along the route, and 2500 at the finish—a total of 6650. Portable toilets need to be available for competitors at the start, along the course and at the finish (total of 950 in London 2006 race). First Aid stations (39) and First Aid staff (1200) are required to assist those who get into difficulties with suitable equipment (500 stretchers) and transport (68 ambulances) to cater for the more serious cases.

In events of this sort, the needs of the elite athletes and those of the amateurs may be completely different and provision will need to be made for both groups separately.

Other Olympic sports

All the 29 summer and 7 winter sports run regular events on an annual basis. Many of these will be classified as big events (World Championships) and appropriate medical cover will be needed. The general principles outlined earlier can be applied to all these events, but a number need to be emphasised.

Table 14.8 Checklist medical staff.

Medical staff	Pre-event	During event
Planning	How many days How many competitors How many spectators How many venues Location and scope of the Polyclinic	Review and update daily
Appointment of staff	How many medical staff needed Selection of core staff for venues, Polyclinic and spectator duties Make provision for extra staff in case of illness or domestic crisis Obtain documentary evidence that all medical staff are suitably qualified, currently registered with their professional organization and have appropriate malpractice insurance	Review and update daily Communicate with on-call staff daily to ensure availability at short notice
Training	Ensure that all staff have appropriate qualifications for the duties they have been assigned Arrange appropriate specialist training for some staff (see Major Incident Medical Management and Support—later) Training to use the communication system	
Rehearsal	Ensure that all staff are familiar with the venues and have had an opportunity to rehearse the extraction of an injured player or spectator Ensure all staff are familiar with and can use the chosen communication system	
Arrival and attendance	Organize a rota for every member of the medical staff with appropriate rest periods and days off	Review and update daily
Venue cover—athletes	Number of expected athletes and times of attendance at venue Ensure that all staff are familiar with venue and the sports (events) that will take place in that venue Establish the means of communication at the venue and ensure that it works in all parts of the venue Establish if the event will involve disabled competitors—wheelchair access required	Review and update daily Monitor all injuries and attendance Daily debrief meetings of all venue staff after event has finished Daily report to Chief Medical Advisor or nominated deputy every day
Venue cover—spectators	Number of expected spectators and times of access to venue Ensure that all staff are familiar with the venue and the times that spectators will be on site Establish if the event will involve disabled spectators—wheelchair access required	Review and update daily Monitor all injuries and attendance Daily debrief meetings of all venue staff after event has finished Daily report to Chief Medical Adviser or nominated deputy every day
Polyclinic cover	Number of staff Times of opening	Review and update daily Monitor all injuries and attendance Daily debrief meetings of all staff Daily report to Chief Medical Advisor or nominated deputy every day
VIP cover	Designated staff to deal with VIP problems throughout event—provide 24 h emergency contact number	Review and update daily
Equipment and communication	Establish exact levels of equipment to be located at each venue, to be carried by each doctor and first aider, to be available in the Polyclinic Obtain sufficient walkie-talkies for all medical staff	Review and update daily

(Continued)

Table 14.8 (Continued)

Medical staff	Pre-event	During event
A+E and transport	Number of ambulances and Paramedics needed Location of nearest A+E department Mechanism of referral to A+E department Capacity and waiting times of A+E department Specialist investigations available at this hospital (neurosurgery unit?)	Review and update daily
Outpatient services	Establish the system for outpatient referral (ophthalmology, urology, gynecology) and how to obtain other investigations (MRI, X-ray, pathology) Establish who will be responsible for payments (the individual athlete or spectator, the organizing committee, National Health Service, Insurance company)	Review and update daily
Education	Meetings with all medical staff prior to event Briefing literature for all medical staff with maps and contact details for senior staff and emergency services	Daily medical staff meeting after venue or clinic closed Update daily by e-mail, text, or website
Legislation	Ensure that all medical staff are aware of the Government Legislation relating to medical cover at the event (reporting of accidents, fatal incidents, etc.)	Ensure that all medical staff comply promptly with the Government Legislation relating to medical cover at the event (reporting of accidents, fatal incidents, etc.)
Insurance	Ensure that all medical staff are covered by appropriate insurance in case of accident of injury and have appropriate malpractice insurance (copies of all the current malpractice insurance certificates should be kept on file by the organizers)	
Financial issues	Establish number of paid staff and volunteers needed Prepare and agree budget (signed letter of agreement) Method and timing of payments to medical staff agreed—to include training and rehearsal days (venue visits)	Review and ensure that agreed payments are made

Standing Orders

Standing Orders must be prepared for every event and must include the deployment and duties of all medical staff. Prior to every event, these must have been read and understood by all staff on duty at an event. It is strongly advised that all medical staff are required to sign a declaration that they have read and understood the Standing Orders prior to officiating at an event.

Supplies and equipment

Medical staff must be familiar with all the supplies and equipment that they are carrying or have access to. These must be checked daily and before every event, all items must be in working order and not out of date. A list of all the supplies and equipment held on site, and those carried by the medical staff, must be listed in the Standing Orders.

Briefing

Before every event, a detailed briefing should be carried out by senior medical staff. This may include input from the Senior Medical Officer on duty, the emergency services (paramedic and ambulance crews), and the First Aid providers. *It cannot be emphasized how essential this is to the efficient running of an event.*

Communications

All staff must have access to a central communication system, they must be trained in using this

Table 14.9 Checklist high-risk sports.

Specific issues in high-risk sports	Pre-event	During event
Winter sports (Alpine and Nordic skiing, Luge, Skeleton and Bobsleigh)	Establish the medical criteria mandated by the governing body for medical cover at the event In skiing events these may also include criteria prohibiting the event from taking place in inclement weather (low temperate, high wind speed) Ensure that appropriate rescue equipment and personnel are recruited (blood wagons, ski patrols) Ensure that staff who are on site can rapidly reach all parts of the area they are responsible for (that they can ski or have the use of a snowmobile) Ensure that medical staff are familiar with the personal protective equipment used by participants Establish process whereby the event can be delayed or halted if a serious injury occurs	Monitor and review the management of every injury and adapt medical support as necessary Halt event if medical support staff are required to leave the site and resources are limited Daily debrief meeting essential
Outdoor water sports—including multi-sport events with a swim element (sailing, windsurfing, triathlon, Iron man)	Establish the medical criteria mandated by the governing body for medical cover at the event Ensure that a suitable water-based rescue system is in place which enables medical staff to rapidly reach all parts of the area they are responsible for Ensure that rescue staff can swim and have suitable safety equipment allocated Ensure that medical staff are familiar with the personal protective equipment used by participants Establish a process whereby the event can be delayed or halted if a serious injury occurs	Monitor and review the management of every injury and adapt medical support as necessary Halt event if medical support staff are required to leave the site and resources are limited Daily debrief meeting essential
Equestrian sports (horse racing, 3-day eventing, polo)	Establish the medical criteria mandated by the governing body for medical cover at the event Ensure that medical staff are familiar with the personal protective equipment used by participants Establish a process whereby the event can be delayed or halted if a serious injury occurs	Monitor and review the management of every injury and adapt medical support as necessary Halt event if medical support staff are required to leave the site and resources are limited Daily debrief meeting essential
Motor sports (Formula 1, motor cycle racing, drag racing, NASCAR)	Establish the medical criteria mandated by the governing body for medical cover at the event Establish a process whereby the event can be delayed or halted if a serious injury occurs	Monitor and review the management of every injury and adapt medical support as necessary Halt event if medical support staff are required to leave the site and resources are limited Daily debrief meeting essential
Events taking place at high temperature or altitude	Specialist staff (physiologists) must be recruited to advise medical staff and competitors of the particular risks involved in due advance and publish recommendations on adequate preparation	Daily distribution of expected weather conditions
Emergency transport—ambulances and helicopter	Ensure that additional emergency transport is on site or on immediate call to evacuate the expected major trauma cases	Monitor and review daily

(Continued)

Table 14.9 (Continued)

Specific issues in high-risk sports	Pre-event	During event
Communications	Highest priority All staff must be given suitable equipment and trained to use it All communications equipment must be able to function in inclement weather and across the whole venue site (many kilometers)	Monitor and review daily
Training	Ensure that all staff are suitably qualified and trained to deal with the injuries that they will encounter. This may include ATLS training in cases where major trauma is expected (equestrian and motor sports)	
Insurance	Ensure that all medical staff are covered by appropriate insurance in case of accident of injury and have appropriate malpractice insurance (copies of all the current malpractice insurance certificates should be kept on file by the organizers)	

Table 14.10 Checklist disability staff.

Disability sport	Pre-event	During event
Athlete support staff	Ensure that adequate provision is made for additional individuals—accommodation, medical support	Obtain daily feedback from athlete support staff Review existing arrangements and adapt as necessary
Transport	Ensure that suitable transport is available at all times	Review daily and arrange for deficiencies to be rectified
Access	Ensure that access to all areas needed by disabled athlete's is easy and safe	Review daily and arrange for deficiencies to be rectified

equipment and the equipment must be tested before the event starts. To preserve confidentiality, it is essential that the network used for medical communication is not shared with other non-medical staff.

Training and Major Incident Medical Management and Support

All medical staff must be appropriately trained and qualified to undertake the duties they have been allocated. In events that include large crowds, this may include additional training in major incident management.

Security and accreditation

All medical staff must be able to move freely from venue to venue and from area to area (spectators, athletes, training, etc.) within each venue. Careful consideration needs to be given to the levels of accreditation needed under these circumstances.

The unexpected event

It is clearly not possible to predict the unpredictable but the need for flexibility and having a contingency strategy for sudden unforeseen problems is essential in the preparation for any major event. History has a habit of repeating itself and the need to review similar sporting events that have taken place in the past, to plan for the unexpected, and to pay meticulous attention to detail cannot be emphasized enough.

On 27th July 1996, a bomb in the Centennial Olympic Park in Atlanta killed one spectator and injured 111 others.

In 1998 during the Sydney to Hobart yacht race, 6 boats sank or had to be abandoned in atrocious weather, 50 sailors had to be rescued from the water by helicopter and 6 sailors died. Only 2 fatalities had previously been recorded in the 54 race history.

The Paris-Dakar rally has resulted in at least 48 competitor deaths in its 28-year history with an even larger number of spectators' deaths. Organization of a race that takes place over 10,000 km in some of the most inhospitable terrain on the globe is a significant challenge.

Competitors have been assaulted by members of the public (Monica Seles).

Assaults involving spectators are more frequent in soccer and rugby when the national team wins and the number of assaults increases as the crowd gets larger, irrespective of the location of the game (home or away) (Sivarajasingam et al., 2005).

Alcohol is frequently associated with disturbances amongst spectators and some events ban the sale or consumption of alcohol on site. Well-documented sporting disasters have involved stands collapsing, stampedes, spectators being crushed, fires, and locked exits. Events taking place in remote locations can easily overwhelm the local emergency infrastructure, including the local district hospital which may have very limited specialist cover and no neurosurgical or burns unit on site.

Sub-zero temperatures result in ice formation and spectators will be at considerable risk when walking on this surface. At the ski jumping at Lillehammer 1994 Olympics, fine sand was used to prepare the paths used by spectators but this was rapidly incorporated in a layer of ice as the day progressed. This resulted in a large number of spectators falling and suffering fractures when returning to the village after the event. Coarse gravel was used on subsequent days and the incidence of fractures plummeted.

Post-event activities

Following any major event, an audit should be undertaken to review the positive and negative experiences and make recommendations about future events of this sort. These results should be published whenever possible to enable other organizers to share your experiences (Budgett et al., 1997; Junge et al., 2004; Junge et al., 2006; Dvorak et al., 2007). In certain circumstances these may form the basis of guidelines for the organization of major sporting events (*Guide for Managing risk in Motor Sport*, 2007).

Conclusion

The challenges presented in planning a major event are virtually unlimited. However, by carefully identifying the basic requirements and by using the specific planning tools outlined in this chapter, the organizers will find that the process becomes manageable. A structure can be imposed on the event and medical planning can be positively channeled to minimize the risk of injury or disaster.

References

Budgett, R., Harries, M., Aldridge, J., Jaques, R., Jennings, D.E. (1997) Lessons learnt at the 1996 Atlanta Olympic Games. *British Journal of Sports Medicine* **31**, 76.

Dvorak, J., Junge, A., Grimm, K. and Kirkendall, D. (2007) Medical report from the 2006 FIFA World Cup Germany. *British Journal of Sports Medicine* **41**, 578–581.

Ekeland, A. (1995) Proceedings of the 11th International Congress on Ski Trauma and Skiing Safety, Voss, Norway, April 23–29, 1995. *Scandinavian Journal of Medicine and Science in Sports* **5**, 110–124.

Guide to Safety at Sports Grounds. 5th Edition (2008) ISBN: 978 0 11 702074 0. Health and Safety Executive (HMSO UK).

Guide for Managing Risk in Motor Sport (2007) HB 192-2007. ISBN: 0733781454. Standards Australia, Sydney.

Junge, A., Dvorak, J., Graf-Baumann, T. (2004) Football injuries during FIFA Tournaments and the Olympic Games, 1998–2001. *American Journal of Sports Medicine* **32**, 80–89.

Junge, A., Langevoort, G., Pipe, A., Peytavin, A., Wong, F., Mountjoy, M., Beltrami, G., Terrell, R., Holzgraefe, M., Charles, R., Dvorak, J. (2006) Injuries in team sport tournaments during the 2004 Olympic Games. *American Journal of Sports Medicine* **34**, 565–576.

Sivarajasingam, V., Moore, S., Shepherd, J.P. (2005) Winning, losing and violence. *Injury Prevention* **11**, 69–70.

Further reading

Major Sports Events: The Guide. (2005) UK Sport, London (http://www.uksport.gov.uk/pages/major_sports_event_the_guide/)

Index

abdominal muscles, 91, 96, 105, 106–7, 110, 112
Accident Compensation Corporation (ACC), 198, 200, 201, 202, 203, 204
Achilles tendon, 187, 188, 190, 191, 192, 193
acromioclavicular joint injury, 135–6, 141
Act Respecting Safety in Sports, 205, 206, 207, 208
active versus passive measures, in sports, 15
acute injury, 160, 161
   versus chronic injury, 97, 105
   targeting, 164–5
acute traumatic injuries/repetitive stress, 120–21, 153, 164
adductor muscles, 91, 94, 95, 99, 105, 107, 109, 111, 112
age and sport experience, 93–4
alpine skiing, 5, 10, 14, 17, 49, 50, 146, 153, 182
   knee ligament injury mechanisms in, 56–7
American Academy of Orthopedic Surgeons, 150
American College of Sports Medicine (ACSM), 199
American football, 2, 31, 33, 51, 61, 72, 78, 80, 121, 124, 135, 138, 141, 146, 176, 178, 180, 182, 183, 212
American Sports Medicine Institute, 173
ankle braces, 7, 40
   versus tape, 44–5
   types, 43–4
ankle injuries, 531
   epidemiology, 30
      American football, 31
      basketball, 31
      gymnastics, 32
      hiking, 31
      jogging, 31
      racquet sports, 32
      rugby, 31
      running, 31
      sport-specific injury, 30–31
      volleyball, 32
   injury mechanisms for
      anatomical and biomechanical aspects, 36–7
      specific sports, examples from, 37–8
   preventive measures for, 38
      balance training, 45–7
      braces, 40, 43–5
      player skills, improving, 39–40
      rule changes, 38–9
      take-home message, 47
      taping, 40, 41–2
   risk factors for
      ankle joint laxity, 34–5
      ankle ligament sprain, 32
      foot type, foot size, and anatomic alignment of lower extremity, 34
      gender, 32–3
      generalized joint laxity, 34–5
      height and weight, 33
      limb dominance, 34
      muscle strength, 35
      play setting, 35
      playing position, 35–6
      postural sway, 32, 34
      range of motion, of ankle, 33
      shoe type, 35
      take-home message, 36
   training and competition program, risk identification in, 38
ankle joint laxity, 33, 34–5
ankle ligament sprain, 32, 33, 35
ankle sleeves, 40, 43
ankle sprain, 30, 31, 32, 33, 40, 45, 72
   injury mechanisms for, 36–8
   injury prevention matrix for, 39

anterior cruciate ligament (ACL) injuries, 2, 5, 11, 49, 51, 55, 60, 66, 67, 69
  and osteoarthritis (OA) prevalence, 4
  plyometrics, 63
  prevention program, for team handball, 66–7
  risk, 50
  and single leg balance training, 67–8
  strength training effects on, 68
  targeting participation in, 61–3
Athens Paralympic Games (2004), 213
athlete-related crash measures, in sports, 14
athletes at risk
  identifying, 32, 50, 74, 83, 92, 96, 119, 136, 138–9, 155, 177
  targeting, 166–7
athletic hernia, *see* incipient hernia
athletics, 91, 92, 198
Australian Rules football, 2, 5, 31, 72, 73, 74, 75, 77, 78, 82, 85, 86, 94, 176, 178, 182, 183, 184
awareness exercises, 126, 127

badminton, 31, 32, 143, 187
balance test, 34
balance training, 45–7, 68
Bankart lesion, 141, 142
baseball, 2, 8, 19, 124, 134, 135, 136, 137.138, 146, 153, 154, 155, 157, 166, 168, 176, 182, 183–4, 187
  and overhead throwers, 168, 170–73
basic planning, 214, 215
basketball, 2, 5, 11, 31, 35, 37, 38, 49, 50, 55, 56, 57, 58, 154, 187
basketweave method, 40, 41
behavioral adaptation, 28
biomechanical load, 79
body building, 136, 142, 144, 147
body mass index (BMI), 33, 51, 94, 193
bodychecking injuries, in minor ice hockey
  evaluation, 206
  facts and belief structure, 205–6
  injury problem, 205
  preventive measures for, 206
  stakeholders, identifying, 206
boxing, 2, 153, 154, 155, 160, 163, 177, 200
British Standard, 183
Bundersliga 1 soccer, 213

Cam impingement, 111
Canada, 204, 205, 207, 210
Canadian Community Health Survey, 204
Canadian Hockey Association, 205, 206, 207

Canadian Province of Québec model, 198, 204–5
Canadian Standard Association, 182, 207
catastrophic head and spinal cord injury, 176–7
Centennial Olympic Park, 226
Centers for Disease Control and Prevention, 199
cervical orthoses, 146
chronic disease, 193–4
chronic elbow injury, 163
chronic overuse injuries, 155
chronic versus acute injury, 97, 105
closed head injury, *see* non-penetrating brain injury
competition versus training, 78
competition venue, checklist of, 217
competitors
  checklist, 217
  provisions for, 214, 215
compression loads, 121
concussion and mild traumatic brain injury, 175–6
contracting hamstring muscles, force length curve of, 81
contusions, 2, 140–41, 161, 165
core instability, 62
core stability training, 118–19, 147
  evidence for, 68
crash measures, in sports, 14–15
cycling, 141, 153, 184

deep spine muscles, 118, 119
direct impact injuries, 161
direct traumatic injuries, 140–41
disability sport and spectators, in wheelchairs, 220, 225–6
disability staff, checklist of, 226
disc degeneration, 116, 117, 118, 120
diving and acrobatic sports, injury mechanisms in, 123
dominant leg imbalance, 62
dynamic instability, 138
dynamic neuromuscular analysis (DNA) training program, 64–5
dynamic strength training, 129–31
  see also strength training
dynamic stretching, 195
dynamometer, 77

eccentric strength training program, 84, 195
  using Nordic hamstring lowers, 85
effectiveness versus efficacy, 15–16
elastin, 189
elbow injuries
  epidemiology, 153

elbow injuries (*Continued*)
    high demand versus low demand sports, 153, 154
    high energy injuries, 153–4
    low energy/overuse injuries, 155
  injury mechanisms for, 160
    direct impact injuries, 161
    fall on an outstretched hand (FOOSH), 161
    overuse injuries, 161–3
    throwing sports, injuries in, 163–4
  preventive measures for, 164
    acute injuries, targeting, 164–5
    athlete at risk, targeting, 166–7
    baseball and overhead throwers, targeting, 168, 170–73
    early recognition, targeting, 167–8
    environment, targeting, 165
    golf, targeting, 168
    overuse injuries, targeting, 165–6
    take-home message, 173
    tennis, targeting, 168, 169–70
    training, targeting, 166, 166
  risk factors for, 155, 156
    external risk factors, identifying, 157–9
    forces, transfer of, 156–7
    mature and masters athletes, 155–6
    racquet sports, risk factors in, 159–60
    repetitive compressive loads, across elbow, 160
    take-home message, 160
    young athletes and growing bones, 155
  training and competition program, risk identification in
    skeletal maturity and training, 164
emergency management, 27
England, sport-related fatalities in, 177
English Football Association, 2
environment, 165, 182
environmental crash measures, in sports, 14
environmental pre-crash measures, in sports, 14
epidemiology, 153
  of ankle injuries, 30–32
  of elbow injuries, 153–5
  of groin injuries, 91–2
  of hamstring injuries, 72–4
  of head and cervical spine injuries, 175
  of knee injuries, 49–50
  of low back pain, 114–17
  of shoulder injuries, 134–6
equestrian, 153, 182, 183, 184, 212, 220, 225
equipment, 14, 28–9, 61, 62, 98, 144–5, 146, 181, 182–4, 215, 216, 217, 219, 223, 224
equipment-related crash measures, in sports, 14–15

equipment-related pre-crash measures, in sports, 14
eye injuries, 2, 206, 207, 208

face shields, 183
facial fractures, 2
fall on an outstretched hand (FOOSH), 153, 161
familial tendency and ethnicity, 51
fatigue resistance, improving, 83
fibronectin, 189
FIFA World Cup (2006), 212
FIFA's Medical and Research Committee (F-MARC), 203
figure-eight method, 40
figure skating, 117, 153
Finland, 4
FIS Injury Surveillance System (FIS ISS), 18
flexibility
  in hamstring injuries, 77
  in muscle strain injuries, 84–5
flexion and extension compression loads, 121–2
foot pronation, 52, 54
football, 2, 8, 124, 135, 176, 177, 180, 187, 202, 203, 204
  see also soccer
football codes, 2, 21, 72, 79, 82, 83
full-face protection, for ice hockey players
  discussion, 208
  evaluation, 207–8
  facts and belief structure, 207
  injury problem, 206–7
  preventive measures for, 207
  stakeholders, identifying, 207
functional performance tests, for sport, 97

gait cycle, stage of, 80–81
generalized joint laxity, 33, 34–5
glenohumeral internal rotational deficit (GIRD), 138, 151
golf, 154, 155, 162, 166, 167, 168
"grapple tackles", in rugby league, 178
groin injuries
  epidemiology, 91–2
  injury mechanisms for
    acute versus chronic injury, 97, 105
    mechanism by structure injured, 105–9
    training and competition program, risk identification in, 109–10
  preventive measures for, 110
    hip ROM, increasing, 111
    previous groin injury, rehabilitation of, 110–11
    strength training, 111–12
    take-home message, 112
  risk factors for, 92

age and sport experience, 93–4
body composition, 94
gender, 94
modifiable intrinsic risk factors, 94–5
muscle strength and function, 95–6
non-modifiable intrinsic risk factors, 93
sport specificity, 94
take-home message, 96–7, 98–104
training background, 95
ground hardness, 182
Guide to Safety at Sports Grounds, 218, 220
gymnastics, 31, 32, 50, 114, 115, 117, 120, 121, 123, 124, 153, 154, 155, 160, 162, 163, 165

hamstring injuries, 5, 72, 95
epidemiology, 72
diagnosis, 73
time loss, 73–4
injury mechanism for
excessive biomechanical load, 79
gait cycle, stage of, 80–81
hamstring muscle injured, 80
musculotendinous junction, 80
principles, 79
reduced load tolerance, 79–80
take-home message, 81
preventive measures for, 82
athletes at-risk, identifying, 83
fatigue resistance, improving, 83
flexibility, 84–5
hamstring injuries, rehabilitation of, 85–6, 87, 88
hamstring muscle injury prevention, current trends in, 89
injury management, current trends in, 86–8
sport, changing, 88–9
strengthening, 83–4
take-home message, 89–90
thermal pants, 88
training specificity, improving, 83
warm-up, 88
with resultant posterior thigh bruising, 73
risk factors for, 74
competition versus training, 78
flexibility, 77
hamstring muscle strain injury, size of, 76–7
hamstring muscle strength, 77
hamstring/quadriceps strength ratio, 77
insufficient warm-up, 78
level of competition play, 78
muscle fatigue, 78
older athletes, 75

player position on field, 78
previous hamstring strain injury, 74–5
race, 77
take-home message, 78–9
training and competition programs, risk identification in, 81–2
hamstring muscle strain injury, 74–5
MRI investigations, 76
prevention, 89
rehabilitation program, 86, 87
risk, 72
size, 76–7
hamstring muscle strength, 75, 77, 82, 83
hamstring/quadriceps strength ratio, 77, 89
handball, 1, 2, 5, 11, 31, 37, 49, 50, 51, 66, 187
head and cervical spine injuries
epidemiology, 175
injury mechanisms for, 177–8
head injury, biomechanics of, 178–9
spinal cord injury, biomechanics of, 179–80
pathophysiology, 175
catastrophic head and spinal cord injury, 176–7
concussion and mild traumatic brain injury, 175–6
preventive measures for, 180
administrative controls, 180–81
environment, 182
equipment, 183–4
neck muscle strengthening, 184
personal protective equipment, 182–3
preparticipation screening for, 181–2
secondary injury prevention, 184
training, 182
risk factors for, 177
take-home message, 184–5
head-first and diveback sliding techniques, 146
head injuries, 2, 4, 5, 8, 17, 27, 176, 182, 183
biomechanics, 178–9
in soccer, 12, 180
heavy loads, 121, 124, 147, 153
helmets, 15, 180, 182–3, 184
hierarchy of controls, 20
high demand versus low demand sports, 153, 154
high energy injuries, 153–4
high intensity and strength training, 195
high-risk events, 220
high-risk sports, checklist of, 225–6
hiking, 31
hip and knee control, 67
hip muscles, stretching program for, 98–9
hip ROM, 111

hyperlordosis, 119
ice hockey, 2, 15, 49, 50, 91, 92, 93, 95, 105, 110, 115, 124, 135, 141, 154, 176, 178, 180, 182, 183, 184, 205, 206, 209

iliopsoas muscle, 91, 105–6, 107, 112
incipient hernia, 91, 106
inciting event, 10, 12
indirect traumatic injuries, 141–3
injury
  causation, 10
  causes, 9
    etiology, 9–11
    injury mechanism, 11–14
    modifiable and non-modifiable risk factors, 11
    risk factors, 9, 10
  classification, 8
  definition, 8
  exposure, 9
  loading patterns, associated with, 121–3
  recurrence, 9
  severity, 8–9
  surveillance, 8
injury management
  current trends in, 86–8
  and prevention, 26–7
injury mechanisms, 10, 11–14, 140
  for ankle sprains, 36–8
  categories, 13
  for elbow injuries, 160–64
  general, 177–8
  for groin injuries, 97, 105–10
  for hamstring injuries, 79–81
  head injury, biomechanics of, 178–9
  for knee injuries, 56–60
  for low back pain, 120–24
  for shoulder injuries, 140–45
  spinal cord injury, biomechanics of, 179–80
  for tendon overuse injuries, 191–2
injury prevention, in sport, 1, 19
  agreement on, 20
  evidence base for, 3–4
  future, 5
  importance, 1–3
  sports participation, 4–5
  systematic approach, 7
    injury, causes of, 9–14
    injury prevention programs, implementing, 15–16
    injury prevention research, sequence of, 7–8
    injury surveillance, 8–9
    intervention methods and programs, developing, 14–15

injury prevention matrix, 14
  for ankle sprains, 39
  applied to ACL injury prevention, 62
  applied to shoulder injury prevention, 146
  applied to sporting head and neck injury prevention, 181
  for elbow injuries, 165
  for groin injuries, 98
  for hamstring strains, 83
injury prevention program, developing and managing, 17
  equipment and facilities
    behavioral adaptation, 28
    inspection and maintenance, 29
    international and national standards for, 28
    training, 29
  implementing, 15–16
  medical staff, roles of, 20
    emergency management requirements, identification of, 27
    injury management and prevention, education regarding, 26–7
    injury risk management, coordination of, 27–8
    injury surveillance program, developing, 21–2
    monitoring, 25–6
    preseason screening, 24–5
    return to play, following injury, 26
    season analysis, 22–4
  risk management, principles of, 17
    agreement, on injury prevention, 20
    risk control, 19–20
    risk identification and assessment, 18–19
injury prevention protocol, for tennis, 169–70
injury prevention research
  model, 8
  sequence, 7–8
  steps, 198
injury prevention strategies, 146
injury problem, analyzing, 197, 208
injury risk management, coordination of, 27–8
injury risks, 17, 156–7
injury surveillance program, developing, 21–2
Injury Surveillance System (ISS), 198
inspection and maintenance, of equipment and facilities, 29
intercondylar notch width, 53
intermediate spine muscles, 118
"internal impingement", 137, 138
internal tibial rotation, 60
international and national standards, for equipment and facilities, 28
International Skiing Federation (FIS), 18, 29

interspinous ligament sprains, 116
interval rehabilitation program, 167
interval throwing program, 166
intervention methods and programs, developing, 14
  active versus passive measures, 15
  crash measures, 14–15
  post-crash measures, 15
  pre-crash measures, 14
IOC Medical Commission, 1

javelin, 154, 155, 163, 166
jogging, 31
joint laxity, and ligament material properties, 54

Kentucky Derby horse racing, 213
knee injuries, 49
  epidemiology, 49–50
  injury mechanisms for
    internal tibial rotation, 60
    knee ligament injury mechanisms, in alpine skiing, 56–7
    non-contact ACL injury situations, description of, 56, 57, 58
    quadriceps-induced anterior tibial drawer, 59–60
    take-home message, 60
    valgus loading, 58–9
  preventive measures for, 60
    core stability training, evidence for, 68
    movement biomechanics, technique and education components, 63–7
    plyometrics, 63
    safety equipment, 61
    single leg balancing component and ACL injury risk, 67–8
    strength training effects, on ACL injury risk, 68
    take-home message, 69
    targeting participation, in ACL injury interventions, 61–3
    training dosage, 68–9
  risk factors for, 50, 51–2
    age, 51
    anatomical factors, 51, 53–4
    body composition, 51
    external risk factors, 51
    familial tendency and ethnicity, 51
    foot pronation, 54
    hormonal factors, 54
    internal risk factors, 51
    ligament material properties and joint laxity, 54
    movement patterns, 55
    neuromuscular measures, 55
    patella tendon-tibia shaft angle, 54–5
    take-home message, 55–6
    tibial plateau slope, 54–5
    training and competition program, risk identification in, 60
knee ligament injury mechanisms, in alpine skiing, 56–7

La Liga soccer, 213
lacerations, 2
lacrosse, 35, 135, 154, 155, 165
laminin, 189
large-scale injury prevention programs, implementing, 197
  American National Collegiate Athletic Association model, 198
  back-up technological systems, developing, 198, 209
  bodychecking injuries, in minor ice hockey
    evaluation, 206
    facts and belief structure, 205–6
    injury problem, 205
    preventive measures for, 206
    stakeholders, identifying, 206
  Canadian Province of Québec model, 204–5
  coalitions, developing, 198, 209
  facts on injury problem, 168, 208–9
  full-face protection, to prevent facial injuries
    discussion, 208
    evaluation, 207–8
    facts and belief structure, 207
    injury problem, 206–7
    preventive measures for, 207
    stakeholders, identifying, 207
  injury problem, analyzing, 197, 208
  NCAA Wrestling Weight Management Program, 199
    components, 199–200
    discussion, 200
    evaluation, 200
    facts and belief structure, 199
    problem, 199
    stakeholders, identifying, 199
  New Zealand model, 200–201
  Québec Sports Safety Board summit, on sports safety, 210
  RugbySmart program
    evaluation, 202
    facts and belief structure, 201
    injury problem, 201
    stakeholders, identifying, 201–2
  safety, 198, 209
  SoccerSmart program, 202
    evaluation, 204

large-scale injury prevention (*Continued*)
    facts and belief structure, 203
    injury problem, 202–3
    stakeholders, identifying, 203
lateral ankle ligaments, 30, 36
  mechanism, for injury, 38
ligament material properties and joint laxity, 54
limb dominance, 33, 34
"Little Leaguers Shoulder", 137
load tolerance, of muscles, 79–80, 81
loading patterns, associated with injury, 121–3
  compression loads, 121
  flexion and extension compression loads, 121–2
  rotation compression loads, 122–3
London Marathon, 213, 220
lordotic lumbar back, *see* hyperlordosis
low and high load tests, for assessment of scapular stability, 140
low back pain, 114
  anatomy and function, of spine
    core stability/neuromuscular control, 118–19
    development, 117–18
    lumbar spine, muscles of, 118
  epidemiology
    adult athletes, low back pain in, 115–16
    increased training levels, 114
    radiological abnormalities, in spine of athletes, 116–17
    spondylolysis, 117
    young athletes, low back pain in, 114–15
  injury mechanisms for
    acute trauma or repetitive stress, 120–21
    in diving and acrobatic sports, 123
    loading patterns, associated with injury, 121–3
    for spine injuries, 123–4
  prevention methods, 124
    principles, 125–31
    secondary prevention, 132
    take-home message, 132
  risk factors for
    age, 120
    hyperlordosis or excessive curvature, of lower spine, 119
    improper technique, 119
    posture, 119
    previous injury, 120
    sex, 120
  training and competition program, risk identification, 124
low demand versus high demand sports, 153, 154
low energy/overuse injuries, 155

lumbar spine, 115, 116, 117, 122, 124
  muscles, 118

magnetic resonance tomography (MRI), 54, 73, 76, 115, 116, 117, 121, 123
major events, planning for, 212
  events requiring special attention
    disability sport and spectators in wheelchairs, 220, 225–6
    high-risk events, 220
    marathon, 220–22
    Olympic sports, 222, 224, 226
  factors, 213–14
  participants, 213
  post-event activities, 227
  spectators, 212–13
  tools
    basic planning, 214, 215
    medical cover, for spectators, 218, 219, 221
    medical indemnity and international competition, 218
    provisions, for competitors, 214, 215, 217
    selection and training, of medical staff, 219–20, 223–4
    teams traveling with medical staff, 216–18
    venue medical cover, 214, 216, 217
    very important people (VIP), 218–19, 222
  unexpected event, 226–7
Major Incident Medical Management and Support, 218
Major League Baseball, 213
marathon, 220–22
  climate, 221–2
  education, 221
  health questionnaire and medical clearance, 221
  media, 222
  venue preparation, 222
mechanics of sports, 138
medial collateral ligament (MCL) injuries, 49, 58, 61
medial elbow ligaments, anatomic drawing of, 157
medical attention injuries, 8
medical indemnity, and international competition, 218
medical staff
  checklist, 223–4
  roles, 20
    emergency management requirements, identification of, 27
    injury management and prevention, education regarding, 26–7
    injury risk management, coordination of, 27–8
    injury surveillance program, developing, 21–2
    monitoring, 25–6
    preseason screening, 24–5
    return to play, following injury, 26

season analysis, 22–4
selection and training, 219–20
teams traveling with, 216–18
Melbourne Commonwealth Games (2006), 213
Melbourne Cup horse racing, 213
modifiable intrinsic risk factors, 11, 92, 94–5
mouthguards, 183
movement biomechanics, technique and education components, 63–7
movement patterns, 55
multi-national events, 213
muscle fatigue, 75, 78
muscle strains, 116
muscle strength, 33, 35, 53
and flexibility, 194
and function, 95–6
musculoskeletal preparticipation examination, 96, 97

NASCAR, 213
National Collegiate Athletic Association (NCAA) model, 18, 198
National Federation of State High School Associations (NFHS), 200
National Football League, 135
National Hockey League, 18, 92, 93, 95
National Soccer Leagues, 213
National Wrestling Coaches Association, 199
NBA basketball, 213
NCAA Committee on Competitive Safeguards and Medical Aspects of Sports, 18
NCAA Sport Rules Committees, 18
NCAA Wrestling Weight Management Program, 199
components, 199–200
discussion, 200
evaluation, 200
facts and belief structure, 199
problem, 199
stakeholders, identifying, 199
neck muscle strengthening, 184
net-line rule, 39
neuromuscular control training, 118–19, 126, 128–9
neuromuscular training, 45, 60–61, 63, 69
New York Marathon, 213
New Zealand model, 200–201
New Zealand Rugby Union (NZRU), 201, 202, 203, 204
NFL American football, 213
NHL ice hockey, 213
NOCSAE standards, 182
non-contact ACL injury situations, description of, 56, 57, 58
non-modifiable intrinsic risk factors, 11, 92, 93
non-penetrating brain injury, 175

non-rigid ankle braces, 40
Nordic hamstring lowers, 84, 85
nordic skiing, 153
notch width index, 54
NPB baseball, 213

Olympic Games, 1, 2, 60
Olympic sports, 49, 50, 56, 91, 222, 224, 226
briefing, 224
communications, 224, 225
security and accreditation, 226
standing orders, 224
supplies and equipment, 224
training and major incident medical management and support, 226
Olympic summer program, 2
Olympic winter sports, 49
optimal throwing or serving technique, 158
osteitis pubis, 91, 94, 95
overhead athletes, 137, 167
overuse injuries, 143–4, 161–3, 164
preventing, 147–50
targeting, 165–6

padded headgear, 182, 183, 184
Panjabi's model, of stability, 118
Paris-Dakar rally, 227
passive stability, 137–8
passive versus active measures, in sports, 15
patellar tendon, 54–5, 187, 190, 192
patella tendon-tibia shaft angle (PTTSA), 52, 54–5
personal protective equipment, 182–3
"phantom foot mechanism", 56, 58
Pincer impingement, 111
pitch count guidelines, in youth baseball, 173
plyometrics, 63, 69
post-crash measures, in sports, 15, 184
post-traumatic osteoarthritis, 2
postural sway, 32, 33
pre-crash measures, in sports, 14
Premier League soccer, 213
preparticipation examinations, *see* preseason examinations
preseason examinations, 24–5
for head and neck injury, 181–2
pre-season training programs, 82, 95
preventive measures
for ankle injuries, 38–47
for elbow injuries, 164–73
for groin injury, 110–12
for hamstring injuries, 82–90
for head and cervical spine injuries, 180–84

preventive measures (*Continued*)
    for knee injuries, 60–69
    for low back pain, 124–32
    for shoulder injuries, 145–51
    for tendon overuse injuries, 194–5
preventive training, principles of
    awareness exercises, 126, 127
    dynamic strength training, 129–31
    stability training/neuromuscular control, 126, 128–9
previous groin injury, rehabilitation of, 110–11
primary injury prevention, 7, 175
proprioceptive training program, 45, 46
protective equipment, 144–5
proteoglycans, 188–9
PubMed search, 3

Q-angle, 53
quadriceps dominance, 62
quadriceps tendon, 188
quadriceps-induced anterior tibial drawer, 59–60
qualitative risk matrix, in community rugby, 19
Québec Sports Safety Board summit, on sports safety, 210

race, 52, 75, 77
racquet sports, 32, 162
    risk factors in, 159–60
racquetball, 32, 155, 165
randomized controlled trials (RCTs), 3, 4, 8, 112, 182, 183
repetitive compressive loads, 160, 162
repetitive overuse injuries, 155, 159
risk assessment, 17, 18–19
risk compensation, *see* behavioral adaptation
risk control, 17–18, 19–20
risk factors, 9, 10
    for ankle injuries, 32–6
    for elbow injuries, 155–60
    for groin injury, 92–7, 98–104
    for hamstring injuries, 74–9
    for head and cervical spine injuries, 177
    for knee injuries, 50–56
    for low back pain, 119–20
    for shoulder injuries, 136–40
    for tendon overuse injuries, 192–4
risk identification, 18
risk management, 21
    principles, 17
        agreement, on injury prevention, 20
        risk control, 19–20
        risk identification and assessment, 18–19
risk of concussion, in elite sports, 176
rotation compression loads, 122–3
rowing, 115, 124, 200

rugby, 2, 4, 31, 72, 73, 78, 80, 176, 177, 178, 182, 183, 184, 203, 204, 227
rugby scrum, 180
Rugby Union football, 176, 183
Rugby World Cup, 180, 213
RugbySmart program, 201
    evaluation, 202
    facts and belief structure, 201
    injury problem, 201
    stakeholders, identifying, 201–2
running, 31, 80, 105, 124, 182, 187

safety equipment, 61
Salt Lake (2002) Winter Games, 213
season analysis, 22–4
secondary impingement, mechanism of, 143, 144
secondary injury prevention, 7, 132, 175, 184
semi-rigid braces, 44
shoe–surface interaction, 51
shot put, 153
shoulder injuries, 134
    epidemiology, 134–6
    injury mechanisms for, 140
        direct traumatic injuries, 140–41
        indirect traumatic injuries, 141–3
        overuse injuries, 143–4
        pain, 144
        protective equipment, 144–5
    preventive measures for, 145
        getting back after shoulder injury, 151
        overuse injuries, preventing, 147–50
        strength training, 150–51
        take-home message, 151
        traumatic injury, preventing, 146–7
    risk factors for, 136
        age, 136–7
        anatomical factors, 137
        athletes at risk, identifying, 138–9
        dynamic instability, 138
        external factors, 138
        gender, 137
        mechanics of sports, 138
        passive stability, 137–8
        take-home message, 139–40
    training and competition program, risk identification in, 145
side-arm motion of delivery, 159
single leg balance training, and ACL injury risk, 67–8
single load, 121
skeletal maturity and training, 164
SLAP lesion, 137, 141, 142

snowboarding, 5, 15, 49, 146, 160, 176, 182, 184
soccer, 1, 5, 8, 11, 12, 30–31, 35, 37, 39, 49, 50, 55, 72, 73, 74, 75, 78, 82, 91, 92, 93, 115, 117, 124, 154, 176, 177, 180, 183, 184, 227
  see also football
SoccerSmart program, 202
  evaluation, 204
  facts and belief structure, 203
  injury problem, 202–3
  stakeholders, identifying, 203
softball, 19, 134, 135, 146, 151, 154, 155, 156, 159, 166, 182
specific sports, 37–8
spectators, 212–13
  checklist, 219
  medical cover for, 218, 219, 221
speed skating, 91, 92, 153
spinal cord injury
  biomechanics, 179
    rugby scrum, 180
  mechanisms for, 123–4, 179
spine
  anatomy and function
    core stability/neuromuscular control, 118–19
    development, 117–18
    lumbar spine, muscles of, 118
    radiological abnormalities in, 116–17
spondyloarthropathy, 193–4
spondylolysis, 116, 117, 119, 120
sport-specific injury, 30–31
sport specificity, 94, 109–10
sports concussion, 175–6
  intrinsic and extrinsic risk factors in, 177
sports hernia, *see* incipient hernia
sports participation, from public health perspective, 4–5
SportSmart model, 201, 202, 203
squash, 32
stability, 119
stability exercise program, 128–9
standard neuro-musculoskeletal examination, 96
standard shoulder training program, 147
static stretching, 195
sternoclavicular joint injury, 141
strength training, 111–12, 150–51
  effects on ACL injury risk, 68
  and high intensity, 195
stress strain curve, 190
superficial spine muscles, 118, 119
suprascapular nerve injury, 137
supraspinatus tendon, 144, 187
swimming, 91, 92, 134–5, 137, 144
Sydney 2000 Olympics, 213

Sydney to Hobart yacht race (1998), 226
systematic approach, to sport injury prevention, 7
  injury
    causes, 9–14
    classification, 8
    definition, 8
    exposure, 9
    recurrence, 9
    severity, 8–9
    surveillance, 8
  injury prevention programs, implementing, 15–16
  injury prevention research, sequence of, 7–8
  intervention methods and programs, developing, 14
    active versus passive measures, 15
    crash measures, 14–15
    post-crash measures, 15
    pre-crash measures, 14

taping, 40
  versus braces, 44–5
  methods for, 41–2
team setting, 17
10-point action plan, 201, 202
10-step rehabilitation program, 26
tenascin-C, 193
tendinopathy, 187–8, 192, 193
tendon
  architecture, 189
  mechanics and strength, 190
    adaptation to loading, 190–91
    pathology, 191, 192
  structure, 188
tendon matrix proteins, 188–9
tendon overuse injuries, 187
  mechanics and strength, of tendon, 190
    tendon adaptation, to loading, 190–91
    tendon pathology, 191, 192
  mechanism, 191–2
  preventive measures for
    adaptation to loading, 194
    eccentric training, 195
    high intensity and strength training, 195
    stretching, 195
    take-home message, 195
    training load, adjusting, 195
  risk factors for
    age, 192–3
    body composition, 193
    chronic disease, 193–4
    genes, 193
    muscle strength and flexibility, 194
    range of joint movement, 193

tendon overuse injuries (*Continued*)
    sex, 193
    take-home message, 194
  tendon structure, 188
    architecture, of tendon, 189
    tendon matrix proteins, 188–9
tennis, 32, 115, 117, 120, 123, 124, 134, 135, 137, 145, 154, 155, 156, 157, 159, 160, 166, 167, 168, 169–70
tertiary injury prevention, 7, 203
"The 11" program, 203, 204
thrower's 10 exercise prevention program, 170–72
throwing sports, injuries in, 163–4
tibial plateau slope, 54–5
timeloss injuries, 8
torso muscles, exercises for restoring recruitment of, 99–104
Tour de France cycling, 213
training, 29, 126, 182, 215, 223, 226
  background, 95
  versus competition, 78
  dosage, 68–9
  levels, 114
  load, 195
  of medical staff, 219–20
  program, 148–50
  and skeletal maturity, 164
  specificity, 83
  venue, 216
training and competition program
  review, 22–4
  risk identification in
    ankle injuries, 38
    elbow injuries, 164
    groin injuries, 109–10
    hamstring injuries, 81–2
    knee injuries, 60
    low back pain, 124
    shoulder injuries, 145
traumatic injury, prevention of, 146–7
trunk/pelvis instability, *see* core instability
type I collagen fibrils, bundles of, 188
type II muscle fibers, 75
type V collagen, 193

unexpected event, 226–7
United Kingdom, 176, 183, 218
United States, 1, 31, 134, 175, 176, 183, 198, 200, 207
US Catastrophic Injury Registry, 176
US College football, 213
USA baseball, 173
USA Wrestling, 199

valgus loading, 58–9, 155, 157, 163
valgus-extension overload, 162, 163, 168
van Mechelen's approach, 7, 14
venue medical cover, 214, 216, 217
very important people (VIPs), 215, 217, 218–19, 222
volleyball, 2, 5, 30, 31, 32, 33, 35, 37, 38, 39, 50, 55, 58, 135, 154, 187
volleyball-specific proprioceptive program, 46–7

Wales, sport-related fatalities in, 177
water polo, 2, 124, 135, 137
weight lifting, 114, 115, 117, 124, 136, 137, 138, 143, 144, 153, 154, 155, 160, 162, 163, 167
World Cup, 18, 181
wrestling, 50, 114, 115, 117, 121, 123, 124, 135, 153, 154, 166, 177, 199, 200, 208, 209
wrist injuries, 5

X-rays, 115, 116, 123